Integrative Chinese Herbal Therapy

The Correspondences of

Dr. Lee Chen-Yu and **Dr. Juno Yang**

Volume I

Beyond the Being

Cancer, Autoimmune Diseases, and Other Conditions

Compiled, Translated, and Authored by
Scott L. Herbster, OMD, LAc

Edited by Marc Wasserman, PhD, LAc
& Seth Shamon, LAc

The teacher should never be concerned that a student might surpass him in ability; rather, the teacher should only worry that he doesn't guide the student well enough.

The more complex the pathocondition, the more imperative it is to provide an effective resolution. Though the etiology and pathomechanism may appear opaque at first, you must remain resolute in your efforts to accurately identify the pattern as the basis for administering the optimal treatment. That's the only way to advance the pursuit of scientific discovery and progress—continually striving to improve your fortitude and capacities in the art of medicine.

Dr. Lee Chen-Yu (李正育)

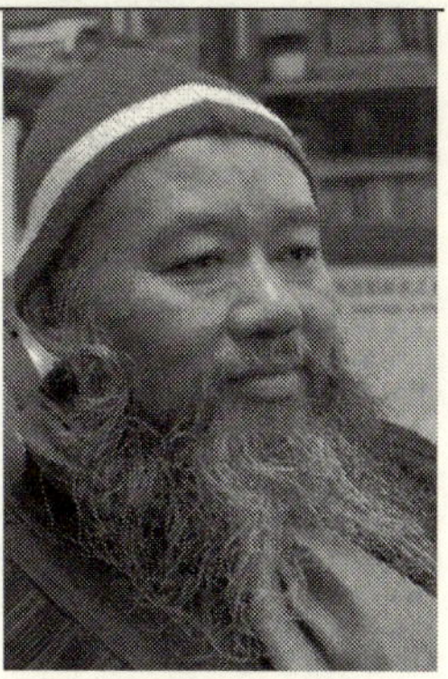

Dr. Lee Chen-Yu (李政育), OMD, LAc, PhD

Dr. Lee Chen-Yu is an acclaimed traditional Chinese medicine physician who has practiced and conducted research for over 40 years. Renowned as a pioneering innovator at the forefront of integrative medicine, he is actively engaged in all specializations of clinical medicine. However, he is best known for his seminal research on neurology and oncology, receiving numerous U.S. patents for Chinese medicine formulas that promote nerve tissue regeneration and inhibit cancer cell growth. Dr. Lee is currently the Director of Yu Sheng Chinese Medicine Clinic (founded in 1980) and also serves as the Honorary Chairperson of the Taiwan Chinese-Western Medicine Neurology Association and Honorary PhD Advisor for Liaoning University of Traditional Chinese Medicine. He has authored more than 30 books, coauthored 10 others, written hundreds of professional papers, and been the subject of many masters and PhD dissertations. Dr. Lee has personally instructed hundreds of students from around the world and inspired the pursuit of new vistas in the applications of Chinese medicine.

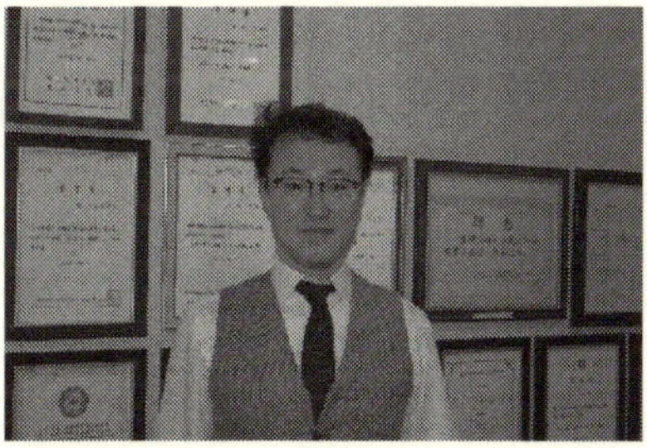

Dr. Juno Yang (梁珠勞), OMD, LAc, PhD

Dr. Juno Yang graduated from the prestigious College of Oriental Medicine at Kyung Hee University in 1998. He later went on to complete his Master of Science in Traditional Korean Medicine Pathology in 2003, and earned a PhD in Radiation Oncology from Ajou University in 2008. After his early years studying with Dr. Lee Chen-Yu, he has been very active writing innumerable professional papers, engaging in experimental research on integrative medicine, and presenting case studies at oriental medicine conferences worldwide. He has also authored three books titled Traditional Korean Medicine Therapies for Miscellaneous Diseases Vol. I (2008), Vol. II (2013), and Vol. III (2017). Dr. Yang is now the director of his own successful medical practice, Kyungheeyedang Oriental Medicine Clinic in Suwon City, near Seoul, South Korea.

ISBN:
ISBN-13: 978-0-9600303-0-9

TABLE OF CONTENTS

LIST OF CASE STUDIES

I. Cancer

Section 1: Brain Tumors

Section 2: Respiratory Tract Cancers

Section 3: Stomach Cancer

Section 4: Colorectal Cancer

II. Autoimmune Diseases

Section 1: Rheumatoid Arthritis

Section 2: Systemic Lupus Erythematosus (SLE)

Section 3: Idiopathic Thrombocytopenic Purpura

Section 4: Behcet's Disease

Section 5: Other Autoimmune Disorders

III. Neurological Disorders

Section 1: Stroke

Section 2: Other Cerebrovascular Disorders

Section 3: Concussion

Section 4: Parkinson's Disease

Section 5: Essential Tremor

IV. Cardiovascular Disease

VI. Head & Neck Disorders

ACKNOWLEDGEMENTS

Immeasurable appreciation and gratitude must be afforded to Dr. Lee Chen-Yu (李正育), whose unwavering guidance and dedication to his student Dr. Juno Yang (梁珠勞), to the compiler/translator/author and editors of this book, and to the hundreds of other traditional Chinese medicine (TCM) students he has personally instructed and mentored has made this project possible. Dr. Lee's nearly 40 years of clinical practice; clinical and laboratory research endeavors in both TCM treatment and integrative TCM and Western medicine; extensive affiliations and cooperation with Western medicine physicians; countless lectures, presentations, and papers; numerous books (both academic and mainstream); and health advocacy radio broadcast programs have reached out to touch the lives of millions of people worldwide. Much gratitude and respect must be given to Dr. Juno Yang, whose quest for knowledge and commitment to the clinical practice and research of TCM has made it possible for us to compile, translate and elucidate this invaluable material.

Further thanks goes out to these fellow students and preceptees of Dr. Lee's: Frank Delaigue (an accomplished TCM practitioner with over 20 years of clinical experience) and Cyril Oswald (an aspiring TCM educator and practitioner), who together compiled and translated excerpts of this material for a French language book they co-authored titled *Les Hommes de l'Art*, which served as a valuable reference for this book; Dan Altschuler, EAMP, PhD (an acclaimed TCM educator and clinical practitioner with over 25 years of experience and currently a faculty member at the Seattle Institute of Oriental Medicine and Bastyr University), whose *Neuropathy: Traditional Chinese Herbal Treatment in a Modern Medical Environment* (English edition) served as a reference and inspiration for this book; Chen, Ching-Hui (陳璟徽), OMD, MSc (aka "Big Brother Hui"), who has studied and served as an assistant of Dr. Lee's for nearly 30 years and has been an inexhaustible source of clarifying details about the clinical application of both TCM and integrated TCM and Western medicine; Paulo Fonte, a talented physiotherapist and TCM practitioner, now practicing at Estoril Wellness Center in Estoril, Portugal, whose professionalism and optimism is always a motivating influence on everyone; and Matthew Stampe, a massage therapist and

TCM student at the Virginia University of Oriental Medicine, for providing critical analysis for this book.

FOREWORD

"The teacher should never be concerned that a student might surpass him in ability; rather, the teacher should only worry that he doesn't guide the student well enough." As a pupil of Dr. Lee's, this is something you hear him say often. He doesn't keep secrets and he'll gladly share all of his wisdom with those willing to make a sincere effort.

This book is an extension of his mission to spread knowledge and healing. Readers will face the same challenges as those traveling thousands of miles to study in his clinic. The knowledge available from the case studies in this collection provides limitless opportunity for gaining clinical experience and opens ongoing opportunities for the practical application of integrated traditional Chinese medicine (TCM) and Western medicine in our modern medical environment.

The familiar nature of the correspondences, the focus on difficult cases, the meticulous translation of source text, and the scrupulous compilation of supplemental material all make for an ideal ongoing learning companion. You'll find it challenging, often getting stuck with questions of your own. This is part of the learning process; it allows for exploration of concepts and growth of new ideas. Anyone who has studied and worked with Dr. Lee has gone through it. Be patient, clarify questions in your mind, and continually search for answers both in this text and beyond.

TCM has always been a system that grows and evolves with each generation. This book will give you a substantive framework to build upon and find your own ways to innovate. You'll see the way Dr. Lee has updated classical prescription formulas to serve as effective treatments for the severe and intractable diseases of our current times. The balance between classical wisdom and adapting to modern medical trends is his expertise.

If you were to step foot in his clinic, you'd see someone who has mastered his craft. You'd see his ability to diagnose and treat difficult cases. You'd see the comfort and guidance he provides to patients. And you'd see smiles on the faces of patients and staff. The brightness of his work compared to the gloominess of many medical settings speaks for itself.

I'm excited that this book makes a small part of the Yu Sheng Chinese Medicine Clinic available for everyone to experience.

Marc Wasserman PhD, LAc
September 2018

PREFACE

TCM Applications & Acceptance

Traditional Chinese medicine (TCM) continues resonating with potential—through a diversity of therapeutic modalities and vast pharmacopoeia, there are few limitations for its efficacy. The starkest limitations are from the institutional confines of academia and modern medicine in step with the pharmaceutical and insurance industries that seem more than often to be holding the reins. Of course, cultural factors also play a role in the acceptance of so-called "alternative" therapies, but based on the perpetual exchange of ideas, adaptation of peoples, and acculturation of societies throughout history, the viability and resounding efficacy of TCM has the persuasive power to overcome.

TCM Education and Status in Societies of Chinese (Han) Cultural Heritage

In societies influenced by Chinese culture (such as China, Taiwan, and South Korea) certified TCM (referred to as traditional Korean medicine (TKM) in South Korea) physicians are required to complete formal TCM medical school programs and pass national licensure examinations authorized by the respective nation's education oversight agency.

In China, 5- and 7-year bachelor's, master's, and doctoral programs are designed for students to receive a doctor of clinical medicine and doctor of integrated medicine with the option of practicing both Western medicine and TCM and eligibility to take the respective national licensure examinations. In Taiwan, a 5-year post-baccalaureate and an 8-year bachelor's program are designed for students to receive a TCM degree in the former and the option of a dual degree in Western medicine and TCM in the latter and eligibility to take the respective national licensure examinations. In South Korea, a 4-year post-baccalaureate and a 6-year bachelor's degree program are designed for students to receive a TKM degree and eligibility to take the national licensure examination.

The dual Western medicine and TCM degrees in China and Taiwan require students to fulfill all basic coursework in biomedicine and Western medicine specializations along with clinical internships in both Western medicine and TCM. For TCM (TKM) programs in Taiwan and South Korea, two-thirds of the curriculum focuses on coursework in basic biomedicine and specializations, comparative to the requirements for students in dentistry programs, and one-third on TCM, along with a clerkship in a Western medicine hospital and a clinical internship in the TCM department of a Western medicine hospital.

The relative emphasis on modern biomedicine and Western medicine specializations in the coursework load is balanced out by an intensive TCM curriculum that includes the classics and contemporary texts and their clinical applications. Based on my TCM academic pursuits in Taiwan and relationships with many TCM students, practitioners, and scholars, who have either received TCM educations or are educators themselves in countries such as China, South Korea, the United States, Australia, New Zealand, Israel, France, England, and Canada, I am confident that the depth and breadth of TCM curriculums in East Asian university TCM programs (at least in Taiwan, China, and South Korea) go far beyond that of TCM programs in other countries. To a large extent, this is due to an inherent cultural affinity that accepts this traditional medicine heritage as viable and effective.

There is no question that the institution of modern medicine is synonymous with Western medicine, but despite the enormous amount of funding and energies devoted to research and development, there are still glaring deficiencies. In Taiwan, China, and South Korea, this has opened up the opportunity for TCM to play a role as part of a unified medical system. Just as a major hospital may have dentistry and physiotherapy departments, they also have a TCM department. Indeed, this inclusion within the mainstream institution of modern medicine has in some ways been a boon, ensuring the perpetuation of this form of traditional medicine. However, there has been a price to pay with TCM serving a subservient role—recognized as more of a neoadjuvant, adjuvant, complementary, or palliative therapy—as opposed to primary and secondary care and first-line treatment.

There are still a few TCM physicians with clinical practices outside of the institutional healthcare system who embrace the powers of integrated TCM and Western medicine and have been able to achieve success at providing primary and secondary care and first-line treatment beyond adjuvant, complementary, and palliative therapy roles. Physicians such as Dr. Lee who have been dedicated to a lifetime of research, clinical practice, and educating have gained due respect and elevated status within the medical community.

Backed by clinical experience and a thorough understanding of the advantages and disadvantages of Western medicine drugs and procedures, in certain cases Dr. Lee may advise patients to consult with their Western medicine physician about gradually reducing the dose and eventually discontinuing a given drug, or holding off on surgery if the side effects and potential complications outweigh the benefits—particularly if TCM offers a better therapeutic solution. Dr. Lee may also advise patients admitted to the hospital receive decocted TCM formula through their nasogastric (NG) tube, which requires both the consent of the patient (and/or family members) and the physician in charge.

Obviously, this type of consent and coordination requires a high degree of trust and communication. This poses significant challenges even in East Asian societies with the legal ramifications that may arise if something unexpected happens. There is still a lot of work that needs to be done in establishing protocols and fostering universal acceptance. Evidence-based medicine research involving integrated TCM and Western medicine treatment is still sparse. However, based on both the results of evidence-based medicine studies and thousands of years of empirical clinical evidence, there is growing impetus towards recognizing the efficacy of TCM and integrated TCM and Western medicine in the treatment of a broad spectrum of diseases.

Know Your Medicinals and Define Your Paradigm

There is no single TCM medicinal or formula that *must* be administered for a specific symptom, pathocondition, or disease pattern. Classical and contemporary texts and the experience of mentors provide the foundations for the practitioner to clinically apply methodologies, but it is only through experience that dedicated physicians may develop their own paradigm. Medicinals of various properties and chemical constituents are grouped together in pairs and combinations—opposing and complementing, restraining and empowering, accentuating and corresponding—to form a formula composition whose overall action will resolve symptoms and promote the return of homeostasis. In addition to personal preference based on clinical experience, a variety of factors may influence a TCM physician's selection of medicinals for a formula composition, such as availability, quality, price, storage, legal regulations, and patient preferences (taste, religion, customs, diet, etc.).

Medicinal processing plays an integral role in procuring the intended action, storage life, and mitigation of toxicity. If preparation methods are not tightly monitored and controlled, there could be potentially severe side effects (possibly even fatal). In times of antiquity, it was standard practice for TCM physicians to have their own raw medicinal processing facilities (or have a close cooperative relationship with a licensed medicinal dispensary that specializes in preparing and processing medicinals) and herbal dispensaries stocked with decocting pieces (medicinals) of their choice.

Nowadays, even in China, Taiwan, South Korea, and other Asian nations where TCM is a part of mainstream culture, the majority of physicians do not have their own processing facilities, and most do not even have onsite herbal dispensaries stocked with decocting pieces (medicinals). Their herbal dispensaries are more commonly stocked with extract powders/granules for the sake of convenience and regulatory oversight (in Taiwan this is particularly evident in part due to the National Healthcare Plan (a single-payer system) that provides nominal coverage for TCM)).

Dr. Lee is among the remaining TCM physicians who carry on the original spirit of the tradition, believing that you have to really "know your medicinals like the back of your hand" in order to utilize their best qualities, enhance their weaknesses, temper their volatilities, and harness the extent of their capacity for providing therapeutic efficacy.

Throughout the years, Dr. Lee's relationship with his medicinals has evolved as he continues to fine-tune his craft, modifying traditional formulas and designing his own to provide the optimal therapeutic regimen for his patients in Taiwan and across the globe. These formulas are referred to throughout the text, either explicitly or implicitly, as "(Yu Sheng)" formulas. Yu Sheng (育生 yù sh□ng) simply refers to the name of Dr. Lee's clinic.

Perspectives on the Four Examinations

The four examinations—inspection, listening and smelling, inquiry, and palpation—were first recorded in the Warring States period (475–221 BC) nearly 2,500 years ago. Patient examinations are conducted to determine the correlation of all four examinations and identify the pattern as the basis of treatment.

Depending on the type of symptoms, injury, and pathocondition, the four examinations are generally conducted in the following order: *inspection* (including observing skin, gait, mannerisms, complexion, color of stool and urine, and the tongue) offers an initial "look" at the patient and is the natural first step; *listening and smelling* (including listening to the sound of speech and breath, and smelling the body, breath, and excretions) provides additional information and is the next natural step; *inquiry* (including patient history, chief complaint, diagnostic images, and lab test results) allows the physician to collect subjective and objective information and data about the patient's condition, and may often be the most valuable; and *palpation* (including touching and feeling the body to determine the presence of heat, tenderness, and accumulations, and also taking the pulse) enables the physician to get a "feel" for the patient's condition and is the last step.

As is often the case with experienced physicians, over the years Dr. Lee has developed a refined application of the four examinations with a keen sense for observing mannerisms, gait, skin manifestations, temperament, disposition, speech, and odor; discerning the nuances of history taking, performing abdominal palpation, and elucidating the significance of pulse.

Early on in Dr. Lee's clinical practice, he would rely on tongue examination much more, but throughout the years, this reliance has diminished due to natural variations in size, color, texture, and fur among individuals, and the intake of food and beverages that stain the tongue and alter the appearance of the fur. In fact, if one observes Dr. Lee's patient interviews during consultations, you will notice that he rarely examines the tongue except for those cases in which patients have a pathology of the tongue or mouth proper.

Pulse-taking remains a hallmark of TCM examination and diagnostic protocol, and early on in Dr. Lee's clinical practice he authored a reputable academic book on this topic titled *Illustrated Traditional*

Chinese Medicine Pulse Reading (圖解中醫脈學 *Tu Jie Zhong Yi Mai Xue*). Indeed, in its historical context pulse-taking is a vital source that opens up vistas into the discrete inner workings of the human body and reveals information about blood flow, volume, and viscosity; heart rate, cardiac output, and vascular patency; and the organs and physiological systems of the entire body (including the endocrine system, autonomic nervous system, and central nervous system).

However, since the advent of modern biomedicine's diagnostic imaging and lab tests, which offer once unimaginable detail in its tangible images and quantitative data, the significance of pulse examination has in many regards been supplanted. This is compounded by the absence of a set, definable and quantifiable standard for interpreting the quality and nature of the pulse, with each individual potentially defining the *feeling* of a pulse differently. Though many well-intended TCM practitioners and devout patients who still cling to the nostalgia may disagree with this assessment, in my opinion pulse-taking is a relatively ambiguous *art* to practice. It is even more difficult to communicate with others, as one pulse-taker's description of a particular pulse may not be the same as another's, even though they may actually be feeling the same pulse! This doesn't entirely relegate its usefulness for the individual practitioner as a reference for conducting pattern identification, but its subjectivity does limit its function as conveyed to other individuals.

Yet another factor is the widespread administration of Western medicine therapeutic agents for patients with established illnesses and as preventive care. Many of these drugs have a direct affect on the autonomic nervous system and endocrine systems, which regulate cardiovascular blood flow and the feedback mechanisms affecting vasoconstriction and vasodilation. The near ubiquitous administration of pharmaceuticals in our modern society makes the "drug pulse" (藥脈 yào mài) phenomenon that much more of a challenge to objectively discern the *feeling* of a pulse.

That said, just as it was applied traditionally, Dr. Lee takes each patient's pulse and records the reading in the patient's medical record and uses these readings as a baseline for subsequent patient examination. In certain cases where the pulse reading is noticeably inconsistent with the other presenting signs and symptoms, lab tests, and diagnostic imaging findings, then the pulse may play a vital role in pattern identification (e.g., accurately discerning true and false and complex patterns).

TCM Terminology and Usage

Readers familiar with TCM may know that there are several commonly used terminology systems employed in the translation and explanation of TCM concepts. I began studying Chinese contemporary and classical texts on subjects such as literature, philosophy, and religion in 1991. Since 2001, I have been focusing energies on studying TCM. These extensive studies have included graduating from a five-year postbaccalaureate program in a prominent Taiwanese medical teaching college with an affiliated hospital, pursuing studies of classical and contemporary texts in Chinese and English on his own, and also working professionally translating classical and contemporary TCM texts from Chinese to English.

Through these experiences, I have explored the use of the various 'systems,' mixed and matched various 'systems,' and created my own complementary interpretations. At first, this 'trial and error' approach seemed innocuous enough; after all, the objective is simply to get the idea across, right? Well, the more I began to analyze and realize the seamless congruity and irrefutable underlying logic of Prof. Nigel Wiseman's TCM terminology "system," the more I became persuaded to get on board and adopt this lexicon.

Prof. Wiseman's TCM lexicon is the only comprehensive, standardized "system" to date. It is possible that this particular system appeals to my bilingual sensibilities, providing insight into the underlying historical usage and context of particular characters and phrases throughout different eras. I find that this system most accurately articulates the original meaning of the source text.

Naturally, there are limitations in any system and I admit that some of the usage may seem awkward or unorthodox for those not familiar with the system. But as stated above, the advantages of congruity far outweigh the occasional ambiguity and archaic flavor. It is the comprehensive system that I believe is the best format to convey and advance the valuable medical insights and scientific methodology of TCM. It may require a bit of getting used to and looking up some terms at first, but in the end, I am confident you will discover the "rhyme to this reason."

INTRODUCTION

This book comprises the collection of fax and e-mail correspondence between Dr. Lee Chen-Yu (李政育), recognized as one of Taiwan's most accomplished and prominent traditional Chinese medicine (TCM) physicians, and his dedicated student Dr. Juno Yang (梁珠勞) from South Korea. Nearly 40 years of clinical experience and insights are made readily available through these clear and concise interactions, offering practical antidotes for the clinical application of integrated TCM and Western medicine.

In 2000, Dr. Yang came to study under the mentorship of Dr. Lee Chen-Yu at Yu Sheng Chinese Medicine Clinic in Taipei, Taiwan (ROC). Following this period of immersed clinical study, he returned to South Korea where he started his own TCM clinical practice, gradually honing his capacities over the years until becoming confident and competent in treating patients with complex and severe pathoconditions.

At the onset, Dr. Yang lacked experience and thus had many questions about accurately diagnosing and effectively treating the broad scope of pathoconditions for which patients sought consultation. Thus, the student would correspond with his mentor by fax or e-mail seeking advice and guidance. Dr. Lee enjoyed sharing the knowledge gained from decades of study, research, and clinical experience, and further imparted the necessity for maintaining "a balance between prudence and confidence" and the importance of continuing education and developing professional capacities to make a positive impact on the lives of those depending on your medical assistance.

This regular correspondences between Dr. Lee (mentor) and Dr. Yang (student) took place from 2001 up until 2008, and consequently these interactions formed the content and outline for the conception of this book. Rather than presenting this correspondence in its original chronological order, the author has sorted and collated the material by grouping follow-up correspondences of specific patient's cases and associated pathological conditions together as well as modifying some of the letter formatting, making the presentation of each case study concise and informative. It contains troves of information on TCM pattern identification as the basis for determining treatment; clinical application of TCM medicinals, formulas, and acupuncture regimens; classical TCM pathologic terms and their correlating Western medicine pathological nomenclature; background information on symptoms, diagnostic tests, and treatment modalities; and keys to differential diagnosis and prognosis.

The sheer breadth and expanse of this material warranted division into a three-volume series, of which this is the first volume compiled and translated into English. Volume I includes chapters on cancer (and benign tumors) of the central nervous, respiratory, gastrointestinal, lymphatic, circulatory, and genitourinary systems; breast cancer; autoimmune disorders; pathologies of the cerebrovascular, cerebellar, central nervous system, cardiovascular, and peripheral vascular systems; and head and neck disorders.

A wide range of other pathological conditions will be published in the upcoming Volume II and Volume III of this series. Case studies involving pathologies of the following will be included: respiratory, gastrointestinal, musculoskeletal, and genitourinary systems; neurology, endocrinology, dermatology, ophthalmology, nephrology, hematology, gynecology and obstetrics, and pediatrics; and metabolic disorders, infectious diseases, and psychiatric conditions.

By no means does this book attempt to present a comprehensive analysis of all the pathological conditions TCM is capable of treating, either independently or through Western medicine integration. Its precept stems from the candid correspondence and guidance between a promising TCM physician (student) and an innovative spirit at the forefront of integrative TCM and Western medicine development (mentor). The scope of the pathological conditions and the descriptions of the cases presented here are simply derived from the questions a dedicated student has asked seeking guidance from his mentor.

The reader should not expect an unabridged, pedagogical explanation for all of these pathoconditions. However, the compiler/translator/author has made extensive efforts to insert further details and descriptions, including etiology, pathomechanisms, pattern identification, underlying theoretical concepts, medicinal actions, pharmaceuticals, and therapeutic procedures, of topics discussed in these correspondences in hopes of providing more informative and authoritative content.

This material will serve as a valuable reference source for practical application—a catalyst that inspires the TCM practitioner to continue applying and integrating the classical traditions within our modern biomedical environment—and an insightful medium for those interested in learning about the vast potential for both the clinical applications of TCM and integrative TCM and Western medicine therapeutic approaches.

UNIT CONVERTER

In this text, doses of medicinals are given in the traditional Chinese units (fen/qian/liang/jin). This measuring system may be initially less familiar to the Western reader than the metric system commonly used nowadays. Despite this initial learning curve, I have chosen to preserve this element of the text with the consideration of honoring the traditional way still practiced in the East. This unified system also provides a simple reading experience and avoids the need for in-text conversions or decimal points.

The gram (g) equivalencies are as follows:

1 fen = 0.375 g
1 qian (10 fen) = 3.75 g
1 liang (10 qian) = 37.5 g
1 jin (16 liang) = 600 g

I. CANCER

Cancer is among the leading causes of mortality worldwide. Despite the rapid technological advancements in modern medicine and the evolution of new therapeutic modalities, adverse effects and iatrogenic complications remain an overshadowing concern. Many cancer patients experience loss of appetite following chemotherapy, resulting in malnutrition and cachexia (aka wasting syndrome) and essentially wither away. TCM medicinals have been used in the treatment of cancer for thousands of years and remain an effective choice for supplementing the deficiencies and complementing the overall treatment of modern biomedicine, and in some cases alleviating the need for toxic pharmaceutical agents and invasive therapies altogether.

Section 1: Brain Tumors

Case Study #1: Corticosteroids – First-line Treatment of Brain Swelling (Edema) Following Surgery, Radiotherapy, and Chemotherapy

Q: A 50 y/o male patient was administered an injection of vincristine, cyclophosphamide, and procarbazine to treat a brain tumor. He suffered severe adverse effects from chemotherapy and came to my clinic seeking consultation. First, I prescribed You Gui Yin variant to remedy the side effects, but it turns out, in addition to improving energy level and strength, this formula also had an anitcancer action inducing shrinkage of the patient's tumor.

The patient's children were grateful, telling me that I had brought their father back to life and given their family renewed hope. Actually, the credit really goes to my mentor, whose guidance and instruction walked me through this process. From both the family and me, we thank you so much!

I remember you asked me at the time, "Has the patient been administered corticosteroids?" Without verifying to make sure, I told you that he had *not*, and only later on did I find out that he had taken corticosteroids over a period of time. I admit that I wasn't detailed enough while conducting the patient interview and must be more attentive in the future. Now, I have another question: Does You Gui Yin really have an anticancer action?

A: When I talked to you on the telephone, you said that this patient had *not* taken corticosteroids, but the patient's medical records that you faxed me clearly indicated corticosteroid administration. Remember! Every brain tumor patient who undergoes surgery and follow-up radiotherapy and chemotherapy will incur brain swelling (edema), and to alleviate the damaging effects on brain cells caused by increased intracranial pressure (ICP), general protocol calls for the administration of corticosteroids.

Once corticosteroids have been either injected or taken orally, the patient's condition can be identified as kidney yang vacuity pattern. At this time, regardless of the formula prescribed, you must add The Three Great Yang-Supplementers and Ren Shen. If severe swelling and elevated ICP present, mannitol (osmotic diuretic) or glycerin will be administered to reduce ICP levels. At this time, the TCM physician must add Bai Zhu, Fu Ling, Zhu Ling, Ze Xie, Tian Ma, Wu Zhu Yu, The Three Insects, and Yu Sheng Wan to moderate irregular electrical acticity in the brain that might induce seizures. If the patient's condition exacerbates and becomes difficult to control, then add Wan Ling Dan.

Chemotherapy inhibits hematopoietic function in the bone marrow as well as hematopoietic function and growth factor pathways in the kidneys. You Gui Yin improves this condition and promotes hormone secretion and pathway function. Since the administration of corticosteroids puts the patient in a kidney yang vacuity pattern state and the brain (sea of marrow) belongs to the kidney, prescribing You Gui Yin effectively treats this condition, preventing the brain tumor from proliferating and possibly even shrinking or completely eradicating the tumor.

Remember! Once corticosteroids have been discontinued, you should change the formula to (Yu Sheng) Ban Xia Tian Ma Bai Zhu San variant. After 2 to 3 months of administering this formula, you should consider changing to a blood-nourishing blood-quickening, stasis-dispelling pain-relieving, and network vessel-freeing channel-regulating formula, such as Ru Mo Si Wu Tang adding Fu Ling, Bai Zhu, Ze Xie, The Three Yellows, Tian Ma, Wu Zhu Yu, The Three Insects, Chuan Qi, Yu Sheng Wan, and Wan Ling Dan; or a heat-clearing phlegm-damp-transforming and water-disinhibiting formula such as Chai Ling Tang adding Da Huang, Tian Ma, The Three Yellows, Wu Zhu Yu, The Three Insects, Dan Pi, Chi Shao, Qing Hao, Di Gu Pi, Yu Sheng Wan, and Wan Ling Dan.

The principle here is that you want to bring the patient's condition back to the "essential state" of repletion heat and stasis heat pattern, which is the state it was at the onset of disease before the patient received chemotherapy and radiotherapy. The problem with administering yang-supplementing medicinals over too long a period is that it could induce neoplastic differentiation in stem cells peripheral to the tumor, thus accelerating proliferation and deterioration of the patient's condition.

If the patient receives chemotherapy and radiotherapy without administration of corticosteroids, then you should prescribe Da Chai Tang, Chai Ling Tang, or Ru Mo Si Wu Tang variants from the onset. Do *not* administer yang-supplementing formulas such as (Yu Sheng) Ban Xia Tian Ma Bai Zhu San and (Yu Sheng) You Gui Yin. If you feel it is necessary to add The Three Great Yang-Supplementers, then only use small doses adding corresponding amounts of The Three

Yellows, and large doses of Qing Hao, Zhi Mu, Di Gu Pi, and Mu Dan Pi, which combine to counterbalance the heat and protect the yin aspect. You could also consider prescribing Wen Dan Tang or Zhi Bo Di Huang Tang variants instead, depending on the presenting signs, symptoms and pattern. Clearly understanding this basis of reasoning and applying this approach in clinical practice is fundamental to the integrated Chinese and Western medicine treatment of disease.

Case Study #2: Benign Brain Tumor – Postoperative Complications

Q: Thanks for your encouragement and support. Since you gave me the confidence and guidance to treat my classmate's malignant brain tumor, I have gone on to treat several other brain tumor cases. However, I know this is just the beginning and there are so many things for me to learn. I look forward to your continued support, guidance, and instruction.

Now, I have a 39 y/o male patient who underwent surgical excision of a brain tumor (right side) on February 14. Following the surgery, he presented with right-sided facial paralysis and had difficulty rotating his head. The diagnosis was postsurgical complications of benign brain tumor. I also gave the patient acupuncture for over a month without any noticeable effect. He is still taking drugs to lower ICP. What do you think the best course of action is from here?

A: Most surgeries for brain tumors induce postsurgical complications. Facial paralysis is one of these and is similar to the complications of cerebrovascular accident (CVA). First, if the tumor enlarges, it will occupy space and compress nearby stroma and parenchyma causing nerve damage and impairment; second, iatrogenic nerve damage from the surgical procedure may occur; and third, the toxin secreted from the tumor itself may cause nerve damage as well.

Regardless of the specific etiology, TCM medicinals should be administered. Admittedly, efficacy manifests slowly, but the sooner treatment is started the greater the potential for nerve regeneration and functional recovery. As for acupuncture, *only* corresponding distal acupoints should be needled; local acupoints on the affected side will *not* provide efficacy due to the nerve conduction block deep in the parenchyma.

Case Study #3: Brain Tumors – Impact of Chemotherapy and Radiotherapy on Hematopoiesis

Q: A brain tumor patient was first administered chemotherapy and then underwent more than 10 cranial surgeries. This resulted in decreased CBC counts: WBC 1,000, Hb 7, and PLT 6,000. After being administered emergency blood transfusions (whole blood 1x and Hb 6 packs), amounts increased to WBC 2,200, PLT 60,000, and Hb 10.2. As you advised, I prescribed (Yu Sheng) You Gui Yin (including Gan Jiang, Fu Zi, Rou Gui (5 qian each)) adding Ren Shen/Chuan Qi Powder. Two weeks later, levels had increased to WBC 3,800 and Hb 15 (normal range 12-16 g/dl). The entire medical staff couldn't believe this had happened!

The first time the patient received a Procarbazine injection CBC counts dropped: WBC 2,400 and PLT 64,000. After administering the (Yu Sheng) You Gui Yin variant above, his CBC counts increased: WBC 3,800 and PLT 15,000. This time, following injections of anticancer chemotherapeutic agents, WBC levels remained at pretty much normal levels, but the PLT dropped to 48,000, and a week later hit a low of 32,000. Do you think I should add large doses of The Three Great Yang-Supplementers and Ren Shen? Or should I add Lu Rong and Zhu Jie?

I once prescribed (Yu Sheng) You Gui Yin adding Ren Shen to a patient undergoing chemotherapy and the tumor shrunk by 1/3. It appears that it was effective!

A: Inevitably, following chemotherapy and radiotherapy for the treatment of brain tumors, hematopoietic function will be inhibited. (Yu Sheng) You Gui Yin adding Ren Shen/Chuan Qi Powder will improve hematopoietic function and relieve symptoms; so yes, I would continue prescribing this formula. However, if chemotherapy and radiotherapy are no longer being administered, then you could consider changing the original formula to Ban Xia Tian Ma Bai Zhu San or (Yu Sheng) Ru Mo Si Wu Tang adding Huang Qin, Huang Lian, Huang Bo, Bai Zhu, Fu Ling, Ze Xie, Tian Ma, Wu Zhu Yu, Chuan Qi, Yu Sheng Wan, Wan Ling Dan, and possibly small doses of The Three Great Yang-Supplementers. Remember! Administration of these TCM medicinals may not always produce noticeable results overnight, but don't get deterred—just stay the course!

Generally, inhibition of hematopoietic function is most marked during the second week following anticancer agent infusions. In addition to blood transfusions and injections of erythropoietin (EPO) or G-CSF, oncologists commonly administer corticosteroids or autologous stem cell transplantation (ASCT) to improve hematopoietic function. However, adverse effects are severe, because the proliferation of both good and bad cells is greatly increased. This method does kill cancer cells (verified by hematologic and imaging tests), but after some time these neoplastic cells will proliferate again, and once they do these renegade cells run rampant.

TCM medicinals can promote renal secretion of hematopoietic factors and the secretion of hematopoietic stem cells in the bone marrow without the adverse effects of Western medicine drugs. It's best to begin TCM medicinal treatment soon after (about 1 week) administration of chemotherapy to ensure optimal results at preserving hematopoietic function.

You are starting to get the hang of the integrative TCM and Western medicine approach for treating brain tumors. I can tell by the formulas you are prescribing and the questions you are asking. Just remember! 2–3 weeks (at the absolute uppermost limit 2–3 months) after the completion of chemotherapy you need to change formulas.

Yang-supplementing medicinals improve low blood protein concentrations and BUN and Cr levels, thus remedying the side effects of Western medicine drugs, and also prevent tumor growth. However, administration of yang-supplementing medicinals for too long of a period (upper limit of 3–6 months) has the potential of inducing rapid proliferation of the brain tumor. At this time, the condition can be identified as repletion heat and stasis heat pattern, requiring you to change to a formula such as Ru Mo Si Wu Tang, Wen Dan Tang, or Ban Xia Tian Ma Ban Zhu San adding Gan Jiang and Fu Zi.

Note: Chemotherapy side effects in brain tumor patients usually begin about two weeks after treatment, with low complete blood count (CBC) levels and other physical signs and symptoms of decreased hematopoietic function presenting. With this in mind, it is best to begin prescribing TCM medicinal treatment 1 week after administration of chemotherapy.

The administration of TCM medicinals will dramatically shorten the period of time hematopoietic function is inhibited. Of course, it would be even better to coordinate efforts with the hematology-oncology specialist, ensuring that chemotherapy be administered in smaller doses (say 80% or even 50% of the normal dose) spread out over several times. That way the adverse effects can be minimized. (Anitcancer agents are developed in Western countries with people of European descent the primary focus of research studies and clinical trials. The dosage standards are based on this focus group. For the majority of Asians, who tend to be smaller in physical stature, this dosage is too heavy; it is no wonder there are so many adverse effects!)

Case Study #4: Postsurgical Radiotherapy Induces Brain Swelling

Q: The patient is a 46 y/o male with a brain tumor located near Broca's area presenting with symptoms of speech impairment, gait disturbance, limb weakness, and poor appetite. A brief history is as follows:

He underwent his first surgery in April 2007, and following radiotherapy, he incurred massive brain swelling. After receiving chemotherapy his WBC and PLT counts severely decreased and he was admitted into ICU three times. In March of the next year (2008) his condition worsened and his doctors said they couldn't do anything for him.

On June 30, he came to my clinic by referral for consultation. First, I prescribed Ban Xia Tian Ma Bai Zhu San adding Chi Shao, Dan Pi, Gu Sui Bu, Xu Duan (1 liang of each), and Wan Ling Dan (6 pills/3x/day), which proved effective in improving strength. By the end of July, the patient's condition had deteriorated, presenting with symptoms of heightened dysphasia, gait disturbance, and severe; thus, the attending physician decided to perform the second surgery on August 20 (2008).

The strange thing is on August 15 the patient awoke from sleep without a headache and the dysphasia and gait disturbance also gradually resolved, so his doctor decided to cancel the second surgery. How could this have happened?

A: Treatment of brain tumors involves reducing brain swelling, lowering ICP, inhibiting angiogenesis, preventing seizures, averting tumor exacerbation, and stabilizing the overall condition. If there is no improvement after receiving surgery, chemotherapy, and radiotherapy, the administration of TCM medicinals will usually stabilize the patient's condition, even to the extent where the tumor is not visible on an MRI image. This is when you must change back to using the "essential state" formula, otherwise the yang-supplementing medicinals may induce relapse. I have mentioned this many times now—you must remember this!

Case Study #5: Advanced Stage Malignant Brain Tumor Necrosis

Q: I am currently treating an advanced stage malignant brain tumor patient who has already received the full regimen of Western medicine cancer therapies prior to seeking my consultation. I prescribed Ru Mo Si Wu Tang, and after taking the formula for 2 months, an MRI image revealed tumor contrast enhancement along with right-sided motor dysfunction and visual disturbance. Concerned that sections of the tumor had undergone necrosis, his doctors have decided to perform another craniectomy.

A: This could be a sign of liquefactive necrosis in an advanced stage brain tumor. To quickly resolve these symptoms, you can simply add large doses of The Three Yellows, Bai Zhu, Fu Ling, Ze Xie, and Da Huang to your original formula, which will accelerate the clearance of metabolic waste and resolve toxin. Your patient's doctors may also decide to insert a drainage tube, which will also promote resolution of the lesion.

For brain tumors, there are three possible results of treatment: tumor apoptosis, calcification, and necrosis. Your therapeutic approach has accurately identified the pattern and thus has produced effective results. The contrast enhancement in your patient's MRI simply indicates that the tumor has necrosed, releasing profuse amounts of blood and lymph fluids that accumulate due to inadequate resorption. You should advise the patient to have follow-up CT scan and MRI performed to evaluate the amount of fluid and adjust your TCM formula prescription accordingly.

Case Study #6: Bu Zhong Yi Qi Tang Variant "Conquers All Pathoconditions"

Q: Recently, I was invited to the Department of Radiation Oncology at the affiliated hospital of Ajou University to treat patients. Some professors from Kyung Hee University have asked me to collaborate on a research project based on the clinical results from the affiliated hospital. We plan to design several TCM formula compositions within three years to provide the Western medical community with reference sources. The focus of our research is to improve the adverse effects of dry mouth following radiotherapy to the head and neck in cancer patients and the symptoms that mimic menopause syndrome, such as tidal heat and facial sweating, following chemotherapy in breast cancer patients.

The treatment for improving symptoms of dry mouth simply entailed acupuncture treatment (no moxa nor TCM medicinal formulas) needling Ting Gong (SJ19), Yi Feng (SJ17), and He Gu (LI4) (1x/week for 1 month (total of 4 treatments)). This 4-treatment regimen proved effective in improving symptoms (patients were able to naturally produce saliva on their own). Similarly, I needled acupoints San Yin Jiao (SP6), Shui Quan (K5), and Xue Hai (SP10) (1x/week for 1 month (total of 4 treatments)), which proved effective in improving the symptoms that mimic menopause syndrome, such as tidal heat and facial sweating in breast cancer patients.

We are presently conducting further studies on animals and humans, essentially using your three main formulas: Xiao Chai Hu Tang combining Sheng Yu Tang, Shi Quan Da Bu Tang, and You Gui Yin. Additionally, due to the climate and environmental differences here in South Korea, I want to slightly modify these formulas by adding blood-quickening stasis-transforming and heat-clearing toxin-resolving medicinals. What do you think about this project? Do you have any suggestions or advice?

A: Acupuncture is very effective at treating "early stage" salivary gland atrophy. However, if there is lymphatic obstruction or swollen and sclerosed glands and the muscle tissues of the head, face and neck have undergone fibrosis, then warm needling (moxa cubes on the needle) will offer even better results. As for treating menopause symptoms with yin-nourishing heat-abating acupoints and TCM medicinals, these modalities offer excellent efficacy in the treatment of psychosomatic symptoms and autonomic nervous system disorders arising during menopause. Based on my experience, they are also effective at treating the tidal fever and facial sweating induced by chemotherapy in breast cancer patients. Keep up the good work and publish your results. The only way to ensure your efforts make an *enduring* impact is getting these results down in print. Let's go!

Bu Zhong Yi Qi Tang variant is a good formula for treating the adverse effects of chemotherapy and radiotherapy in cancer patients. Adding medicinals such as Huang Qin, Yuan Hu, Mu Xiang, Dan Shen, and Ren Shen/Chuan Qi Powder to this formula promotes wound healing from surgery and repairs the initial liver damage caused by chemotherapy. Large doses of Huang Qi may also be included (anywhere from 1.5–2 liang) for its center-supplementing and blood and flesh-engendering actions. If hematopoietic dysfunction presents add The Three Great Yang-Supplementers and Lu Rong; if low total protein (TP) levels present with edema (e.g., in sternocostal, abdominal, lower leg regions) add Bai Zhu, Fu Ling, and Ze Xie; and for increased BUN and Cr add Ren Dong Teng, Ding Shu Xiu, and Pu Gong Ying. If I had to make a choice of one formula that could "conquer all conditions," an elixir if you will, it would be Bu Zhong Yi Qi Tang variant.

Case Study #7: Dry Mouth and Eyes Following Radiotherapy – Don't Misuse Glaucoma Drug (Pilocarpine HCl)!

Q: A 24 y/o male received radiotherapy for a brain tumor with increased □-HCG levels. Following radiotherapy, the patient suffered from adverse effects of severe dry mouth, dry eyes, insomnia, and irritability, which prompted him to seek my consultation.

The patient said that he was using pilocarpine hydrochloride (prescribed by an ophthalmologist), which provided relief for dry eyes within minutes of application and also improved dry mouth symptoms, but induced side effects of profuse, generalized (entire body) sweating and the relief lasted for only a short time. Is TCM effective at treating this condition?

A: Pilocarpine hydrochloride is an externally applied cholinergic agonist used for treating glaucoma and does *not* contain any active properties that can improve dry eye syndrome (DES). In fact, long-term application of this drug can lead to even drier eyes, a "burning" sensation in the eyes, unstable blood pressure, cataracts, and glaucoma. Elevated □-HCG levels are present in endometrial cancer in women and testicular, prostate, and adrenal gland pathologies in men. For brain cancer patients with elevated □-HCG levels, TCM medicinals that clear kidney and liver heat should be administered.

In cases of severe dryness, you can follow the therapeutic regimen for Sjogren's syndrome by prescribing Hyperactive Immune Formula variant. And if insomnia presents, then add Dai Zhe Shi and/or Sheng Long Gu and Sheng Mu Li. Also, bleed Zan Zhu (UB2), Si Zhu Kong (SJ23), and Da Zhui (DU14); and needle combinations of acupoints such as Feng Chi (GB20), Tian Zhu (UB10), Wan Gu (GB12), He Gu (LI4), San Yin Jiao (SP6), Yin Ling Quan (SP9), Tai Chong (LV3), Shen Men (HT7), Nei Guan (PC6), Xin Shu (UB15) and Shen Shu (UB23).

Administration of cholinergic agonists may induce profuse sweating, and if severe, then you can change to a liver-settling wind-extinguishing and yin-enriching yang-subduing formula such as Jian Ling Tang (including Gan Cao) adding The Three Yellows, Qing Hao, Zhi Mu, and Di Gu Pi.

Case Study #8: Non-healing Wound Following Meningioma Resection

Q: Recently, a female patient diagnosed with meningioma sought my consultation. She has already undergone brain surgery 5 times (including Gamma Knife and CyberKnife) as well as receiving several regimens of radiotherapy. At the time, she presented with right-sided hemiparesis and I prescribed Ru Mo Si Wu Tang variant for 1 month. After her symptoms improved a bit she never returned for consultation and treatment (I heard that she had had a stroke and was consulting another TCM doctor closer to her home).

Well, the meningioma grew back, requiring another surgical resection. After surgery, the wound wouldn't heal and the skin graft didn't take well either. The patient's husband was worried sick about her condition and wanted her to come back to visit me, but she declined, saying, "I want to use the little time I have left to go see things and have fun." Infection set in and she ended up passing away.

When I heard the news, I was saddened and wondered why a person would not cherish their own life. If this were your patient, what would you have done?

A: Meningioma relapse following resection could induce stroke-like symptoms such as hemiparesis, asthenia, seizures, and hallucinations (aural, visual, spatial, olfactory, and gustatory). If the TCM physician is inexperienced and treats this hemiparesis as a stroke (mistakenly administering TCM supplementing medicinals!), the tumor will again likely relapse and grow back at a faster rate and develop into a space-occupying lesion, which requires cranial surgery to reduce the intracranial pressure (decompressive craniectomy).

Following surgery, adjuvant radiotherapy is typically administered. Skin and tissue exposed to radiotherapy is susceptible to damage and necrosis. Failure of the granulation tissue to grow makes it difficult for the wound to heal; and even if skin grafts are performed, success rates are low and infection prevalent.

In cases where infection spreads to the brain, rapid tumor proliferation and expansion readily occurs in the presence of a compromised immune system (from the invasive surgical procedure) often developing into a space-occupying lesion. At this time, corticosteroids must be administered to prevent cerebral swelling (edema) and inflammation. The problem is that long-term administration of corticosteroids will also end up suppressing the immune system, leaving the patient susceptible to infection and resulting in tumerogenesis. On the surface, it appears that the decompressive surgery was successful (decreased ICP levels), but the patient's condition may rapidly deteriorate and eventually result in death due to secondary pathologies.

So remember! You must explain to patients and their families how vital it is to comply with TCM treatment. Even when symptoms improve and the patient appears to be well on the path of recovery, patients must continue with this therapeutic regimen for at least 3–5 months longer, up until the image scans indicate *no* signs of relapse—that's when you can begin to gradually reduce the dosage. In the future, the patient must be vigilant for any signs and symptoms of common cold (external contraction) and immediately seek treatment (preferably TCM); otherwise, the patient is highly susceptible to subsequent infection and brain swelling (edema).

Case Study #9: Intracranial Lipoma – Is Treatment Necessary?

Q: I have a 42 y/o male patient with an 8 cm lipoma on the left side of his brain stem. He has *no* presenting symptoms or signs of impairment or discomfort. Is it necessary to treat this condition?

A: Although this patient with the brainstem lipoma does not have any presenting signs or symptoms right now, the tumor will continue growing slowly over time. If its growth is not inhibited, then it could compress breathing and swallowing nerve centers, resulting in airway obstruction and aspiration pneumonia and possibly causing death.

I recommend prescribing a blood-nourishing blood-quickening, stasis-dispelling pain-relieving, and network vessel-freeing channel-regulating formula such as Ru Mo Si Wu Tang adding The Three Yellows, Tian Ma, The Three Insects, Bai Zhu, Fu Ling, Ze Xie, Chuan Qi, Ma Huang, Xing Ren, Di Long, Yu Sheng Wan, and Wan Ling Dan. This formula will effectively shrink the size of the lipoma and possibly even achieve complete resolution.

Case Study #10: Multiple Primary Tumors – "Popping Up Like Bamboo Shoots After a Rain"

Q: Not long ago a 56 y/o female patient weighing 60kg came to my clinic seeking consultation and treatment for multiple primary tumors. The earliest detection of this condition came during a routine physical examination when a malignant thyroid tumor was discovered. Surgical resection was performed upon the recommendation of her physician. Two years later, tumor cells were discovered in her brain, and ever since then it seems as if malignant tumors have been "popping up like bamboo shoots after a rain." Tumors have grown in all parts of her body, such as her right thigh and right upper arm (deltoid muscle), among other places. The patient and her family are very worried.

After taking TCM medicinals for 2 months, she began to feel improvement. For instance, before she could *not* even walk on her own without assistance from someone and now she can take short hikes on her own. However, the tumors in her right thigh and upper arm continue to enlarge and she was considering having another surgical resection. Recently, she went for a routine examination at the hospital, which revealed metastatic spread to the ovaries and uterus. That's when I really started having reservations about this case.

Am I providing the right treatment? What advice should I give her? Please, as always, offer your invaluable advice and guidance on this case. Thank you for your help!

A: This patient suffers from post-illness depression and dual blood and qi deficiency resulting from chemotherapy and radiotherapy. In addition to prescribing qi-supplementing, yang-supplementing, and dual qi- and blood-supplementing medicinals, you must also be attentive to caring for the patient's emotional well-being and mental health. Prescribing Yu Sheng Wan, starting out at doses of 1 pill/1x/day and gradually adding up to 3 pills/1x/day, should help resolve some of the anxiety and depression.

Case Study #11: Clinical Treatment of Anaplastic Astrocytoma

Q: I have asked you many times about the diagnosis and treatment of brain tumors, but have been apprehensive about getting involved in these cases until I was ready. Well, recently a classmate of mine came to me complaining of frequent headaches and blurred vision in the right eye that began one year ago. A CT scan revealed a 5–6 cm tumor located towards the center of the left cerebral hemisphere below the motor cortex behind the optic nerve.

He was diagnosed with anaplastic astrocytoma, and his doctors told him performing surgery would be a difficult task and not curative. Under the advice of his physician, he spent US$2,700/month on the newest U.S. chemotherapy agent, but after taking the drug for several months results have proven ineffective.

Five days ago, my classmate felt that the vision in his right eye was blurrier and he had a splitting headache. He went to the hospital where mannitol infusions were administered to relieve increased intracranial pressure (ICP). He also had another CT scan performed, revealing the tumor had enlarged to 7 cm, prompting him to make a special visit hoping I could prescribe TCM medicinals that would reduce the tumor size and lower ICP in order to ease the pain. I plan on advising him to undergo surgical resection and then come back to me for follow-up TCM treatment. What do you think I should do?

A: Anaplastic astrocytomas are found towards the middle of the cerebral hemispheres and lower aspect of the motor cortex, which happens to be directly behind the optic nerve. These tumors tend to be deep, infiltrative, and large, making surgical resection extremely difficult. Your best option is to administer TCM medicinals and advise the patient to receive radiotherapy in order to reduce the tumor size and prevent exacerbation of symptoms, and then go from there.

Temodal (Temozolomide) is currently the first-line chemotherapy agent for the treatment of this type of cancer. Following oral administration or injection of this alkylating agent, it is completely absorbed and broken down into small molecules—with the capacity to cross the blood-brain barrier and directly reaching the tumor where it kills off some of the cancer cells and inhibits proliferation. This is why it is the first-line drug for treating this condition. The problem is that it only provides temporary relief of symptoms with a brief respite in proliferation, but does *not* offer an effective cure. If the ICP continues increasing, the best option is to immediately administer injections of corticosteroids and mannitol (osmotic diuretic).

Radiotheraphy treatment using the LINAC system (X-Knife or CyberKnife) should be performed, while also accompanying the administration of TCM medicinals to enhance therapeutic effectiveness. For larger tumors, proton beam therapy (cyclotron) with the radionuclide cadmium 60 will typically be performed along with administration of corticosteroids.

As for the TCM formula, you should prescribe a spleen- and stomach-supplementing, phlegm-damp-transforming, and wind-stabilizing formula such as Ban Xia Tian Ma Bai Zhu San adding Ren Shen/Chuan Qi Powder and Wan Ling Dan. If tics, spasms, or seizures present, then add Quan Xie, Wu Gong, and Bai Jiang Can; if there is constipation, then add Da Huang and Pu Huang; and for severe headache add Tian Ma and Wu Zhu Yu. Once the tumor size shrinks, change the prescription to Ru Mo Si Wu Tang adding heat-clearing toxin-resolving and blood-quickening stasis-resolving medicinals to prevent the tumor cells from proliferating.

If you are still unable to achieve effective control of this patient's condition through this therapeutic regimen, then resulting brain swelling will compress cranial nerves causing abnormalities of vision, hearing, swallowing, breathing, arm and leg motor function, cognitive function, personality, temperament, etc. Severe headache, nausea and vomiting may also present, and eventually severely elevated ICP combined with high doses of corticosteroids may induce death during sleep.

This is an extremely difficult condition to treat, but you should stand up and face the challenge. Obviously, you need to coordinate treatment with your classmate's attending physicians (e.g., neurologist, neurosurgeon, and oncologist). Solely using TCM medicinals to treat this condition will *not* provide effective treatment. If the ICP continues to increase, it's best to perform decompression surgery, and at the least, attach a drainage tube to relieve the symptoms. For patients whom have had surgery, an external ventricular drain or ventriculoperitoneal shunt is commonly inserted. Care should be taken to keep the catheter clean of metabolic waste, and if blockage does occur, then it must be reinserted.

Risky surgery clears away only three-fourths…

Q1: Last week my classmate developed severe brain swelling, and despite the prevailing dangers, surgery was performed in hopes of completely resecting the tumor. The patient's family told me that an MRI was performed prior to surgery revealing an 8 cm tumor; however, during the surgical procedure surgeons found diffuse proliferation of the tumor at a size much larger than 8 cm, making clearance impossible. They ended up only clearing away three-fourths of the tumor about "the size of an adult's fist."

Initial results following surgery were good, as brain swelling and headache resolved, vision improved and motor, mental status, speech, and personality all returned to relatively normal. Unfortunately, the attending physician said that the brain tumor had already metastasized and would definitely relapse sometime in the future. What can I do to help improve this condition and allow him to maintain a better quality of life?

A1: Happy to hear about the success of your classmate's surgery! At this stage, the focus of TCM treatment is still on treating symptoms and improving the condition. You can prescribe the same TCM prescription as before (Ban Xia Tian Ma Bai Zhu San variant), and continue with this formula until his next MRI. If the tumor has shrunk, then change the prescription to Ru Mo Si Wu Tang adding Huang Lian, The Three Insects, Tian Ma, Ren Shen/Chuan Qi Powder, Wan Ling Dan and possibly combinations of medicinals such as Xia Ku Cao, Pu Gong Ying, Lian Qiao, and Jin Yin Hua.

Remember! As a general rule, this type of brain tumor's deep infiltration makes it virtually impossible to completely resect, regardless of location. A clearance of 80–90% is considered a good result, followed up by adjuvant radiotherapy in an attempt to shrink tumor size and eliminate as many of the remaining tumor cells as possible. If ICP presents, then a drainage tube is commonly inserted to drain the fluid that causes swelling. If the cerebral shunt becomes occluded, increased ICP will recur, prompting the need for another shunt placement procedure.

Q2: Thank you for clarifying the principles of using TCM medicinals to treat postoperative brain tumor patients. Due to the critical nature of this condition, prior to consulting with me, the patient had already undergone surgical excision of the tumor.

Following surgery, he has *normal* motor and congnitive function and *absence* of secondary bleeding.

Considering his stable condition, I haven't initiated TCM treatment yet, and quite honestly, I am apprehensive about doing so. According to the information I have found, astrocytomas are extremely difficult to treat, with the outcomes of surgery, chemotherapy, and radiotherapy all very poor. For glioblastomas, the most malignant type of astrocytoma, the average expected life span after diagnosis is just over 1 year. Following surgical excision, about how long will it be before the tumor recurs? Is there any way to prevent relapse? What TCM medicinals should I prescribe?

A2: Regardless of whether surgery is performed on astrocytoma patients, treatment with corticosteroids must be administered. If chemotherapy and radiotherapy are *not* administered, then in the early stage a spleen- and stomach-supplementing, phlegm-damp-transforming, and wind-stabilizing formula such as Ban Xia Tian Ma Bai Zhu San variant can be prescribed, which may induce shrinkage of tumor size. However, it is likely that the tumor may relapse in 3–5 months.

At this time, you can change the formula to Ru Mo Si Wu Tang (nourishes and quickens the blood, dispels stasis and relieves pain, and frees the network vessels and regulates the channels) or Xian Fang Huo Ming Yin (clears heat and resolves toxin, disperses swelling and breaks hardness, and quickens the blood and relieves pain) variants adding medicinals that control seizures and convulsions and lower ICP, such as Tian Ma, The Three Insects, Fu Ling, Zhu Ling, Bai Zhu, Cang Zhu, and Ze Xie. If the ICP remains elevated, prescribe Jian Ling Tang, Wu Ling San, or Chai Ling Tang variants. Long-term administration of these TCM therapeutic regimens may be able to substantially prolong the patient's life. If the tumor does recur, it will be necessary to perform surgery again with follow-up adjuvant treatment as mentioned previously.

Relapse occurs within a year…

Q: My classmate began experiencing headaches and blurred vision last year, so he went for an examination. Results revealed an astrocytoma and his doctors performed surgical decompression (decompressive craniectomy) in August. I saw him after the surgery and his condition was good. I wanted to prescribe TCM medicinals as follow-up and preventive treatment, but wasn't confident it would be effective. I read up on this topic and sought your advice about "How long it usually takes for the astrocytoma to recur?"

With these thoughts still vivid in my mind, my classmate returned for follow-up consultation revealing a single 1 cm large tumor in his brain and the attending physician told him: "During this last surgery we only excised three-fourths of the tumor tissue so the residual tumor cells will likely grow and proliferate. And since you are still relatively young (37 y/o) and physically fit, tumor cell development tends to occur at a faster pace." Thus, the attending physician recommended another surgical resection for my classmate, but this time placed an anticancer agent (capsule) inside his brain. What is your opinion on this case? Is it possible to use TCM medicinals to treat this condition?

A: Despite surgical attempts, the diffuse infiltration of astrocytoma tumerogenesis makes complete resection impossible and the probability of reproliferation highly likely. Chemotherapy, radiotherapy, and "the American elixir" of corticosteroids are administered in full force following surgery to prevent tumor proliferation for as long as possible in hopes of getting the cancer under control. As for TCM medicinals, you can prescribe the original spleen- and stomach-supplementing, phlegm-damp-transforming, and wind-stabilizing formula Ban Xia Tian Ma Bai Zhu San (including heavy doses of Huang Bo) adding Ru Xiang, Mo Yao, Chuan Qi, Niu Xi, Yu Sheng Wan, and Wan Ling Dan. For some cases involving persistent recurrence, I may recommend prescribing the blood-nourishing blood-quickening, stasis-dispelling pain-relieving, and network vessel-freeing channel-regulating formula (Yu Sheng) Ru Mo Si Wu Tang adding Tian Ma, The Three Yellows, The Three Insects, Chuan Qi, Bai Zhu, Fu Ling, Ze Xie, Yu Sheng Wan, and Wan Ling Dan.

If relapse has already occurred, then in my opinion you should prescribe (Yu Sheng) Ru Mo Si Wu Tang adding large doses of The Three Yellows (8 qian each), Bai Zhu, Fu Ling, Ze Xie, The Three Insects, Tian Ma, Wu Zhu Yu, Ren Shen/Chuan Qi Powder, Yu Sheng Wan, and Wan Ling Dan. If the condition improves initially after taking these TCM medicinals, but then declines again or even further deteriorates, add The Three Great Yang-Supplementers. If necessary, you can prescribe Da Huang (incrementally increasing doses to maintain 2–3 stools/day) to loosen the stool and promote excretion. As for Quan Xie, start out with a dose of 3–5 qian adding up to 8 qian. Since Wu Gong is very expensive, start out with 1.5 qian gradually adding up to 3 qian. For the other medicinals such as Bai

Jiang Can and Tian Ma, you can prescribe up to 8 qian, Wu Zhu Yu (5 qian), and for Wan Ling Dan, start out with 8 pills/3x/day gradually increasing as much as threefold over a period of time (the most I have ever prescribed is 28 pills/3x/day).

It's possible that the patient will experience blurred vision (like looking at an object through a dense fog), dizziness, and auditory hallucinations. This is a therapeutic response simply indicating that the potency of the medicinal treatment has reached a level exhibiting efficacy. All you have to do is gradually reduce the dosage until these therapeutic responses resolve, and then, once again, gradually return to the doses originally prescribed. The patient's constitution will develop tolerance and the efficacy will remain at peak levels.

Condition deteriorates and efforts abandoned . . .

Q1: Bad news…recently my classmate's family told me that his condition had deteriorated with a dramatic increase in ICP and left-sided hemiparesis. The attending physician administered mannitol to lower ICP, which was ineffective and also induced repeated vomiting. Another MRI was performed revealing a 20 cm large tumor that could not be resected, and his doctors were planning to give up hopes for treatment. My classmate and his family visited me seeking assistance. I can't just stand by doing nothing. This is why I am seeking your advice.

I am really close to this classmate. We have been friends since our early 20s when we both first came to live in Seoul. We have kept in touch over the years and have gone out for drinks, sharing both the joys and sorrows of life. Three days ago, I went to see him. Due to excessive corticosteroid administration his face was severely swollen, he had hemiparesis, and spoke in a slow, slurred manner (dysarthria). The moment he saw me he struggled to mutter: "Brother, I'm about to die, please save me! I know you studied…a famous Chinese medicine doctor in Taiwan…learning advanced approaches…treating complex diseases…severe cases. But you're…not willing…try helping me…Last year…my first surgery…doctors said I…had six months to live. I listened…to your advice…following…treatment regimen…have lived fairly well…for over a year now. My condition is critical…now, I know…I believe you can still…save me. I'm only 37…old. Please…help me."

After listening to my friend, all I could do was cry and console him saying "Don't worry, everything will be fine." But I knew there was nothing I could do other than rely on your assistance and guidance.

Do you think it is possible to save my classmate? Please help me try to save him!

A1: Coming across a severe illness such as your classmate's in the beginning of your medical career will help you formulate your diagnostic and treatment methods and give you direction for future medical research pursuits. There is a great void to fill in developing methods for the treatment of cerebrovasculature and nerve compressing space-occupying lesions. This is in part due to the broad diversity of conditions that affect the brain, including infectious, autoimmune, metabolic, and chronic diseases, along with the natural process of aging. Most pathological conditions of the body start in the brain centers, specifically the brain's functional capacity of regulating and monitoring the endocrine system, hormones, central nervous system (CNS), and autonomic nervous system (ANS).

Modern biomedicine still lacks the capacity to sufficiently evaluate and diagnose the subtleties and nuances of brain function. The TCM "five orifices" (sense organs) can be interpreted as a functional blueprint of the brain, with exterior pattern infections in the upper, middle, and lower burners almost all deriving from breathing, swallowing, urinary, reproductive, and digestive centers located in and around the brainstem. These centers receive errant signals and transmit false information that leads to intrinsic environmental changes in the respiratory, digestive, and urogenital system, which thus affects or alters adaptation to various bacteria, viruses, and microorganisms.

As stated in *The Yellow Emperor's Inner Canon* (**黃帝內經** *Huang Di Nei Jing*): "Evil will encroach when the qi is vacuous." The term "qi" used here may very well refer to brain centers receiving errant signals and thus transmitting false information that suppresses chelonianin (a protective secretion in the mucous membrane of the oral cavity that secretes leukocyte protein enzyme inhibitors) and thus makes the body susceptible to contraction of external evil.

Based on the information you have provided, it sounds like there is still some hope. Don't allow yourself to become so disheartened and discouraged that you lose confidence. If he wants to take TCM medicinals, then by all means, you should prescribe medicinals for him. You can prescribe the blood-nourishing and -quickening, stasis-dispelling pain-relieving, and network vessel-freeing channel-regulating formula Ru Mo Si Wu Tang adding large doses of The Three Yellows and The Three Insects (8 qian each), Qi Cao (5 qian),

Ren Shen/Chuan Qi Powder (3 qian each), Da Huang (adding incremental doses of 0.5 g up until the patient maintains 2–3 stools/day), The Four Lings, Huang Qi, Yin Xing Ye, Yu Sheng Wan, and Wan Ling Dan (adding incrementally up to as much as 28 pills/3x/day (for maximum total of 84 pills/day)).

These relatively large doses will ensure optimal therapeutic results. You must have confidence! By carefully monitoring your friend's condition and choosing the appropriate medicinals and doses, you will be doing everything you can to take care of him. Keep me updated on how the treatment progresses and contact me if you have any questions or observations.

Q2: Thank you, Professor Lee! The formula you prescribed really did help revive my friend from his critical condition. After taking these medicinals, not only was he able to make it through the crisis, but it seems the tumor has plateaued, maintaining the same size without enlarging. However, he still suffers from hemiparesis, which you explained was a result of brain tissue damage caused by radiotherapy and chemotherapy.

The attending physician thinks the reduction in tumor size (down to 6 cm) and the revitalization of the patient is due to the "effects of chemotherapy." Thus, his oncologists have decided go on the offensive, while the cancer cells appear to be on the defensive, by performing another tumor resection next week followed by a regimen of radiotherapy and chemotherapy.

Since this will induce further brain tissue damage, what preemptive TCM medicinals should I prescribe? How can I prevent the tumor from enlarging?

A2: It's great to hear that the patient's tumor shrunk following administration of TCM medicinals, and so far, his condition is being kept under control. After surgery, you can continue prescribing Ru Mo Si Wu Tang adding The Three Yellows, The Four Lings, The Three Insects, Chuan Qi/Ren Shen Powder, Da Huang, Yu Sheng Wan, and Wan Ling Dan along with small doses of The Three Great Yang-Supplementers. This approach should promote further progress.

3 cm large tumor appears again with the sensation of ants crawling…

Q: The patient's condition has been stable following the most recent surgery and administration of TCM medicinals. On March 6, another MRI was performed revealing an astrocytoma 3 cm in size and the sensation of ants crawling (formication) on the left side of his body. Western medical physicians believed this to be a sign that the tumor was undergoing abnormal differentiation and thus administered additional antitumor agents.

Unexpectedly, the tumor grew in size to 7 cm within a one-month period, and the WBC count decreased dramatically. I was worried he might pass away if things continued to regress, so I prescribed Ru Mo Si Wu Tang variant increasing the amount of Huang Qin from 4 qian to 1.5 liang. The patient's CBC and liver function tests improved and I felt relieved.

About two weeks ago the patient felt numbness and tingling on his left side again, but not complete paralysis, and imaging tests revealed brain edema. I was concerned that the tumor had already begun to proliferate once again. What I couldn't figure out was why there would be brain edema if the tumor had remained the same size (7 cm). His father wanted to have another procedure performed to reduce ICP, but the attending physician deemed the the patient's chance of survival dismal (0.01%) and thus advised against going ahead with decompression surgery. I felt that surgery to lower ICP would give my friend a chance to survive. At worst, dying on the operating table seemed a better option than lying there suffering on an ICU bed, so I strongly recommended performing another surgery.

Surprisingly, the surgeons discovered that 90% of the brain tumor had shrunk and undergone necrosis, and there was still extensive cerebral edema. It seemed that the vicious cycle of relapse and proliferation had somehow been altered, and now the treatment objective was simply to remedy the brain swelling. The physician in charge was shocked by these findings; over his nearly 20 years of practicing medicine, he had never witnessed a neoplasm undergo necrosis and shrinkage like this. I knew TCM treatment was the reason for these results and was so happy that I couldn't sleep the whole night, thinking about the exceptional efficacy and potential of TCM medicinals. I felt like I was floating on clouds and almost started crying from joy!

Soon after, my classmate was moved to a general ward. He cried and thanked me for saving his life, saying that when he is able to leave the hospital he wants to write a book entitled *How I Overcame Astrocytoma!*, and planned to spread the news through the media. Myself, I was thinking about conducting further research and presenting the results that would undoubtedly draw a lot of attention.

The experiment would use your (Yu Sheng) Ru Mo Si Wu Tang variant adding Huang Qin 1.5 liang, Fu Ling 8 qian, Ze Xie 8 qian, Huang Bo 1 liang, Chuan Qi 3 qian, and Wan Ling Dan. What do you think about this idea?

A: I am also excited about the results of (Yu Sheng) Ru Mo Si Wu Tang variant in the treatment of brain tumors. Over the past year, I have been using this formula primarily on brain tumor patients with normal (or slightly raised) ICP whose corticosteroid administration has already been fully metabolized, and those whom have undergone surgery and radiotherapy with ensuing tumor relapse. This formula can also improve brain function and stabilize the condition of patients with iatrogenic brain tissue damage (e.g., hypoxia, scarring, vascuslar injury, necrosis, swelling) resulting from chemotherapy and radiotherapy.

Currently, the Western medicine treatment regimen focuses on improving symptoms with surgery, radiotherapy, and chemotherapy. The problem is there really are *not* any effective chemotherapeutic agents that can treat this pathocondition. Human trials have shown that surgery and radiotherapy can only reduce tumor size, but not completely eradicate it, leaving neoplastic cells behind that rapidly reseed and relapse. The newest LINAC systems (e.g., CyberKnife) that rotate around the lesion at multiple angles are capable of achieving better results. However, regardless of the regimen, to achieve the best results it is essential to use TCM medicinals such as Ru Mo Si Wu Tang variant. Regarding your interest in conducting a study and presenting the research report, I think it would be best to wait for a while to further assess your classmate's condition and then talk about it later.

Moved to general ward and is able to walk…

Q1: Yesterday I went to check up on my classmate. Vision in his left eye was impaired (unable to depict objects) and he had rigidity in his left arm, but a little bit better mobility in his left leg. Basically, he was still afflicted with left-sided hemiparesis.

His radiologist is also my former professor, a very experienced professional who had worked in the U.S. for nearly 15 years, and has used 3D-CRT extensively. Since this was a very large and deep astrocytoma, he couldn't use Gamma Knife; instead, he recommended corticosteroid administration to control the condition. This treatment resulted in the patient developing a red, swollen face.

A1: The treatment of astrocytomas can lead to irreversible loss of peripheral vision. A case like this occurred not long ago in a major hospital here in Taiwan. The accumulated effects of repeated, long-term radiotherapy regimens may induce brain swelling and epileptic seizures. If the positioning and wavelength of the radiotherapy are not strictly controlled, normal cells will be damaged and necrosis may occur. Thus, I recommend administering TCM medicinals during the radiotherapy regimen as a means of mitigating these potentially severe iatrogenic complications.

Generally, for large tumors that compress nerves, resection is the best approach because radiotherapy is *not* ultimately effective regardless of the type (e.g., Gamma Knife, X-knife (photon knife), CyberKnife). TCM medicinals should be administered in the treatment of this condition regardless if corticosteroids are administered—it's just a matter of altering the formula composition.

If corticosteroids are being administered, a commonly used formula is Ban Xia Tian Ma Bai Zhu San combined with Bu Yang Huan Wu Tang (which is essentially (Yu Sheng) Ban Xia Tian Ma Bai Zhu San) adding Chuan Xiong, Chi Shao, Yin Xing Ye, and Ren Shen/Chuan Qi Powder. Once corticosteroid administration has been discontinued, wait about 3 to 5 months up until the side effects have resolved, and then change formulas to Ru Mu Si Wu Tang variant.

Q2: Can malignant brain tumors be cured? My classmate can walk on his own now, but he always worries about the possibility of relapse. This kind of malignant tumor is really a nightmare; it attacks out of nowhere, turning a perfectly healthy young person into an invalid virtually overnight. I remember the first time my classmate's brain tumor relapsed, causing hemiparesis. He received treatment for a time, narrowly avoiding the grasp of death before progressing to recovery. You never know when it will relapse next or what effects it will have on the patient.

Now, my classmate has regained mobility and can get around, but is still weak. I continue prescribing Ru Mo Si Wu Tang adding Huang Qi (1 liang), Huang Qin, Ze Xie, Chuan Qi, Bai Jiang Can (8 qian each), Chuan Xiong, Chi Shao, Yin Xing Ye (4 qian each), and Wan Ling Dan (8 pills/3x/day). Do you think this is a good prescription?

A2: My treatment principle for malignant brain tumors is really quite simple. For patients who have undergone surgery and corticosteroid administration, and two years have elapsed without relapse, then prescribe Ban Xia Tian Ma Bai Zhu San variant. If the tumor has shrunk to the point it is virtually indiscernible from the MRI, PET and CT scan images, then change the formula to Ru Mo Si Wu Tang variant adding The Three Yellows (similar to Wen Qing Yin variant). If relapse does occur, you can still prescribe Ru Mo Si Wu Tang variant adding The Three Yellows, which offers tumor-suppressing action. This is what I have learned from my clinical experience so far. If you have any further discoveries or insights, share them with me, and we can learn from one another!

The anticancer agent Timodol has shown some efficacy in 70% of the subjects in trial studies, but up to now, only animal experiments have been conducted. I am still gathering information on this drug and cooperating with Western medical doctors on experimental studies. If I find out anything new, I will contact you about it.

Q3: Since our last correspondence, in addition to 1/3 of his left eye having visual impairment, my classmate currently presents with mild edema in his left lower leg and a slight gait abnormality, but his mobility is improving and, most significantly, the tumor has not relapsed.

I am considering adding Ren Shen into his current formula (Ru Mo Si Wu Tang) adding Fu Ling, Ze Xie, The Three Yellows, Yin Xing Ye, Dan Shen, Chuan Qi, Da Huang, Pu Gong Ying, and Wan Ling Dan. Do you think this is a good idea? Will it induce tumor proliferation? [4/9/2007]

A3: Ren Shen will not induce proliferation and growth of brain tumors. You don't need to be concerned about that! Ren Shen—supplements original qi, stems vacuity desertion, supplements the spleen and boosts the lung, engenders liquid, and quiets the spirit—is an adaptogen that complements the actions of other medicinals in the overall formula composition. Depending on the dosage and formula it is in, it can serve as a sovereign medicinal as well as a minister, assistant, or envoy.

For instance, added to cold and bitter heat-abating medicinals, it accelerates the heat-abating, swelling-dispersing, and antitumor actions; added to yang-supplementing medicinals, it assumes a great yang-supplementing action; added to blood-quickening stasis-transforming medicinals, it quickens the blood and transforms stasis; and added to other antitumor (especially for brain tumors) medicinals, it serves to suppress proliferation of cancer cells.

In the case of brain tumors, corticosteroids are the first-line treatment administered, regardless if surgery, chemotherapy, and radiotherapy are part of the therapeutic regimen. The administration of corticosteroids inevitably causes the side effects of edema and fat deposition (especially the face and neck). Adding Ren Shen into your TCM formula actually helps prevent brain swelling, atrophy, and marrow failure. You do *not* have to worry about using it!

Tumor shrinks with no signs of relapse…

Q1: An MRI performed on 04/12 confirmed that the postsurgical tumor remnants had shrunk. The attending physician said: "Very odd, usually the tumor will relapse about 3 months after surgical excision. This patient's neoplasm has not spread; on the contrary, it has incurred a marked reduction in size." The patient's parents were grateful and his father was drinking liquor and singing, overwhelmed with tearful joy.

My friend is still young and should be able to look forward to a bright future. Originally, he thought there was no hope and couldn't imagine ever recovering; and now he is ecstatic. I want to change my formula to Ru Mo Si Wu Tang adding Yin Xing Ye and Dan Shen (8 qian each). What do you think about his idea? [4/19/2007]

A1: Yes, this is a good idea, and actually, you could add a small amount of Huang Qi as well. But remember! You only need to use a small dose. Once the tumor has been suppressed, TCM medicinals can be used to promote nerve conduction and functional compensation. This is why I always say that TCM medicinals also have a rehabilitative action.

You do *not* want to inundate the body with supplementing medicinals, prescribe just enough to activate this process and let the body's natural capacity to restore itself take effect. Completely depending on medicinals or other agents will have the deleterious effect of accelerating degeneration of the brain's functional capacities and possibly even result in dementia.

Q2: My classmate has gone two years without malignant brain tumor relapse. This is great, but the problem he faces now is being badly overweight (verging on obesity) due to long-term administration of the tumor cell suppressor drug Tamoxifen and a host of digestants. He has experienced a dramatic weight gain now tipping the scale at 120kg (height: 182 cm). This is troubling, what can I do? [4/17/2008]

A2: The main side effect involving the long-term administration of the tumor cell suppressant Tamoxifen is water amassment (蓄水 xù shuǐ). If not carefully monitored the patient will inevtiably gain weight. I suggest you prescribe either Zhi Bo Di Huang Tang; Ru Mo Si Wu Tang adding The Three Yellows; Wen Dan Tang combining Huang Lian Jie Du Tang; or Xian Fan Huo Ming Yin variant—these formulas will inhibit estrogen receptors and prevent rapid weight gain. If water amassment presents, then add Bai Zhu, Fu Ling, and Ze Xie; and if mild seizures present, then add Tian Ma, Wu Zhu Yu, The Three Insects, and Zhu Ru.

Q3: An MRI performed in July 2009 revealed the presence of a heart-shaped polyp at the site of the original brain tumor lesion. It does *not* appear to be cancerous. Left-side arm and leg mobility, function, and strength has improved and the patient can now easily raise his arm and lift his leg, but the tips of fingers and toes severely ache and tingle. Is this a good or bad sign? I hope it isn't a neoplasm. [7/16/2009]

A3: From what you have described, it sounds like the fortuitous signs of brain cell regeneration. I have seen this before during experiments on animals and in patients here in my clinic. There is no doubt TCM medicinals can induce stem cell regeneration and inhibit neoplastic stem cells. You should compile these results and present them in a paper. The title could be something like "Traditional Korean Medicine (TKM) regenerates normal brain stem cells in astrocytoma patient." You can show the images before and after and explain the recovery process of limb and facial function. I am confident these results will attract international attention and recognition. Don't forget to mention my name in the report!

Q4: On a related topic, a senior traditional Korean medicine doctor says that the administration of Dao Tan Tang will reduce tumor size within 2 months. Is this possible?

A4: Dao Tan Tang (dries dampness and eliminates phlegm and moves qi and opens depression) has a similar action as Wen Dan Tang (clears heat and transforms phlegm). These types of formulas can definitely reduce tumor size, but it depends on the size and type of tumor. If the tumor is large causing severe compression, patients with increased ICP must first have surgical decompression, resection, and then adjuvant radiotherapy.

As for oral administration of TCM medicinals, you must accurately identify the pattern. If it is indeed phlegm-heat pattern or cold-phlegm (rheum) pattern, then these types of formulas will be effective. You could consider formulas such as Er Chen Tang, Wen Dan Tang, Di Tan Tang, Dao Tan Tang, Meng Shi Gun Tan Wan, Xiang Sha Liu Jun Zi Tang, Gan Jiang Ren Shen Ban Xia Wan, and Ban Xia Tian Ma Bai Zhu San variants.

I remember telling you about my animal experiments and how the most effective formulas were Ban Xia Tian Ma Bai Zhu San, Da Chai Hu Tang, Long Dan Xie Gan Tang, Huang Lian Jie Du Tang, Wen Dan Tang, and Qing Xin Niu Huang Wan variants adding Yu Sheng Wan and Wan Ling Dan. However, in cases involving iatrogenic brain tissue damage (e.g., hypoxia, scarring, vascuslar injury, necrosis, swelling), or if chemotherapy and/or radiotherapy are a part of the therapeutic regimen with initial tumor shrinkage or resolution but then grows back again, then this can be identified as repletion heat and stasis heat pattern. For this pattern, it is best to prescribe Ru Mo Si Wu Tang, Da Chai Hu Tang, or Chai Ling Tang variants adding large doses of The Three Yellows, The Three Insects, Da Huang, Chuan Qi, Tian Ma, Yu Sheng Wan, and Wan Ling Dan.

I am still in the exploratory stages of treating brain tumors myself. I wish there were some "golden elixir" that I could share with you, and if there is, I have not found it yet. This is an intensely involved and multifaceted pathocondition posing immense challenge, but also a lot of promise. Next year, I will be collaborating with Dr. Ma Hsing-yi, Director of the Division of Neuro-Oncology, Department of Neurological Surgery at Tri-General Services Hospital (Taipei, Taiwan), on an integrated TCM and Western medicine national cancer research project.

The project involves CTS, MRI, and PET diagnosis, surgical procedures, biopsies for conducting gene research, and treatment using radiotherapy and Timodol accompanied by administration of TCM medicinals. This research is very expensive, requiring the acquisition of funding and assistance from the pharmaceutical manufacturer of Timodol. I hope this research will propel my clinical work into the international spotlight, advancing the administration of TCM medicinals as a part of the conventional therapeutic regimen for brain tumors. The good news is that we have already applied for and are currently in the patent pending phase for nine TCM formulas that treat brain tumors. If accepted, patent licensing will be issued in 3 months, and plans are being made for conducting further research in the future.

Section 2: Respiratory Tract Cancers

This section encompasses pathological conditions extending from the nasal cavity to the lungs—the respiratory tract. Cases primarily involving nasopharyngeal carcinoma and lung cancer will be presented.

Case Study #1: Nasopharyngeal Carcinoma

Q: Recently, I treated a patient with nasal lymphoma. Following radiotherapy, the patient experienced side effects of dry mouth and tongue, middle ear effusion, and loss of olfactory sense. He wanted to try acupuncture for treating these symptoms, but in my opinion TCM medicinals have the capacity to offer much better results. Please explain your approach for treating this condition.

A: Atrophy of the salivary glands, olfactory nerve, and auditory nerve are all common side effects of radiotherapy treatment for nasopharyngeal carcinoma (NPC). Some patients may present with obstruction of the Eustachian tube and middle ear effusion (purulent discharge) that causes dizziness and vertigo, and others may incur lymphatic swelling, which when severe may result in the patient looking "like a toad with eyes swollen shut."

This pathocondition requires patience and compliance from the patient, with the administration of both TCM medicinals and acupuncture necessary to achieve the quickest and best efficacy. For patients with lymphatic swelling that resembles "elephantiasis," prescribe (Yu Sheng) Wu Ling San (Nephritis Formula) adding heavy doses of Huang Qi, Gan Jiang, and Rou Gui along with Yin Xing Ye (8 qiang–1 liang) and Ren Shen/Chuan Qi Powder. At the onset, the affected area will begin to soften up and become even more swollen, but after taking the formula for 1–2 months, the swelling will begin to disperse. Marked improvement will continue with complete resolution occurring in roughly 6 months to 1 year.

If there is no lymphatic swelling, then simply follow the principles of my book *Cancer Therapy: New Approaches in Integrative Chinese-Western Medicine* (中西醫結合治癌新法 *Xi Yi Jie He Zhi Ai Xin Fa*), using

Xiao Chai Hu Tang combining Sheng Yu Tang adding Ma Huang, Xi Xin, Bai Zhi, and Xin Yi (pounded). For Ma Huang start out at small doses, gradually adding up to 5–6 qian (or even more if the patient's sleep isn't affected); for Xi Xin start out at small doses gradually adding up to 3 qian; and for the remaining medicinals you can prescribe doses of up to 8 qian. Once the middle ear effusion has gradually been reabsorbed, you can begin adding The Three Great Yang-Supplementers. If after adding these yang-supplementing medicinals hematopoiesis is still insufficient, then you should change the prescription to a formula such as Shi Quan Da Bu Tang or You Gui Yin adding Ma Huang, Bai Zhi, Xin Yi, and Xi Xin.

As for acupuncture, you can consider warm needling combinations of the following acupoints: the Trigeminal Nerve Special Points corresponding with the pathways of the trigeminal nerve (CNV) and facial nerve (CNVII) (starting at a point about 1 cun out from Ting Gong (SI19) below the zygomatic arch, transversely insert 3 needles joining Si Zhu Kong (SJ23), Quan Liao (SI18), and Jia Che (ST6) respectively), Feng Chi (GB20), Feng Fu (DU16), He Gu (LI4), Zu San Li (ST36), Bai Hui (DU20), Da Zhui (DU14), Ying Xiang (LI20) joining Qing Ming (UB1), San Yin Jiao (SP6), Yin Ling Quan (SP9), and Xue Hai (SP10). Of course, you could choose Fei Shu (UB13), Ya Men (DU15), and Jing Chuan Dian (aka Bai Lao (EX-HN15)) as well, but due to their anatomical location, you must be very careful when needling these points, only inserting at shallow depths. Remember! Warm needling and electroacunpuncture (though I do *not* use this method myself) generally offer better results compared to just needling without moxa.

Case Study #2: Lung Cancer – Can TCM Provide Effective Treatment?

Q: Recently, a 59 y/o male with lung cancer visited my clinic accompanied by his wife. Two years ago, he was diagnosed with Stage III lung cancer, and over the past three months, he has experienced shortness of breath, persistent cough, dysphagia, frequent heat sensation, and weight loss.

While conducting the patient interview, I found out that he has a brother with lung cancer who went through 8 years of Western medical treatment, describing it as a very unpleasant process *without* very effective results. His brother's experience made him want to give

TCM a try. What is the best approach for treating lung cancer?

A: For lung cancer patients already presenting with neoplastic fever, I recommend prescribing a heat-clearing phlegm-damp-transforming water-disinhibiting formula such as Chai Ling Tang (including large doses of Fu Ling and Ze Xie) adding large doses of Qing Hao, Zhi Mu, and Di Gu Pi (enrich yin and downbear fire and clear vacuity heat and eliminate steaming bone); Ting Li Zi, Ma Huang, Xing Ren, and Fang Ji; Shan Zha and Ji Nei Jin (aid digestion); Ren Shen/Chuan Qi Powder; and Yu Sheng Wan. This prescription should effectively provide relief for these symptoms.

Once symptoms have been relieved, then subtract Qing Hao, Zhi Mu, and Di Gu Pi. If the above symptoms once again return, then consider adding combinations of the following medicinals: The Three Great Yang-Supplementers; Zi Yuan, Kuan Dong Hua, and Wu Wei Zi; or Xu Duan, Gu Sui Bu, Qian Cao, and Huai Niu Xi. The guiding principle is to apply pattern identification as the basis for determining treatment, adjusting your formula accordingly based on the presenting signs and symptoms.

Case Study #3: Lung Cancer – TCM Treatment and Medicinal Foods

Q: I have a 60 y/o male patient with advanced lung cancer who drinks three bottles of soju (Korean rice wine) and smokes three packs of cigarettes every day. Recently, he had been feeling tired and lacked energy, so he decided to stop smoking cigarettes.

Two days after he quit smoking, he started coughing, so he went to a family medicine doctor who prescribed some drugs for the cough. One week later, he began coughing blood (hemoptysis). He went to get it checked out by a pulmonologist at a hospital and discovered widespread proliferation of cancer cells in his lungs.

The patient said he did *not* want to take TCM medicinals because "it tastes bad," but he wants to try eating medicinal foods. What kind of food is good for patients with lung cancer?

A: Unfortunately, at this stage, medicinal foods are not going to be enough to prevent lung cancer from proliferating and spreading. Medicinal foods, though beneficial, are *not* the most important part of the therapeutic regimen. Right now, it is critical that you have a serious discussion with him and his family, clearly explaining the need to take TCM medicinals and potentially be open to Western medical intervention—that is, if he "really values life."

If the patient incessantly shuns your compassionate attempts of concern, then you could resort to a more prodding approach by saying something like this: "Can't eat this, don't want to take that…if you are no longer living, then we won't even need to have this conversation." Yes, I know, this may *not* be the ideal approach, but for some patients, it may be the *only* way to make them recognize the gravity of this situation.

TCM medicinals are an essential part of the therapeutic regimen for lung cancer patients, administered either as a first-line therapy or as accompanying Western medicine intervention. I recommend prescribing a heat-clearing phlegm-damp-transforming water-disinhibiting formula such as Chai Ling Tang or possibly a blood-breaking channel-freeing formula such as Tong Jing Fang. For patients presenting with qi vacuity, you can continue prescribing Chai Ling Tang adding Ren Shen/Chuan Qi Powder, Huang Qi, and The Three Great Yang-Supplementers; or change the formula to Bu Zhong Yi Qi Tang variant.

These are formulas with proven efficacy. I have used this approach to treat innumerable lung cancer patients over the years and all have shown improvement in their conditions, with some going into sustained remission. Sometimes the institution of modern Western medicine simply gives up and is *not* willing to treat these types of patients, not even with radiotherapy or chemotherapy.

Time and again, I have successfully administered Chai Ling Tang variant to improve their condition and remedy troubling symptoms, thus dramatically increasing their quality of life and longevity. One 80 y/o patient was told by doctors that he wouldn't make it 3 more months, but he began taking TCM medicinals and it's already been over 1 1/2 years now, and the patient is still going strong and feels healthy!

If the patient insists on just eating medicinal foods and *not* taking TCM medicinals, then you can advise him to stew some of the TCM medicinals prescribed in the formulas above, with his choice of fish or meat. This is the best kind of medicinal food. It will help his body maintain the physical strength and stamina to overcome the trials and travails of this chronic life-shortening condition.

Case Study #4: Non-Small Cell Lung Cancer

Q: I have a 34 y/o male patient with advanced lung cancer. Just 6 months after getting married, he went for a regular checkup that eventually led to a diagnosis of non-small cell lung cancer (NSCLC) with pleural invasion. He is currently undergoing chemotherapy with the anticancer agents Gemzar and Cisplatin. To date, there have not yet been any adverse effects arising from the treatment.

What I don't understand is how this pathocondition could have gone unnoticed by the patient for so long without any signs or symptoms presenting? Please share your advice and guidance on this condition.

A: Typically, lung cancer is *not* discovered until the later stages of disease. Prior to clinical diagnosis, the majority of patients have healthy appetites and lead normal, active lives. But after diagnosis...bam!...everything changes.

This is in fact one of the major topics of debate going on in medical ethics: Lung cancer is discovered during a routine physical examination and metastases has occurred. But the patient has a healthy appetite, and no symptoms or any discomfort whatsoever—Should the patient be informed about his or her illness? Should treatment be obligatory?

Nowadays, Western medical physicians in many advanced nations are advocating that the best approach is to *monitor* the patient's condition taking a "wait and see" approach, instead of telling the patient about the diagnosis. I agree with this approach, because being diagnosed with cancer more often than not leads to a traumatic psychological impact on patients, with many losing confidence and the will to survive.

The formula I prescribe for metastatic lung cancer is still Chai Ling Tang variant, making the appropriate modifications based on the degree and extent of hematopoietic, hepatic, and renal function impairment induced by chemotherapy. Once the patient has weathered the storm of chemotherapy's adverse effects, then you can either make the appropriate modifications to Chai Ling Tang or consider changing to a formula variant such as Shen Ling Bai Zhu San, Xiang Sha Liu Jun Zi Tang, Wu Wei Yi Gong San, or Si Shen Tang. As always, you adjust the formula based on presenting signs and symptoms and pattern identification.

Section 3: Stomach Cancer

There are four main types of stomach (gastric) cancer—adenocarcinoma (90%), lymphoma, stromal, and carcinoid. Gastric cancer has a relatively high incidence rate in East Asia, and this section introduces those cases that the student Dr. Yang has sought advice and direction from his mentor, Dr. Lee. Cases involving the diagnosis and treatment of regional and distant metastases will also be presented.

Case Study #1: Stomach Cancer Treatment – Xiang Sha Liu Jun Zi Tang

Q: A 34 y/o male patient visited his doctor 3 months ago due to poor appetite. Further examination with gastroscopy revealed gastric cancer. The hospital advised him to immediately undergo laparoscopic exploratory surgery, which revealed widespread proliferation of neoplastic cells (end-stage). Thus, they decided it would be best to go ahead and resect as much of the tumor as possible and administer adjuvant chemotherapy and radiotherapy to prevent the continued proliferation of the cancer cells.

However, this approach would inherently have its limitations. The patient eventually developed a mild case of pyloric stenosis, presenting with ascites along the left hypochondrium, constipation, loss of appetite, weight loss, acid regurgitation, and belching. This is when he sought my consultation for treatment.

Since there were *no* abnormalities in his complete blood count (CBC) and other lab test results, I prescribed Xiang Sha Liu Jun Zi Tang. Do you think this is the correct approach for this case?

A: Yes, the qi-boosting spleen-fortifying and qi-moving phlegm-transforming actions of this formula is a good choice, but it would be best to also add Gan Jiang, Fu Zi, Da Huang, Lai Fu Zi, Ze Xie, Ren Shen/Chuan Qi Powder, Yi Yi Ren, and Wan Ling Dan. For Da Huang, you should gradually add incremental doses (as much as 7–8 qian) up until the patient is able to pass 2–3 stools/day. If the patient still cannot pass stool, then you can try adding larger amounts of The

Three Great Yang-Supplementers; and if the patient *still cannot* pass stool, then add Mang Xiao (moistens dryness and softens hardness and drains heat and frees the stool), or even consider changing to a blood-breaking and channel-freeing formula such as Tong Jing Fang adding combinations of the above medicinals.

Case Study #2: Stomach Cancer – A Difficult Condition to Treat

Q: A 37 y/o male patient who was recently married just two months ago explained that he used to have bad eating habits and gastrointestinal discomfort for many years (usually only taking 1 or 2 meals a day and drinking alcohol almost every evening). After getting married, his wife convinced him to get a check up at the hospital, where an endoscopy could be performed. The endoscopic image showed that he had a grain size lump growing in the submucosa of his stomach, and the biopsy confirmed it to be malignant.

Not long after, he underwent a follow-up examination revealing that the cancer cells had spread rapidly and extensively throughout the lymph nodes and distant areas of the body. His physicians deemed his condition so dire that they informed him he might only have about 6 months to live. In his disappointment and despair, he decided to try novel "natural healing" methods and immunotherapy (biologic therapy), which are very popular in Japan. But his condition did *not* improve and he lost even more weight. That's when he decided to try TCM treatment instead and came to see me.

This is the most serious case of gastric cancer I have attempted to treat, and if I understand correctly, gastric cancer with submucosal invasion is very difficult to treat! Usually, upon discovery it has already proliferated to the advanced stages. Please provide me with your invaluable insights. Is there any chance of improving this patient's condition, or at least relieving his symptoms?

A: Gastric cancer with metastases is particularly difficult to treat because of the broad scope of symptoms and complex pattern types. According to TCM theory, gastric tumors can be classified into four main patterns: 1) Yang Ming exterior with stomach heat pattern; 2) stasis heat, static blood, and stasis obstruction pattern; 3) spleen qi and yang vacuity pattern; and 4) spleen qi and yang vacuity with cold stasis pattern. Remember! This is just a generalization for the purpose of categorization and simplification, whereas in actual clinical practice these stages and patterns blend together into complex and overlapping patterns.

1) The early stage of gastric cancer can be identified as Yang Ming exterior with stomach heat pattern, requiring the administration of either a dual exterior- and interior-resolving and heat-clearing diarrhea-checking formula such as Ge Gen Qin Lian Tang or a heat-clearing toxin-resolving, swelling-dispersing hardness-breaking, and blood-quickening pain-relieving formula such as Xian Fang Huo Ming Yin. For instance, if endoscopic examination reveals a tumor growing on the surface of the stomach lining (stromal tumor) with a bright, fleshy color of cinnabar (vermilion), then this can be identified as Yang Ming exterior with stomach heat pattern, requiring the administration of Ge Gen Qin Lian Tang adding Pu Gong Ying, Lian Zhao, Jin Yin Hua, Da Huang, Wan Ling Dan, and Yu Sheng Wan.

2) The stomach is continually exposed to the external environment via solid foods and liquids, bringing legions of bacteria and viruses (evil qi) along for the ride. Continual bombardment by this evil qi (邪氣 xié qi) may induce stasis heat, static blood, and stasis obstruction pattern. For this pattern you can prescribe a blood-nourishing and -quickening, stasis-dispelling pain-relieving, and network vessel-freeing channel-regulating such as Tong Jing Fang, Ru Mo Si Wu Tang, or Xuan Fu Dai Zhe Shi Tang adding combinations of medicinals such as Huang Qin, Chuan Qi, Pu Huang (if heat presents), Shan Dou Gen, Liang Jiang, San Leng, E Zhu, Yan Hu Suo, San Nai, Yu Jin, Yu Sheng Wan, and Wan Ling Dan.

3) Stasis heat, static blood, and stasis obstruction taxes the stomach and spleen's functional capacity, and thus leads to a condition that can be identified as spleen qi and yang vacuity pattern. For these patients you should prescribe a qi-boosting spleen-fortifying and qi-moving phlegm-transforming formula such as Xiang Sha Liu Jun Zi Tang, Bu Zhong Yi Qi Tang, Shen Ling Bai Zhu Tang, or Dang Gui Shao Yao San adding combinations of medicinals such as Shan Dou Gen, Liang Jiang, Chuan Qi, Ru Xiang, Mo Yao, and Gu Sui Bu.

4) In the later stages of this condition, spleen qi and yang vacuity may evolve into spleen qi and yang vacuity with cold stasis pattern, requiring the administration of a qi-boosting spleen-fortifying and stomach-harmonizing dampness-percolating formula such as Xiang Sha Liu Jun Zi Tang combining Shen Ling Bai Zhu Tang

adding Liang Jiang, Fu Zi, and Rou Gui.

If you are treating a gastric tumor in its early stages when the true heat pattern still predominates and there has been no Western medicine intervention, then you should prescribe Xian Fang Huo Ming Yin variant. Nowadays, in my clinical practice more and more patients are presenting with static blood and stasis obstruction pattern types.

Case Study #3: Adenocarcinoma

Q: The spouse of an acquaintance of mine, Professor Cui, visited me a couple of days ago explaining that she had just gotten back results from a physical examination that revealed a gastric tumor. A biopsy confirmed it as gastric carcinoma, and though the tumor is very small, doctors recommended that she undergo surgical resection. What's the best TCM formula I can prescribe for treating this condition?

A: In the early stages of adenocarcinoma, this condition can be identified as stomach heat with Yang Ming exterior pattern. You can consider prescribing a dual exterior- and interior-resolving and heat-clearing diarrhea-checking formula such as Ge Gen Qin Lian Tang adding Ban Xia, Shan Dou Gen, Gao Liang Jiang, Hai Piao Xiao (controls acid and relieves pain and astringes and secures and stanches blood), Zhe Bei Mu, Chuan Qi, Yu Sheng Wan, and Wan Ling Dan.

Keep me updated on this case throughout the treatment process. Maybe I can be of assistance.

Case Study #4: Postoperative Vomiting – How Can I Administer TCM Formula Decoction?

Q: A 49 y/o female patient experienced stomach discomfort and went in for a thorough examination. Her gastroenterologist diagnosed her with early stage gastric cancer (not even at T0) and advised her to undergo total gastrectomy to "cure her once and for all."

About 3 hours after surgery, the patient vomited continuously for 10 minutes, and these vomiting attacks continued occurring at about the same interval (every 3 hours) and duration (for 10 minutes). Drug treatment was ineffective and her doctors didn't know what to do, telling her, "We've never seen this type of complication before."

This is when the patient's family came to see me, hoping I could prescribe TCM medicinals to remedy the patient's condition. Initially, I prescribed Ban Xia and Fu Ling 1 liang each, but it wasn't effective. What do you think about adding Ding Xiang, Shi Di, Dai Zhe Shi, and Yu Sheng Wan?

A: Hmm! Vomiting 3 hours after eating would typically be caused by either duodenal stenosis or obstruction. Since the patient is able to pass stool, we know that food is being digested, which thus suggests either duodenal stenosis or partial obstruction. It cannot be complete obstruction, because the patient would not be able to absorb nutrients and defecate.

Generally, when total gastrectomy is performed the patient would *not* be allowed to eat or drink right away. So, if vomiting presents at regular intervals (e.g., vomiting every 3 hours), I suspect this case may involve some degree of psychosomatic etiology.

With this in mind, I would try prescribing a qi-moving counterflow-downbearing, center-harmonizing agitation-calming, and stagnation-dissipating phlegm-transforming formula such as Gan Mai Da Zao Tang Combining Ban Xia Hou Po Tang adding Yu Sheng Wan (3 pills/day, taking 1 pill after every meal or eating the pill with meals).

You can instruct the patient to casually sip or drink this decoction like a beverage throughout the course of the day. This prescription will serve the dual function of remedying the physical symptoms and calming the heart spirit (心神 xīn shén) at the psychological level.

Case Study #5: Gastric Tumor Resection – What TCM Formula Should I Prescribe?

Q: A 31 y/o male patient was diagnosed with advanced stage gastric cancer, and has already undergone surgical resection and received chemotherapy. Now, the tumor is virtually imperceptible. He is happily married with a 2-month old newborn and really has a strong will to survive.

What TCM medicinals should I prescribe for this patient? Should I prescribe a formula to boost appetite and promote digestion? Or, should I just wait until symptoms present and prescribe medicinals accordingly based on pattern identification?

A: Regardless of the device (e.g., endoscopy, laparoscopy) used for examination, the type of surgery (e.g., endoscopic resection, subtotal or total gastrectomy), or if the imaging scans reveal the presence of a tumor or not, *all* gastric cancer patients should be administered TCM medicinals as soon as possible following surgery. The purpose of treatment is to regulate the function of the stomach, resolve symptoms, and minimize the chance of progression, recurrence, and metastasis.

There are a wide selection of qi-boosting spleen-fortifying, qi-moving phlegm-transforming, and food-dispersing digestion-promoting formula variants that can achieve this goal, such as Xiang Sha Liu Jun Zi Tang, Si Jun Zi Tang, Si Shen Tang, Yue Ju Wan, and Bao He Wan. Based on presenting signs, symptoms and pattern identification, you should also add combinations of the following medicinals: Yi Yi Ren (fortifies the spleen and dries dampness and clears heat and expels pus) and Shan Dou Gen (clears heat and resolves toxin and disperses swelling); Gao Liang Jiang (dissipates cold and relieves pain and warms the center and checks vomiting), Mu Xiang (moves qi and relieves pain), and Yuan Hu (quickens the blood, moves qi, and relieves pain); San Leng and E Zhu (break blood and move qi and disperse accumulations and relieve pain); Gu Ya, Mai Ya, Ji Nei Jin, and Shan Zha (disperse food and promote digestion and fortify the spleen and open the stomach); The Three Yellows (clear heat and resolve toxin), Mu Dan Pi (quickens and cools the blood), and Chuan Qi (transforms stasis and stanches bleeding); and Zhe Bei Mu and Hai Piao Xiao (astringe and secure, control acid, and stanch bleeding).

Remember! Yu Sheng Wan and Wan Ling Dan are essential medicinals for the treatment of cancer and should be included as a part of your therapeutic regimen regardless of which formula you choose to prescribe. This approach will offer exceptional overall anticancer efficacy.

For gastric cancer patients ≥ 75 y/o, the Western medical standard protocol does not advocate surgery, and in many cases, doctors are *not* willing to provide aggressive treatment for this condition. In these situations, you can prescribe a qi-boosting spleen-fortifying and stomach-harmonizing dampness-percolating formula such as Shen Ling Bai Zhu San variant, which will help remedy symptoms. If heat presents, you can add The Three Yellows and Mu Dan Pi; and if anemia presents, then add yang-supplementing medicinals.

Remember! You must understand that Cu Lu Rong offers greater efficacy for treating tumors and Xi Lu Rong offers greater efficacy for promoting hematopoiesis. Thus, for de novo neoplasms and in younger patients, unless there is severe malnutrition or if chemotherapy and radiotherapy has induced hematopoietic dysfunction, then Cu Lu Rong should be administered and *not* Xi Lu Rong. If Xi Lu Rong *is* administered, it could lead to the acceleration of tumerogenesis, and we obviously do *not* want that!

Case Study #6: Cerebral Infarction Patient Diagnosed with Gastric Cancer

Q: A 63 y/o male patient explained that one day 4 years ago he suddenly began salivating profusely and continuously. Upon examination, an MRI revealed signs of a cerebral infarct in the upper left hemisphere. However, he did *not* undergo aggressive treatment and simply began taking antihypertensive medication.

About 2 years ago, he was diagnosed with gastric cancer, underwent a complete gastrectomy, and subsequently has suffered from dysphagia since the procedure. Meanwhile, complications caused by the cerebral infarct have worsened. During his last visit, he presented with dysphagia, weakness in his right leg, and normal stool and urine. Do you think it is a good idea to prescribe Bu Yang Huan Wu Tang with Huang Lian Jie Du Tang?

A: Cerebral infarction patients commonly incur progressive cerebral atrophy. Once degeneration begins, there is an even greater possibility for another infarct and hemorrhage, which cause more complications for the patient.

Since the patient has already had a total gastrectomy to remove the gastric tumor, you can go ahead and prescribe a blood-quickening qi-supplementing formula such as Bu Yang Huan Wu Tang adding Huang Lian Jie Du Tang, Gao Liang Jiang, Sha Ren, Shan Dou Gen, Ban Xia, San Leng, E Zhu, Ren Shen/Chuan Qi Powder, Yu Sheng Wan, and Wan Ling Dan. This approach will offer better results.

Case Study #7: Stomach Cancer – Multiple Metastases

Q: Recently, I have been treating a 59 y/o male patient with gastric cancer. About 3 years ago, he was diagnosed with gastric cancer. Following several less invasive surgical procedures, in October of that year he underwent gastrectomy and colectomy.

In February of the following year, metastatic spread was discovered in the lymph nodes below the pancreas. Resection was immediately performed and 10 sessions of chemotherapy were administered. Three months later (mid May), inguinal lymph nodes on both sides were resected; and in August, malignancies were resected in the abdomen and left lung. In January of the following year (third year), abdominal lymph node metastases had occurred, but with subsequent shrinkage in size, while the left lung tumor had gradually enlarged.

Now, I am treating him with the heat-clearing phlegm-damp-transforming water-disinhibiting formula Chai Ling Tang adding The Three Great Yang-Supplementers (1 qian each) to control WBC levels; and also Bai Zhu, Fu Ling, Ze Xie, Huang Qin (8 qian each), and Wan Ling Dan (4 pills/3x/day). Do you think this is a good approach? Should I advise him to discontinue chemotherapy?

A: Yes, this formula should be effective. The patient must be a very strong-willed person to continue pushing on in the face of such adversity. He will have even better results under your care receiving integrative TCM and Western medical treatment.

The only thing I would suggest is to consider adding Ma Huang, Ting Li Zi, Fang Ji, and Bai Bu to help relieve the complications arising from the lung and lymph node tumors, along with larger doses of Wan Ling Dan (resolves toxin and disperses welling-abscesses, soothes the sinews and quickens the blood, and dispels wind and relieves pain). You can also consider adding Ren Shen/Chuan Qi Powder (supplements the spleen and boosts the lung, engenders liquid, transforms stasis, and stanches bleeding).

As for chemotherapy, if the cancer has already reached the advanced stage, the most important aspect is for the patient to maintain a relatively high quality of life and enjoy himself as much as possible during this final period. Though ultimately it is the patient's decision (after consultation with his oncologist), in my opinion, it may be the best choice to forego chemotherapy.

Case Study #8: Stomach Cancer – Postoperative Regional and Distant Lymph Node Metastases

Q: A 51 y/o male patient was diagnosed with gastric cancer in 1993 (14 years ago) and underwent a complete gastrectomy for it at that time. In 2006 (last year), after seeking care for a swelling on his right arm, an examination revealed that the cancer had relapsed.

His doctors suspected regional and distant lymph node metastases from gastric cancer and the patient received chemotherapy, which was *not* very effective and dramatically weakened the patient's physical condition.

Now, the patient presents as follows: lymphoma in the right arm and both legs, mild ascites, and normal CBC. What formula do you think would be most effective?

A: Patients are consistently seeking your consultation and treatment for relapse of gastric cancer and lymph node metastases. This proves that you have gained some notoriety and the trust of South Korean patients. Keep up the good work!

For this patient, you can prescribe a heat-clearing phlegm-damp-transforming water-disinhibiting formula such as Chai Ling Tang adding Qing Hao, Zhi Mu, Di Gu Pi, Shan Dou Gen, Gao Liang Jiang; Huang Qin and Huang Lian (large doses); Chuan Qi, Yu Sheng Wan, and Wan Ling Dan; Ma Huang and Xing Ren (small doses); and also Cang Zhu, Fu Ling, Ze Xie, Ting Li Zi, and Fang Ji for ascites, pleural effusion, and lung metastases.

Just remember! Most adenocarcinomas (and lymphomas) can be identified as Shao Yang pattern. If the above formula does *not* effectively reduce ascites, then you can consider adding Ren Shen (supplements original qi and stems vacuity desertion and supplements the spleen and boosts the lung). If the blood tests show normal levels of Hb, PLT, LDH, and CPK with only CA72-4, CEA, and CA19-9 elevated, then you should continue monitoring the condition; and if necessary, add larger doses of Huang Qin, Huang Lian, and Wan Ling Dan. If the tumor markers are normal, but T-PRO and ALB are low, then add Yi Yi Ren, Shan Yao, Qian Shi, and Bai Guo; Gan Jiang and Fu Zi (small doses); or consider adding Sha Ren and Cao Dou Kou (Rou Dou Kou or Hong Dou Kou).

Case Study #9: Do Tumor Markers Correlate with Pulmonary Tuberculosis?

Q: I have a female gastric cancer patient with regional metastatic spread to the lymph nodes in the abdomen. The patient had undergone treatment for 2 years at a major hospital, receiving several regimens of chemotherapy prior to seeking my consultation.

To regulate and strengthen her physical constitution, I started out by prescribing Chun Ze Tang adding Bai Zhu, Fu Ling, Ze Xie, Huang Bo, Chi Shao, Mu Dan Pi, Chuan Qi (large dose), and Wan Ling Dan (large dose). I also advised her to *temporarily* discontinue taking Western medicine drugs. Western medical doctors were still prescribing the anticancer agent fluoroucil (5-FU) via rapid injection and slow infusion, and after completion of the second cycle, the secondary cancer in the lymph nodes virtually disappeared. However, a follow-up examination revealed a 1 cm opacity in the right lung with elevated CA19-9 100 U/ml, and there was concern the patient may have pulmonary tuberculosis as well.

Thus, doctors decided to go ahead with 2 doses of chemotherapy, which resulted in a mild reduction of the opacity size and CA19-9 dropped to 50 U/ml. Do tumor markers correlate with pulmonary tuberculosis? What are the best TCM medicinals to treat this condition?

A: High CA19-9 tumor marker levels may have correlations with gastrointestinal cancers and hence lymph node malignancies, but *not* with pulmonary tuberculosis. I have a liver cancer patient who had percutaneous ethanol injection (PEI) performed 3 times. Follow-up examinations showed CA19-9 tumor marker levels at 69 U/ml, confirming the presence of metastatic spread to the lymph nodes with a high degree of probability.

The administration of 5-FU to treat lymph node malignancy may be effective in reducing the size of the tumor or even making it disappear. However, if TCM medicinals are *not* a part of the treatment regimen, then the anticancer agent 5-FU will inhibit hematopoiesis, resulting in low PLT count, prolonged PT, and activated APTT, which likely will lead to cancer progression and accelerated mortality.

If it *is* determined that the increase in tumor marker level reflects the presence of tumor growth, proliferation, or further spread to the lymph nodes (can be identified as Shao Yang heat pattern) and the diagnosis of pulmonary tuberculosis is also confirmed (can be identified as steaming bone taxation heat pattern), then you can simply prescribe a formula such as Xiao Chai Hu Tang (harmonizes and resolves Shao Yang), Di Gu Pi Yin (nourishes the blood and enriches yin), or Hyperactive Immune Formula (clears heat and resolves toxin and clears vacuity heat and enriches yin) adding Yuan Shen, Sha Shen, Bai He, Bai Bu, Tian Men Dong, and Mai Men Dong (nourish yin and moisten the lung and boost the stomach and engender liquid).

Case Study #10: Stomach Cancer – Colonic and Brain Metastases

Q: A 34 y/o male patient with gastric cancer and metastatic spread to the brain suffered from dysphagia and underwent exploratory laparoscopy, which revealed a 3 cm tumor in his stomach and the presence of regional lymph node metastases.

Following surgery, he received a regimen of Leucovorin, Oxaliplatin, and 5-FU, and after 1 cycle, the tumor shrunk from 3 cm to 2 cm, while the lymph node metastases remained the same.

The patient then decided to discontinue chemotherapy and took Jie Geng extract powder instead. Two months later, an emergency surgery was performed on an acute intestinal obstruction. Another regimen of chemotherapy (5-FU and Cisplatin) was then administered, with dissatisfactory results.

Now, he has 1 bowel movement every 1–2 days with variable consistency (sometimes loose), and his blood tests are normal. What formula would you use to treat this condition?

A: In gastric cancer patients with metastatic spread to the small intestine causing obstruction, you can consider prescribing a qi-boosting spleen-fortifying and qi-moving phlegm-transforming such as Xiang Sha Liu Jun Zi Tang adding Yi Yi Ren, Liang Jiang, Shan Dou Gen, Huang Qin, Huang Lian, Tian Ma, Ze Xie, Fu Ling, Da Huang (wine-steeped), Chuan Qi, Yu Sheng Wan, and Wan Ling Dan. For Da Huang, you can start out at 5 fen, gradually increasing the dose up until the patient passes 2–3 stools/day. This formula will help relieve symptoms and improve the patient's condition over time.

Case Study #11: Advanced Stage Stomach Cancer – Proper Care and Diet

Q: A 35 y/o male with advanced stage gastric cancer had a stent inserted to relieve intestinal obstruction and not long after suffered from nephritis and scrotal edema (both gonads). Recently, examination revealed metastatic spread to the stomach, peritoneum, and adrenal gland (right). He has severe ascites (daily drainage of 2.1 liters) and still has difficulty passing stool (1 stool every 2–3 days).

I prescribed Ban Xia, Mang Xiao, Fu Ling, and Sheng Shi Gao, but his condition did *not* improve (still unable to pass stool daily). Western medical doctors informed his family "to be prepared," but the patient is strong-willed and refuses to give up hope. What is the best way going forward?

A: Caring for an advanced stage cancer patient is most certainly a difficult endeavor. That is why so many hospitals admit these patients into hospice care units. The purpose is to allow the conditions of terminally ill patients to decline gradually with as little pain as possible until they peacefully pass away. A similar approach is chronicled in a TCM classical text: "Disperse accumulations and gatherings as much as possible (70–80%) and rely on food and drink for the rest."

However, there is still a rift right now between TCM and Western medicine about what type of diet is best for advanced cancer patients. Many hospitals in Taiwan and South Korea serve a Western (European/U.S.) style diet (the entire meal including the relatively large portions) without any consideration of the patient's body type, weight, and customary dietary habits. There is a lot of food on the plate that the patient does *not* have a palate for and thus does *not* eat, leading to a lack of nutrients and poor physical condition.

For example, most South Koreans have eaten kimchi all their lives and have grown so accustomed to the chili peppers that their bodies actually become physically reliant on the capsicum to function properly. Once the patient is diagnosed with cancer, the doctors and dieticians may claim that eating spicy foods had something to do with it, and specifically advise advanced stage cancer patients *not* to eat chili peppers. Instead, the amount of animal proteins and dairy products (e.g., milk, cheese) are increased. They don't realize that chili peppers are vital for stimulating these patients' gastrointestinal system.

Of course, they don't have an appetite! If the appetite control center in the brain is *not* stimulated, digestive secretions are *not* produced. This leads to a poor appetite and also compromised gastrointestinal immune function, and is the main reason advanced stage cancer patients lack physical strength and energy. Just like Taiwanese (people throughout East and Southeast Asia as well) have the habit of eating steamed rice, taro, and steamed buns, and all of a sudden you want them to change their diet to leavened bread. Naturally, it would *not* feel right so they do *not* want to eat!

TCM emphasizes the concept of "local foods," with "local" having the connotation of "most suitable." This means the kinds of food eaten and the times that they are eaten should be based on local eating customs in order to maintain the healthiest diet. This concept diminishes the appeal of the now popular overseas dietary supplements, especially those claiming to have medicinal effects, sold on the local market. The individual's digestive system and microbiome has already grown accustomed to a specific style of diet and the GI tract must have these types of foods in order to effectively absorb nutrients and receive sustenance that will boost the immune system's natural disease fighting mechanisms.

TCM emphasizes the patient's physical constitution and the severity of the pathocondition. Prescribing mild medicinals to treat serious conditions offers no beneficial value, while prescribing potent medicinals to treat mild conditions may inadvertently harm the constitution, further compromising homeostasis and leading to the manifestation of other diseases. This premise is evident in the TCM materia medica classic *The Essential Herbal Foundation* (本草備要 *Ben Cao Bei Yao*), where under the template for Chuan Xiong this quote from the *The Yellow Emperor's Inner Canon* (黃帝內經 *Huang Di Nei Jing*) cautions: "Frequently taking large doses and for long durations [of Chuan Xiong] will cause overabundance of one organ, leading to sudden collapse and death."

The approach Western medical hospitals commonly take in the treatment of disease typically transpires like this: The patient feels ill or has discomfort and goes to the hospital, where the patient is most likely immediately administered high-dose infusions or intravenous injections (IV), resulting in edema for those patients with poor metabolic function.

Once malignancy is confirmed in patients with tumors, they will inevitably be advised to first have surgery to resect the lesion, then follow-up with adjuvant radiotherapy and/or chemotherapy, or possibly use targeted drugs and therapies in an attempt to eradicate all of the cancer cells. This is tantamount to "clearing the fields and leaving nothing behind" and "killing off the bad along with the good," since chemotherapy eradicates both cancer cells and healthy cells in the process.

During treatment, patients mainly eat a diet recommended by a dietician. Though this diet "technically" meets the nutritional needs of the patient, patients often find these foods unappealing, lose their appetites, and just do *not* eat enough. After the completion of several chemotherapy regimens, this vicious cycle spirals out of control, with patients continuing to lose more and more weight. And in the end, they just get "burnt out" and die.

TCM advocates the approach: "Disperse accumulations and gatherings as much as possible (70–80%) and rely on food and drink for the rest." For advanced stage cancer patients whose physical conditions are already extremely compromised and weak, you should start out prescribing small doses of relatively mild TCM medicinal, and then assess the patient's condition to determine if incrementally larger doses of more potent medicinals should be prescribed. Remember! Trying to expedite the process with large doses is fundamentally contraindicated!

For treating accumulations, gatherings, concretions, and conglomerations (nomenclature that includes both benign and malignant tumors), you only need to eliminate about 70–80% of the cancer cells and tumor mass. It is *not* necessary to achieve complete clearance; in fact, it is technically impossible to completely eliminate all of the cancer cells! The rest of the treatment involves maintaining a healthy diet, which will open the stomach and spleen so that the remaining pathogenic qi can be eliminated, allowing the patient to live a long life in harmony with the condition.

Thus, it's a good idea to prescribe advanced stage cancer patients small doses of Gu Ya, Mai Ya, and Ji Nei Jin, along with Shan Yao and Ou Jie, to open the stomach (increase the appetite). If the patient has a craving for their favorite foods, it would be fine to go ahead and eat small amounts, and even if they wanted to drink a few glasses of Jinro soju, that's ok too! Advanced stage gastric cancer patients lead exceedingly bland lives "dried up like dead wood."

In this stage of their condition, there is no decisive evidence that a healthy diet will have anything but a marginal effect at best, so let the patient eat the foods they like and feel a sense of joy and satisfaction. It may not be very long until they pass away, and they won't have any regrets about it. In fact, these savory foods just might increase their appetites, like "dried up twigs and wilted leaves" on a tree receiving nourishment and moisture, to once again flourish and become vibrant.

Taking TCM medicinals will only be effective if the patient has a good appetite, moderate physical strength, and adequate hematopoietic function. This is a quintessential principle you must always remember as you treat patients.

Before, you told me of a patient whom you prescribed large doses of Huang Lian Jie Du Tang for the treatment of chronic active hepatitis, which conversely led to an increase in AST and ALT. At that time, I thought you should have prescribed Zhi Zi Bo Pi Tang (pulverized powder) instead (with each medicinal at 2–3 qian) adding Shan Zha, Mai Ya, and Ji Nei Jin. This is an example of the principle I just mentioned above.

Remember! For patients with chronic illness, serious disease, or advanced stage cancer, you must prescribe small doses of TCM medicinals, otherwise you may "outsmart yourself," making matters worse instead of better. Just remember the principle: "Disperse accumulations and gatherings as much as possible (70–80%) and rely on food and drink for the rest." You must first "moisten" and "nourish" the intestines and stomach (treat the tip) and then prescribe TCM medicinals to treat the root of the pathocondition. This is the most effective approach.

Section 4: Colorectal Cancer

Case Study #1: Granulomatous Polyp Following Surgical Resection

Q1: A 64 y/o male colorectal cancer patient visited me with a history of undergoing 3 partial colectomies and 1 right-sided nephrectomy during the past 10 years, and now a recent periodic examination revealed the presence of a granulomatous polyp. The patient's oncologist told him that since he had already undergone colectomy there wasn't much left to remove, so the best option was to perform endoscopic laser therapy.

Feeling disappointed and frustrated, the patient sought my consultation for TCM treatment. I prescribed Ru Mo Si Wu Tang variant. Please offer your guidance on this case.

A1: Colorectal cancer patients with metastatic spread to the kidneys and recurring polyps and granulomas following surgical resection can be identified as damp heat and stasis heat pattern. Prescribing a blood-nourishing and -quickening, stasis-dispelling pain-relieving, and network vessel-freeing channel-regulating formula such as Ru Mo Si Wu Tang variant should be effective, or you might also consider a blood-breaking and channel-freeing formula such as Tong Jing Fang variant as well. Just make sure to add Huang Qin, Huang Lian, Huai Hua, Di Yu, Bai Zhi, Chuan Qi, and Wan Ling Dan to your formula.

If the patient is physically weak, then consider prescribing a spleen-fortifying qi-supplementing formula such as Bu Zhong Yi Qi Tang adding the aforementioned medicinals (equivalent to Ti Gang San variant).

After taking the above formula for 1–2 months, the patient should have another endoscopy and CT scan performed to determine if the granulomatous polyp has disappeared. Even if the polyp has disappeared, the patient should *continue* taking TCM medicinals for 2–3 more months.

Q2: The colorectal cancer patient said he had another endoscopy performed about 3 weeks after starting TCM treatment confirming the granulomatous polyp had indeed disappeared. Thank you so much for your guidance. Could you please further elaboborate on your approach to treating colorectal cancer?

A2: The physical constitution of Asians makes it less likely for colorectal polyps to manifest into cancer. Therefore, the presence of granulomatous polyps on inspection should *not* cause too much alarm, and there is no rush to immediatley peform biopsy or undergo surgical resection. In some patients, these polyps are simply the swelling and distention arising from stasis, depression, dampness, or heat in the large intestine channel; and their condition will improve after taking TCM medicinals.

If the polyp does turn out to be colorectal cancer, then at the onset you should prescribe a heat-clearing toxin-resolving, swelling-dispersing hardness-breaking, and blood-quickening pain-relieving formula such as Xian Fang Huo Ming Yin adding Huai Hua, Di Yu, Da Huang, Chuan Qi, and Wan Ling Dan. Doses of Da Huang should be incrementally increased up until the patient maintains ≥ 3 bowel movements per day.

Even if the patient presents with loose stools, slightly bloody stool, or even anorectal mucosal prolapse and lymphocytic-rich exudates, there is still no need to be alarmed. Simply change the formula to a blood-nourishing yin-enriching dryness-moistening formula such as Blood Desiccation Formula adding Bai Zhi (resolves the exterior, dries dampness, and disperses swelling and expels pus), Fang Feng (effuses the exterior, overcomes dampness, and outthrusts papules and heals sores) Tian Men Dong, Mai Men Dong, Dang Shen, Huang Qin, Huai Hua (stanches bleeding), Ren Shen/Chuan Qi Powder, and Wan Ling Dan.

Case Study #2: Recurrence After 7 Years of Remission

Q: Seven years ago, a 63 y/o female patient was diagnosed with colorectal cancer and received radiotherapy and chemotherapy (surgical resection was *not* performed).

Recently, there was recurrence and the patient followed the advice of her oncologist by receiving targeted therapy with EGFR inhibitor. During a follow-up examination, elevated carcinoembryonic antigen (CEA) was discovered, but she did *not* present with any other noticeable signs or symptoms. How should I interpret these findings?

A: As long as hematopoietic function is *not* compromised, then she should be all right. This pathocondition can be identified as blood heat and blood-aspect stasis heat pattern. Thus, you should prescribe a formula that contains heat-clearing with cold and bitter, blood-quickening stasis-transforming, and blood-cooling medicinal. Just make sure to include Huang Qin, Cang Zhu, Bai Zhi, Fang Feng, and Chuan Qi (all Yang Ming channel medicinals), Fu Ling, Ze Xie, and Wan Ling Dan.

Case Study #3: Colorectal Cancer – Liver and Abdominal Cavity Metastases

Q1: This case is similar to another patient of mine [Case Study #2 above] that I asked you about before.

A 58 y/o female patient was diagnosed with colorectal cancer 7 years ago and received radiotherapy, chemotherapy, and targeted therapy with EGFR inhibitor. Recently, she had felt distension, discomfort, and occasional dull pain in her right flank, occasional sharp pain in the left lower abdomen, and pain in the left inguinal region upon walking.

I prescribed Ru Mo Si Wu Tang adding Huang Qin and Huang Lian (8 qian each), Fu Ling and Ze Xie (5 qian each), Yu Sheng Wan, and Wan Ling Dan. After taking this formula for 1 1/2 months (though *not* fully in compliance with the prescribed dosage), one day she suddenly incurred a small amount of anal bleeding.

She immediately went to the hospital for examination, which revealed CEA over 100 and a PET-CT scan confirmed the presence of metastatic spread to the liver and abdominal cavity. However, the two tumors in the abdominal cavity, 5 cm and 3 cm in size, shrank to 4 cm and 2 cm respectively; and the liver tumor remained the same size, but there were also numerous small cystic growths of varying sizes (all < 1 cm). Liver function tests (e.g., AST, ALT, and BIL) were normal, and the flank distension and pain in her abdomen and inguinal region has resolved.

What kinds of cystic growths are precancerous? Do you think the unspecified growths (< 1 cm) revealed on the PET-CT scan are metastatic spread from the existing colorectal cancer? Or, do you think they are new liver cancer growths?

One week ago, the patient visited me again explaining that she had followed the advice of her oncologist and received chemotherapy, but the treatment has *not* been effective. Now, she is scheduled to receive radiotherapy on the large intestine, liver, and cervix. What are your perspectives on this case?

A1: CEA over 100 does *not* necessarily indicate cancer progression; elevated levels most likely arose from tumor cell necrosis and release of metabolic enzymes during the breakdown process. The cystic growths likely are a blood-filled cysts resulting from the process of tumor necrosis, which first liquifies, then forms a cyst, and will eventually be resorbed. A PET-CT scan will be able to confirm if the growth is malignant or benign. Typically, metastasis involving the celiac artery (trunk) can be identified as stasis heat pattern, so you should simply add Xu Duan, Gu Sui Bu, and Chuan Qi to your formula above.

Overall, administration of radiotherapy and chemotherapy to treat patients with colorectal cancer metastases to the liver rarely, if ever, offers effective results. The types of radiotherapy currently used are CyberKnife, photon knife, or Gamma Knife. Radiotherapy treatment of liver cancer with any of these systems will lead to complications of liver stasis and swelling, sudden onset of hepatitis, cirrhosis, and liver failure (though these complications are usually less severe compared to the adverse effects of conventional cobalt 60 irradiation!).

If these complications present, then prescribe formula variants such as Chai Ling Tang, Tong Jing Fang, or Ru Mo Si Wu Tang, and monitor for any changes in AST/ALT, T-Pro, A/G, T/D-Bil, Hb, PLT, BUN/Cr, and ammonia.

Q2: Cancer has spread to the patient's lungs and she presents with cough (dry cough or with very little phlegm), constipation, pain in the left inguinal region, and sore back. I suspect that the lung metastasis was a result of radiotherapy, but since the hepatic cancer enlarged, she still is scheduled to receive another round of radiotherapy.

As adjuvant TCM treatment, I prescribed Ru Mo Si Wu Tang adding The Three Yellows, Da Huang, Fu Ling, Ze Xie (8 qian each), and Yu Sheng Wan (2 pills/day). What is your perspective on this case?

A2: There is no doubt about it; patients with colorectal cancer that has metastasized to the liver, lung, spine, and pelvis really deserve a lot of sympathy! The 'good' thing is that the administration of TCM medicinals still offers effectiveness and hope.

I would prescribe Ru Mo Si Wu Tang adding The Three Yellows,

Da Huang, Fu Ling, and Ze Xie (8 qian each); Cang Zhu, Qing Hao, Di Gu Pi, and Ting Li Zi (8 qian each); Fang Ji, Ma Huang, Xing Ren, and Chuan Qi (3 qian each); Xu Duan, Gu Sui Bu, and Niu Xi, Gou Ji, Zhi Mu, and Di Long (5–8 qian); Sheng Du Zhong (4 qian); Lu Jiao (1 liang); Wan Ling Dan (incrementally increase the amount week-by-week starting out with 12 pills/3x/day and adding up to 26–30 pills/3x/day); and Yu Sheng Wan (up to 6–9 pills/day).

If the patient has dry mouth following radiotherapy and doesn't drink enough water, you can advise the patient to regularly drink fresh vegetable and fruit juices (carrot, pear, apple, etc.) or drink Kudzu (Ge Gen) root juice. Keep working hard and making headway!

Case Study #4: Chemotherapy-Induced Watery Diarrhea – Wu Ling San Variant

Q: I have a colorectal cancer patient who has suffered from watery diarrhea ever since starting chemotherapy. How should I treat this and how long will it take to remedy? If the patient doesn't have a lot of faith in TCM treatment, what can I do to convince the patient? Unfortunately, this is the situation with most cancer patients in South Korea!

A: Following chemotherapy, colorectal cancer patients may incur side effects such as burns and edema of the intestinal mucus membrane that causes iatrogenic mucositis (resembling Behcet's syndrome and Stephens-Johnson syndrome) and most commonly manifests in watery diarrhea. When treating these patients, you must determine the extent of the mucositis, with the first priority being to check diarrhea.

In the TCM classic *Essential Prescriptions of the Golden Coffer* (**金匱要略方論** *Jin Gui Yao Lue Fang Lun*), diarrhea is treated with Ge Gen Qin Lian Tang and Bai Tou Weng Tang. If these formulas are unable to check diarrhea (heat dysentery), and you are certain the patient hasn't eaten contaminated food or contracted an infection (putrid-smelling stool), then the condition can be diagnosed as unable to astringe the intestines watery diarrhea, requiring the administration of Chi Shi Zhi Yu Yu Liang Tang variant.

If this is ineffective, then prescribe Wu Ling San variant, utilizing its separation of the clear and turbid action to restore the absorption capacity of the large intestine, so it can regulate water flow from the cecum to the kidney and bladder and thus promote excretion. This approach is quite simple, just prescribe Wu Ling San (Cang Zhu, Fu Ling, and Ze Xie as the sovereign medicinals) and add Huang Qin and Huang Lian.

Cast Study #5: Metastatic Colorectal Cancer

Q: A 58 y/o male patient had surgical resection performed on metastatic colorectal cancer, and at the time, inflammation of the cecum was discovered (it turned out to be metastatic spread to the cecum).

Two years later, the cancer spread to the rectum and he underwent partial surgical resection; but only 3 years later, it recurred resulting in another partial resection with adjuvant chemotherapy (anticancer agents Xeloda and Oxaliplatin). This treatment was ineffective, and 1 year later, it spread to the lymph nodes near the abdominal aorta and pelvis, resulting in another surgical resection and chemotherapy (this time changing to Xeloda and Irinotecan, and then Erbitux).

One year after that, the patient's condition deteriorated once again, and the family insisted upon changing hospitals, where a different chemotherapy regimen (5-FU, Oxaliplatin, and Leucovorin) was administered. Up to now, the patient's condition has remained stable without additional metastases, but he is very weak, and if it spreads again, there aren't any other drugs available.

This is when he came to me seeking TCM treatment. I prescribed Chai Ling Tang variant. Do you have any advice on treatment from here on out?

A: This case offers a prime example of the difference in approach between TCM and Western medicine. We can see in this case that the Western medicine protocol is still to "eliminate the lesion" as the only option. TCM prioritizes its therapeutic approach in this way:

1) Treat and prevent iatrogenic vasculitis, circulatory system disorders, and myocardial disease.

2) Prevent iatrogenic hepatitis and nephritis and hypertrophy, and iatrogenic cerebral and peripheral nerve damage.

For this patient, as long as the hematopoietic function and serum protein levels are normal, the treatment principle is to open the spleen and stomach (promote appetite) and increase the absorption of nutrients. Doing so will help the patient regain strength, activate immune response, and stablize the condition, thus fostering a physiological environment that enables the patient to proceed into remission.

As for the TCM principle: "Disperse accumulations and gatherings as much as possible (70–80%) and rely on food and drink for the rest." This "rely on food and drink for the rest" refers to nutrient supply and includes the absorption of nutrients by the small intestine (receptor sensitivity and responsiveness), the liver's storage and conversion function, and the kidney's capacity of producing essence (essential physiological substances).

As for TCM treatment, I would start out by prescribing variants of Chai Ling Tang (clears heat and transforms phlegm-damp and disinhibits water), Xiang Sha Liu Jun Zi Tang (boosts qi and fortifies the spleen and moves qi and transforms phlegm), Shen Ling Bai Zhu San (boosts qi and fortifies the spleen and harmonizes the stomach and percolates dampness), Bao He Wan (disperses food and abducts stagnation and fortifies the spleen and harmonizes the stomach), Bu Zhong Yi Qi Tang (fortifies the spleen and supplements qi and upbears yang), or Gui Pi Tang (supplements blood and boosts qi and fortifies the spleen and nourishes the heart) adding medicinals accordingly based on pattern identification and presenting signs and symptoms.

For instance, if water amassment presents, then add Bai Zhu, Fu Ling, Ze Xie, Ting Li Zi, and Fang Ji. If serum protein levels are low, then add combinations of medicinals such as The Four Lings, Shan Yao, Lian Zi, Qian Shi, Yi Yi Ren, Bai Guo, Da Jin Ying, Huang Qi, and Ren Shen. If iatrogenic hepatitis presents, for the acute stage prescribe The Three Yellows and Mu Dan Pi; and for the chronic and remission stages, prescribe Qi Bao Mei Ran Dan or Blood Desiccation Formula adding Wu Wei Zi and Nu Zhen Zi. If hematopoietic bone marrow function is suppressed, then add Tu Si Zi, Rou Cong Rong, Du Zhong, and Niu Xi along with The Three Great Yang-Supplementers, Xi Lu Rong, and Huang Bo. If there is nerve damage, then prescribe Bu Yang Huan Wu Tang adding Ma Huang, Di Long, and Tian Ma. If tidal fever presents, then add Qing Hao, Zhi Mu, and Di Gu Pi.

Metastatic spread to the lympatic system can be identified as Shao Yang heat pattern and is similar to the Shao Yang heat pattern of osteomyelitis, nephritis, and neuritis. These types of "steaming bone" and drug-induced (iatrogenic) fever symptoms (unless there is low WBC count and/or hematopoietic dysfunction) can all be identified as Shao Yang heat pattern. Treatment involves first supplementing the spleen and stomach, and if the cancer relapses, then add The Three Yellows, Mu Dan Pi, Chuan Qi, Yu Sheng Wan, and Wan Ling Dan.

The main channel-conducting medicinals for colorectal cancer are Bai Zhi and Sheng Ma; Fang Feng is an essential medicinal for intestinal wind bleeding; and Huai Hua and Di Yu are both essential blood-cooling and blood-stanching medicinals for the large intestine channel.

Case Study #6: Colorectal Cancer with Fecal Incontinence

Q: Following a partial colectomy, a 64 y/o male patient with colorectal cancer and metastatic spread to the liver visited me, complaining of poor appetite and inhibited defecation. I prescribed Xiang Sha Liu Jun Zi Tang variant. After taking this formula, he said the symptoms had improved a bit and that he had gained a little weight.

Recently, he came back for another visit, this time complaining of fecal incontinence. Examination by a gastroenterologist discovered muscular hyperplasia in the rectum near the anus. His doctor said this was a very difficult condition to treat, and the only thing the patient could do is wear adult diapers or change his underwear frequently (about 10 times/day).

I am thinking this might be caused by yang vacuity pattern (similar to crab's-foot swelling (keloid)). How would you treat this patient?

A: Colorectal cancer with fecal incontinence can be identified as qi vacuity with stasis obstruction pattern, requiring administration of a spleen-fortifying qi-supplementing yang-upbearing formula such as Bu Zhong Yi Qi Tang variant. If the patient has *not* received radiotherapy or chemotherapy, then you can add Ru Xiang, Mo Yao, Huang Qin, and Ze Xie. If he *has* received RT and CT, then add Gan Jiang and Fu Zi instead.

Section 5: Pancreatic Cancer

Case Study #1: Vomiting Following Chemotherapy and Radiotherapy

Q: A 61 y/o female patient with pancreatic cancer has recently suffered from vomiting following chemotherapy and radiotherapy. She also has poor intestinal motility and has lost a lot of weight (down to 33kg). If this were your patient, what formula would you prescribe?

A: For pancreatic cancer patients you can prescribe formula variants such as Da Chai Hu Tang, Chai Ling Tang, or Xie Xin Tang; Xiang Sha Liu Jun Zi Tang; or Wen Dan Tang or Ban Xia Tian Ma Bai Zhu San adding Shan Dou Gen, Liang Jiang, and Da Hui Xiang.

If persistently increased CEA and CA19-9 levels present, add large doses of The Three Yellows, Yu Sheng Wan, and Wan Ling Dan. TCM (Kampo) practitioners in Japan often prescribe Yan Nian Ban Xia Tang adding Ren Shen and Chuan Qi for this condition, and you could consider this formula as well.

Case Study #2: Pancreatic Cancer – It's Really Difficult to Treat!

Q1: I have a 62 y/o female patient with a pancreatic tumor near an artery at the center of the pancreas. Radiotherapy was performed on one occasion and results of recent lab tests are as follows: blood—BUN 5.1 mg/dL (normal 8–25), TP 5.6 g/dL (normal 6–8.5), and S-Alb 3.1 g/dL (normal 3.5–5.3); and liver function—AST 18 u/L (0–40) and ALT 6 u/L (1–30).

Results of a CT scan reveal the tumor has shrunk and there is mild ascites. Later on, metastatic spread to the peritoneum was discovered and the oncologist at the hospital said: "Now, it will be tough to administer aggressive treatment." They could *not* prescribe diuretics or perform aspiration of ascites.

Please help me understand this pathocondition better. Is ascites a result of low serum Alb (s-Alb)? Or, is it caused by peritoneal metastases? Is it possible for her condition to improve? How should I treat this patient?

A1: The way I see it is that ascites is caused by low s-Alb along with low BUN/Cr. Therefore, you can consider prescribing large doses of Ren Shen, Bai Guo, Huai Shan, Da Jin Ying, Fu Ling, Ze Xie, Qian Shi, and Yi Yi Ren. If T-Pro and A/G levels do *not* increase, then add Tu Si Zi; and if levels still do *not* rise, then add small doses of Gan Jiang, Fu Zi, and Huang Qin.

Remember! You should *not* prescribe Gan Jiang and Fu Zi too early in the therapeutic regimen for this condition, but you *can* prescribe medicinals such as Gao Liang Jiang and Xiang Fu.

Second, if peritoneal metastases has already occurred, then the ascites will usually be rapid and profuse, and regardless of the method employed (e.g., paracentesis, automated pump system), attempts at eliminating this fluid buildup are typically *not* successful. The sooner you administer the TCM medicinals mentioned above the better; this will help relieve symptoms and improve the patient's condition.

Typically, unless it is repletion heat pattern ascites (e.g., acute fulminant heptatitis complicated by liver failure with the administration of too much IV fluid), then you should prescribe a heat-clearing phlegm-damp-transforming water-disinhibiting formula such as Chai Ling Tang adding incremental doses of medicinals that address the presenting signs and symptoms. If T-Pro, A/G, Hb, and C3/C4 levels are low and BUN/Cr high, then add The Three Great Yang-Supplementers, Ren Shen, and Huang Qi. For all of these medicinals, start out with small doses and gradually increase as needed (don't overdo it all at once!).

Even in the case of acute ascites, you can still prescribe Chai Ling Tang combined with water-expelling with drastic precipitation formulas such as Da Xian Xiong Tang, Shi Zao Tang, Dan Dong Shen You Wan, or Shu Zuo Yin Zi. In cases of low T-Pro and A/G, then add spleen-fortifying and essence-securing medicinals such as Bai Guo, Huai Shan, Qian Shi, Yi Yi Ren, Lian Zi, Da Jin Ying, and Xiao Jin Ying.

Typically, after pancreatic cancer has been treated and calcification occurs, the symptoms will improve. But remember! Even if CA19-9, amylase, lipase, and GLU all test out at normal levels, the patient should continue taking TCM medicinals for a minimum of 6 months–1 year with periodic lab tests being monitored. You must be vigilant!

Q2: Unfortunately, this pancreatic cancer patient has passed away. At the onset of administering TCM medicinals her symptoms did improve, but towards the end, it didn't seem to matter how strong of a dose I prescribed—it still wasn't enough to prevent the progression of cancer and ascites.

Do you think it would have been helpful for the patient to continue with CT and RT when her condition was in remission? For cases like this, what do you think is the best approach for treatment?

A2: Pancreatic cancer is always difficult to treat. Once a diagnosis has been confirmed, many doctors will tell the patient's family: "The patient can do whatever she or he wants to do." This implies that the hope for a cure is exceedingly dismal.

Administering TCM medicinals for this condition and having the patient survive for 6 months is in itself a commendable accomplishment. Only TCM physicians with exceptional skills can achieve results of having patients survive for more than 1 year.

Thus, if you have a similar patient in the future, I would stick to the same therapeutic approach. Don't feel discouraged and lose confidence in yourself! After all, doctors are only human; the capacity of the medicinals we use and the institution of modern medicine as a whole has inherent limitations.

Through thick and thin, we as doctors must continue striving for development and progress. The day you are able to cure a severe illness such as pancreatic cancer is the day you will be acknowledged as a "master physician," a luminary respected throughout the medical community.

Case Study #3: Advanced Stage Pancreatic Cancer

Q: There is a 74 y/o male patient with pancreatic cancer. Since the diagnosis, he has been administered anticancer agents in an attempt to control the condition, but results have been poor. The patient has a sallow complexion and often feels nauseated with occasional dry heaving. He also has been diagnosed with cirrhosis and maintains 1 stool per day.

The family has decided to give TCM a try, since all their Western medicine options have been exhausted. Can you give me any advice on this case?

A: The pancreas is anatomically located at the back of the abdominal cavity behind the stomach. It is among the body's silent organs, and thus when afflicted with disease (e.g., cancer, inflammation), detection and diagnosis remains difficult in the early stages.

Pancreatic cancer typically goes undiscovered up until the tumor has already enlarged to the point where it presses down on the bile duct, obstructing the bile flow, resulting in bile entering the bloodstream, and causing hyperbilirubinemia, sallow facial complexion, and light-colored stools. Some patients will have nausea, vomiting, poor appetite, tidal fever, fatigue, weight loss, constipation, and severe hemilateral pain between the nipples and diaphragm (these symptoms are most pronounced after eating deep-fried foods or drinking hard liquor.) Once the diagnosis of pancreatic cancer has been confirmed, it is usually already in the advanced stages. Really a tough situation!

The most common causes of mortality from this condition are from hyperbilirubinemia and hepatic coma. However, poor nutrition and low levels of T-Pro, ALB, and Hb will induce generalized edema, cerebral hypoxia, and cerebral edema, which may also lead to mortality.

My formula of choice for treating this condition is typically Chai Ling Tang (clears heat and transforms phlegm-damp and disinhibits water) or Da Chai Hu Tang (resolves exterior evil and frees interior repletion). Just make sure to include Da Huang, Gao Liang Jiang, and Shan Dou Gen. However, you could also consider the Xie Xin Tang series, Yan Nian Ban Xia Tang, or Gui Pi Tang variants. If T-Bil levels drop and then rise again, you should add The Three Great Yang-Supplementers (starting out at small doses and adding incrementally).

Section 6: Liver Cancer

Case Study #1: Hepatocellular Carcinoma (HCC)

Q: I have a 73 y/o male hepatocellular carcinoma patient whose lab test results are as follows: T/D Bil: 0.6/0.2, AST: 86, ALT: 42, ALP: 805 (normal range 102–333), r-GT: 162 (normal range 11–78), PT: 11.9 (normal range 11–14), R-Feto protein: 159.73 (normal range 0–13.4), CA19-9: 49.5 (normal range below 33), CEA: 1.49, PLT: 148 (normal range 150–350), CYFRA 21-1: 2.72 (normal range < 3.3ng/ml), HbsAg (+), and HBV (-).

Results of the most recent CT scan reveal:

1. Slight increases in size and number of multiple, variable-sized, conglomerated hepatic masses involving the entire liver, especially L hepatic lobe, and focal adjacent IHBD dilatation.

Slight increase in size and number of multiple intrahepatic metastatic nodules in the R hepatic lobe.

Little interval change of possible focal L portal vein invasion, and some cavernous transformation of the portal vein.

2. No ascites, no varices, no splenomegaly.

3. About 1.5 cm, Bosniak 1 cyst, L kidney.

A: From the CT scan we know that there are multiple HCC tumors. This means Western medicine will *not* be able to perform percutaneous ethanol injection (PEI), transarterial embolization (TAE), or transarterial chemoembolization (TACE), so their only option is administering chemotherapy. The problem is that the available HCC chemotherapy agents are *not* very effective.

For now, the most important thing to do is make sure the patient is getting enough nutrients. I suggest you tell the patient: "Eat whatever you like, but just make sure it isn't too hot." Remember! This is important because liver cancer patients will often have esophageal varices or gastric ulcers and ingesting scalding hot foods (or liquids) could exacerbate an already precarious condition.

As for TCM medicinals, I would prescribe a heat-clearing phlegm-damp-transforming water-disinhibiting formula such as Chai Ling Tang (including large doses of Fu Ling and Ze Xie) adding Ma Huang (small dose), Xing Ren, Da Huang (adding incrementally to maintain

2–3 stools per day), and of course Ren Shen/Chuan Qi Powder. If chemotherapy has *not* been administered, then add The Three Yellows (large doses), Ru Xiang, Mo Yao, San Leng, E Zhu, and Wan Ling Dan. Patients who have received chemotherapy will have suppressed hematopoietic function, so it is beneficial to add large doses of The Three Great Yang-Supplementers to "boost" the metabolism and immune system.

For patients just completing a chemotherapy regimen, as long as their liver function indices (AST/ALT) remain elevated, then continue prescribing Chai Ling Tang variant, but the dose of Huang Qin can be reduced to 3 qian each (down from 5–8 qian). For patients who incur drug-induced hepatitis, doses of Huang Qin can be increased, while concomitantly *lowering the dosage* of the chemotherapy regimen, or *temporarily discontinuing* chemotherapy altogether, until the drug-induced hepatitis has resolved.

For HCC patients with elevated AFP (tumor marker) levels following chemotherapy, you should prescribe the above TCM formula adding large doses of The Three Yellows; and if this is still not effective, then add The Three Great Yang-Supplementers.

Applying an integrative TCM and Western medicine approach (concomitantly administering TCM medicinals throughout the chemotherapy regimen) offers excellent efficacy. Even when the condition has stabilized and the CT scan, MRI, and PET scan reveal no signs of tumor, the patient must still take TCM medicinals for at least 6 months up to 1 year.

Remember! For patients who have been administered The Three Great Yang-Supplementers (Gan Jiang, Fu Zi, and Rou Gui) continously for 3 months or longer, you must *subtract* these medicinals at this time to alleviate the potential for inducing relapse of the tumor. If AFP rises again, then simply add large doses of The Three Yellows (Huang Qin, Huang Lian, and Huang Bo); and if doses of 8–10 qian fail to bring down AFP, then add large doses of The Three Great Yang-Supplementers along with San Leng, E Zhu, and Yu Sheng Wan.

In the event that *none* of these approaches offers efficacy, then change formulas to Ru Mo Si Wu Tang adding The Three Yellows, Cang Zhu, Fu Ling, Ze Xie, Ren Shen/Chuan Qi Powder, San Leng, E Zhu, Pu Gong Ying, Da Huang, Yu Sheng Wan, and Wan Ling Dan; and if this *still* is ineffective, then once again add The Three Great Yang-Supplementers.

Currently, for advanced stage cancer, regardless of the therapeutic approach (TCM, Western medicine, or integrative TCM and Western medicine), the best prognosis that can be hoped for is to extend survival for 6 months (at most up to 1 year). My hope is that we can all work together (TCM and Western medicine) striving for breakthroughs that will result in survival rates of 3–5 years with a good quality of life. This would be a rewarding consolation for the entire field of medicine.

Case Study #2: Three Formulas for Treating Liver Cancer

Q1: I have a 73 y/o male patient who was diagnosed with hepatocellular carcinoma (HCC) with multiple intrahepatic metastases (more than 20 masses). His most recent liver function tests (including T/D-bil levels) were in the normal range.

I prescribed Chai Ling Tang (including Fu Ling and Ze Xie (5 qian each)) adding Da Huang (5 fen); San Leng and E Zhu (3 qian each); The Three Yellows (8 qian each); and Pu Gong Ying (1 liang).

He has taken this formula for 1 week, and I don't have any information about his latest lab test results (AST/ALT, T/D-bil, PLT, T-Pro, and AFP) yet. How would you treat this patient?

A1: For HCC (with or without multiple intrahepatic metastases) you can consider prescribing these formula options:

1) Chai Ling Tang (clears heat and transforms phlegm-damp and disinhibits water) adding large doses of The Three Yellows (at least 8–10 qian each), San Leng, E Zhu, Shan Nai, Yu Jin, and Chuan Qi.

2) Ru Mo Si Wu Tang (nourishes and quickens the blood, dispels stasis and relieves pain, and frees the network vessels and regulates the channels) adding large doses of The Three Yellows (at least 8–10 qian each), Cang Zhu, Fu Ling, Ze Xie, The Three Insects, Chuan Qi, San Leng, E Zhu, Shan Nai, and Yu Jin.

3) Tong Jing Fang (breaks blood, frees the channels and relieves pain, and supplements the liver and kidney) adding The Four Lings and large doses of The Three Yellows (at least 8–10 qian each).

Remember! You should also add Yu Shen Wang and Wan Ling Dan to your formula selection. Make sure to include adequate doses of Da Huang in order to maintain an optimal 2–3 stools/day and thus prevent the formation of hyperdynamic circulation arising from portal hypertension, ascites, and esophageal varices. Additionally, you should advise the patient to maintain a well-balanced diet with plenty of nutrients to prevent ascites.

If liver function indices and AFP levels happen to increase, or if T-Pro and ALT decrease, then you should add The Three Great Yang-Supplementers and Ren Shen along with spleen-fortifying and essence-securing medicinals such as Si Shen Tang (Huai Shan, Qian Shi, Lian Zi, Yi Ren, and Fu Ling), Bai Guo, Da Jin Ying, and Xiao Jin Ying.

If the patient presents with repletion heat pattern, then you should *not* add Ren Shen, The Three Great Yang-Supplementers, Si Wu Tang, or Huang Qi, because these supplementing medicinals may induce accelerated proliferation and tumerogenesis. Instead, you should prescribe heat-clearing toxin-resolving medicinals. Yes, you can also select heat-clearing toxin-vanquishing and swelling-dispersing bind-dissipating anticancer medicinals such as Pu Gong Ying, Lian Qiao, Jin Yin Hua, Ban Zhi Lian, and Bai Hua She Ku Cao. But quite frankly, you may just as well use the most common and widely available broad-spectrum heat-clearing toxin-resolving medicinals The Three Yellows (Huang Qin, Huang Lian, and Huang Bo). In my clinical experience, I have found that the anticancer efficacy of The Three Yellows is comprable to, if not better, especially if prescribed in large doses in combination with other essential medicinals.

Once the patient's condition has stabilized and enters the chronic stage, then you can also add warm and acrid medicinals such as Jiang Huang, Bai Jie Zi, Hua Jiao, Hu Jiao, Bing Lang, Lao Ye, Bi Bo, Liang Gao Jiang, and Sha Ren Gen.

Q2: I didn't realize the survival expectancy for HCC was so short. I have a question about why you would add The Three Insects to Ru Mo Si Wu Tang (formula 2)) in your previous response?

A2: Right now, if only Western medicine treatment is administered, liver cancer will typically relapse in 3–5 months and possibly manifest as proliferation of diffuse pinpoint lesions. Integrating TCM treatment will overcome the insufficiencies of Western medicine treatment and can achieve remission periods of up to two years (as documented in some of my patients).

As for adding The Three Insects, the use of toxic proteins and chitin in TCM medicinal insects is aimed at suppressing tumor proliferation. The combination of these insect medicinals with heat-clearing toxin-resolving medicinals produces the dual action of suppressing tumor proliferation and inhibiting hyperstimulation of the central nervous system. This disrupts the signal frequencies of cancer cell proliferation and prevents recurrence.

Q3: After receiving treatment, the patient's liver function test results remained normal, he gained 1kg, and AFP dropped to 600 (down from a high of 890) (normal range < 10 ng/mL). Now he feels pretty much back to normal and the distending pain in the right hypochondrium has mostly resolved. A CT scan did *not* show any signs of ascites, but *did* reveal that the tumor and metastatic lesions were still there.

The patient's attending physician was surprised to find there were no signs of jaundice. T-Bil has dropped to 0.8 (normal range 0.2–1.2 mg/dL) and the pain in the right hypochondrium has resolved, so the patient does not need to apply lidocaine patches. The patient occasionally feels nausea, but there is no ascites. The patient and I are genuinely grateful for your advice and guidance.

A3: Congratulations, you are starting to see results! Even though the tumor has not disappeared, it hasn't enlarged or spread. Now, we can anticipate that the tumor will gradually become calcified and inactive. Remember! The patient must continue taking the TCM medicinal regimen.

Case Study #3: Transcatheter Arterial Embolism

Q: I have a 43 y/o female patient with a chronic HBV infection, whose condition deteriorated and progressed to hepatocellular carcinoma (HCC). She has already undergone transcatheter arterial embolism (TAE) several times, yet regional metastases to the abdominal lymph nodes still occurred.

The patient has no ascites, has one bowel movement per day, and the CT scan images show numerous diffusely distributed HCC lesions. Liver function tests are as follows: AST/ALT: 150/113, AFP: 192, and T/D Bil: 3.4/1.6. How would you treat this patient?

A: The best option is a heat-clearing phlegm-damp-transforming water-disinhibiting formula such as Chai Ling Tang (including large doses of Fu Ling, Ze Xie, and Huang Qin) adding Mu Dan Pi (large dose), Ma Huang, Ren Shen/ Chuan Qi Powder, Yu Sheng Wan, and Wan Ling Dan. This approach should be able to prevent tumor enlargement and promote dissolution. If necessary, you can also add medicinals such as San Leng and E Zhu (breaks blood and moves qi, disperses accumulations, and relieves pain), Yuan Hu and Jiang Huang (quicken the blood and move qi and relieve pain), and Yu Jin (disinhibits the gallbladder and abates jaundice).

Additionally, you can consider adding a tablespoon of distilled white vinegar into the pot with the other medicinals, soaking for at least 30 minutes up to 12 hours, and then decocting the formula until there is 2.5 or 3 rice bowls (1 bowl = 200 ml) of liquid remaining. Instruct the patient to drink this decoction like a beverage in small amounts throughout the day accompanying the prescribed doses of Chuan Qi (powder) and Wan Ling Dan. And if the patient has a poor appetite, then you can add Shan Zha, Ji Nei Jin, and Da Huang (small dose of 5 fen).

Note: Soaking in distilled white vinegar and then decocting is a way to promote the body's absorption of these medicinals, which may be necessary if the gastrointestinal tract or accessory organs involved in digestion are compromised.

Case Study #4: Elevated AFP and Low T-Pro Following Surgery

Q: I have a 46 y/o male patient with Hepatitis B virus (HBV) that deteriorated into liver hepatocellurar carcinoma (HCC) and an AFP level of 13,000 (< 10 ng/mL). Following partial hepatectomy, AFP levels dropped to 2,000, AST 35 (0–40 u/L), and ALT 50 (1–30 u/L), and T-Pro 5.3 (5.6–8.4 g/dL). What's the best way to handle this case going forward?

A: AFP dropping from 13,000 down to 2,000 following surgical resection in a liver cancer patient indicates that the surgery was successful. However, the low T-Pro level suggests that the liver's function of protein absorption, storage, and release has been impaired. At this time, even if AFP was elevated, it would *not* definitively indicate liver cancer—it could also be a result of the intensive regenerative responses following hepatectomy. Following hepatectomy, the liver will undergo regenerative hyperplasia (benign) and generally will grow back to the original size within about 6 months. The rapidity of regenerative hyperplasia is reflected in the elevated AFP; however, AFP 2,000 is still too high, so you should try bringing it down further.

I receommend the following two approaches:

1) If the patient has *not* been intubated, then you can prescribe a spleen-fortifying qi-supplementing yang-upbearing formula such as Bu Zhong Yi Qi Tang (including large doses of Huang Qin) adding Yuan Hu, Mu Xiang, Ren Shen, Chuan Qi, Dan Shen, Dang Shen, and large doses of Fu Ling, Zhu Ling, Ze Xie, Bai Zhu, and Mu Dan Pi. You do *not* need to add Ma Huang, Xing Ren, Ting Li Zi, and Fang Ji, because patients undergoing this type of surgical resection almost never incur cardiopulmonary dysfunction (e.g., pleural effusion).

2) If the patient *has* been intubated, then you can prescribe a heat-clearing phlegm-damp-transforming water-disinhibiting formula such as Chai Ling Tang (including large doses of Fu Ling and Ze Xie) adding large doses of Dang Shen, Dan Shen, Bai Zhu, and Si Shen Tang (fortifies the spleen, secures essence, and increases T-Pro). Adding large doses of Huang Qin, Mu Dan Pi, and The Four Lings will bring down AFP and increase T-Pro. If AFP drops down to 50–100, then the large doses of these medicinals can be discontinued; but if AFP initially drops to 500–800 and subsequently jumps back up again, then you need to add Ren Shen and The Three Great Yang-Supplementers.

Case Study #5: Diffuse Hepatocellular Carcinoma

Q: I have a patient who has been diagnosed with diffuse hepatocellular carcinoma (HCC). Recent lab results showed normal AST/ALT, T/D Bil, and AFP levels, and the patient sleeps well, but has a poor appetite, and passes 1 stool per day.

I prescribed Chai Ling Tang adding Bai Zhu, Fu Ling, and Ze Xie (8 qian each), Huang Qin (8 qian), Huang Lian and Huang Bo (5 qian each), San Leng and E Zhu (4 qian each), Xu Duan and Qian Cao (4 qian each), Chuan Qi (3 qian), and Wan Ling Dan (6 pills/3x/day). Do you think this is a good formula?

A: Once an oncologist confirms the diagnosis of diffuse HCC, usually a very conservative "wait-and-see" approach will be adopted, as opposed to aggressive treatment. And sometimes this type of "living with the condition" conservative approach really does extend the patient's survival period, while also sparing the patient of senseless, often agonizing, treatment. You could say it is the lesser of two evils!

Recently, I have treated a patient with a similar condition. The patient was admitted to the hospital on March 15, and 2 weeks later, I was called on to make a hospital visit. After overhearing the doctor tell his family "…currently there is no treatment available…he probably only has 3 to 6 months remaining…," the patient was so worried and full of anxiety that he experienced diaphragm contractions, shortness of breath, and distending pain all over his body.

On March 27, I accepted the family's request to treat this patient and the next morning I had a formula decocted, sealed in packets, and sent over to the hospital. The patient only took one packet before suffering an outbreak of drug-induced (from Western medicine!) fulminant heptatitis, with shortness of breath and panting. The attending physician originally diagnosed the condition as pleural effusion and had an x-ray taken in preparation for aspiration, but to his surprise, there was *no* sign of effusion, so he suspected the cause was from excessive administration of drugs. The previous drug regimen was discontinued, and instead, he was administered the opiod analgesic morphine, Thalidomide, diuretics (even though there was *no* edema, only distention!), intravenous amino acid infusions, and interferon.

Unfortunately, the ensuing lab tests revealed a spike in AST to 1,000 and BIL also increased. I had no choice but to call the family and tell them to stop taking the Western medicine drugs, except for interferon (Lamivudine), which should be gradually discontinued as the AST and ALT levels come down, and by all means, start taking TCM medicinals as soon as possible. I prescribed the qi-boosting spleen-fortifying and qi-moving phlegm-transforming formula Xiang Sha Liu Jun Zi Tang adding Si Shen Tang, Huang Qin, Mu Dan Pi, Chuan Qi, The Four Lings, San Leng, and E Zhu.

It was obvious the attending physician lacked experience. Despite the patient having low T-Pro levels, once this doctor saw the elevated ammonia levels he immediately administered Lactulose and contraindicated the use of TCM medicinals. Other lab test results were as follows: AST 800, ALB 3.4, WBC 25,500, PLT 5,000, T-BIL 17–18, BUN 52, and Cr 3; and other presenting symptoms were lower leg edema, petechiae, and ascites. You could tell right away that this patient could very well have sepsis or possibly even drug-induced hepatorenal syndrome, hemolysis, or drug-induced fulminant hepatitis. The patient also received long-term administration of intravenous ALB and diuretics (oral and intravenous), which perpetuated a state of irreversible edema. Obviously, when you see a PLT count of only 5,000, it is clear that it may lead to sepsis-induced disseminated intravascular coagulation (DIC) and possibly even death.

On April 7, the patient's wife came to my clinic seeking consultation and treatment for her husband. Though I knew this would be a tough case, I felt obligated to try my best. I prescribed Chai Ling Tang adding Huang Qin, Ze Xie, Fu Ling, and Mu Dan Pi (8 qian each); Ren Shen (3 qian); Lu Rong (1 qian); Gan Jiang and Fu Zi (3 qian each); and Da Huang (5 fen). I also explained the importance of having her husband continue the life-sustaining Western medicine treatment (e.g., infusions of whole blood and platelets), while discontinuing all the other drugs.

The patient's condition did improve some, but they did *not* take my advice about discontinuing the other drugs. However, since I had clearly stated my position, I didn't feel it was appropriate to keep persisting. This is an experience we can all learn from. For advanced stage cancer patients, taking a conservative approach of "living with the condition" may be better than aggressive treatment. As for your prescription above, for the most part, I approve, but if T-Pro and A/G levels are low, it is best to add Si Shen Tang, Bai Guo, Dang Shen, and Ren Shen. If the tumor undergoes rapid growth, then add large doses of Wan Ling Dan.

Case Study #6: Elevated AFP Levels

Q: I have a liver cancer patient who received a partial hepatectomy and now has an elevated AFP of 2,000. The patient sought consultation from a South Korean TKM doctor of the Sasang Constitutional Medicine School who told him that he had a Tai Yin constitution. The doctor advised him to eat more table salt to restore energy and strengthen his immune system. What are your thoughts on this approach?

A: If 1 month has already elapsed since partial hepatectomy and the AFP has only dropped from 2,000 to 1,000 then this indicates poor efficacy and inability to correctly identify the pattern and administer the appropriate treatment. My approach would be to prescribe a heat-clearing phlegm-damp-transforming water-disinhibiting formula, such as Chai Ling Tang variant, which would improve the patient's condition in less than 3 weeks time.

Remember! Following partial hepatectomy, the liver will regenerate and thus you should expect AFP levels of anywhere from 30–200. Don't misinterpret this as an indication of liver tumor recurrence! And you don't need to add any special medicinals either! Just keep administering Chai Ling Tang variant—or other relevant formula such as Blood Desiccation Formula, Zhi Bo Di Huang Tang, or Xiang Sha Liu Jun Zi Tang variants—as long as it corresponds with the presenting signs, symptoms and pattern identification).

If AFP suddenly jumps to 500, or even higher to 1,000 or 2,000, then this clearly indicates liver tumor relapse. At this time, you must add large doses of anticancer (e.g., Fu Ling, Ze Xie, Mu Dan Pi, Di Gu Pi, Da Huang, Huang Qin, Chuan Qi, Wan Ling Dan) and yang-supplementing (e.g., The Three Great Yang-Supplementers) medicinals.

Case Study #7: Postoperative Hepatocellular Carcinoma with Multiple Metastases

Q: A 29 y/o female hepatocellular carcinoma (HCC) patient underwent a partial hepatectomy. Later on, peritoneal metastases were discovered, which resulted in another surgical resection. The surgeons allowed her father to attend the operation, and that's how he observed firsthand that they had only resected a small piece of tissue "the size of a rice grain." He was astonished by this and made it a point to attend all of his daughter's subsequent surgeries.

A year later, another sugery was performed on her peritoneum for a lesion near her diaphragm and she also received a regimen of the targeted therapy drug Tarceva (erlotinib). Another year passed, and a massive tumor was found in the patient's pelvis for which she received radiotherapy. It wasn't until 4 years and 5 months after the patient was first diagnosed with cancer that she sought my consultation.

I prescribed Chai Ling Tang adding Bai Zhu, Fu Ling, Ze Xie, Gan Jiang, Fu Zi, Huang Qin, and Mu Dan Pi (8 qian each); Ma Huang (1 qian); Tao Ren (4 qian); Lai Fu Zi, Chen Pi, Ci Wan, and Kuan Dong Hua (5 qian each); Chuan Qi; Wan Ling Dan; and Yu Sheng Wan. In July, the patient had another surgery to resect most of the large tumors in the pelvis, but the tumor in the abdomen had grown larger. I suspected that the tumors on the peritoneum and diaphragm were related.

Recently, the patient has presented with ascites and abdominal distension, but liver function tests are normal; stool normal (3–5/day, currently taking the stool softener and the hyperammonemia drug Lactulose); her appetite is down a bit; and her overall daily activities and functioning are relatively normal. Please offer your advice and guidance on this case.

A: Patients having HCC with peritoneal metastases will inevitably present with ascites and abdominal distention. Also, since the surgical resection involved dissection of the abdominal muscles and peritoneum, absorption of nutrients will be compromised, so you must focus on ensuring sufficient nutritional intake. Once T-Pro and Na levels drop, ascites (known as water drum (水鼓 shuǐ gǔ) in TCM classical pathologic terminology) will rapidly develop.

Based on the patient's current condition, I agree with prescribing Chai Ling Tang (clears heat and transforms phlegm-damp and disinhibits water) variant, but it does *not* seem necessary to add Zi Yuan and Kuan Dong Hua. The key here is to monitor the T-Pro level and make sure to keep it in the normal range. Also, at the onset, do *not* prescribe large doses of Gan Jiang and Fu Zi, because doing so may accelerate lymphatic fluid secretion and thus further obstruct the lymphatic system's capacity to reabsorb the fluid (ascites) in the peritoneal space. As for Ren Shen (powder), from the onset you should prescribe 3 g/3x/day and only consider adding larger doses if T-Pro levels persistently remain.

Based on my experience, for abdominal tumors it is best to add Yuan Hu, Mu Xiang, San Leng, E Zhu, Jiang Huang, Yu Jin, Bing Lang, and Sha Ren. Of course, you could also consider prescribing a blood-breaking, channel-freeing, pain-relieving, and liver- and kidney-supplementing formula such as Tong Jing Fang adding Liang Jiang and Shan Dou Gen for the treatment of tumors. Regardless of which formula you choose, it is essential to add Da Huang in order to maintain low circulatory pressure and prevent the formation of blood stasis and hemorrhage in the GI tract.

Remember! For medicinals that accelerate the metabolism and promote blood perfusion, such as Ren Shen, The Three Great Yang-Supplementers, Huang Qi, and Dang Gui, you should start out by prescribing small doses and increase incrementally. If you do *not* do so, this makes the patient susceptible to hemolysis, GI tract varices, and blood stasis of the endothelial cells and mucous membranes along the GI tract; or worse, it could lead to induration with profuse bleeding, shock, and even death. You must be vigilant!

Why is it that virtually all of my cancer treatment formulas contain Fu Ling, Ze Xie, Mu Dan Pi, Di Gu Pi, Da Huang, Huang Qin, and Chuan Qi? It is because these medicinals have anticancer properties and mutually interact (i.e., have a synergistic effect) with the capacity to repair normal cells, vasculature, lymphatics, and fluids; inhibit abnormal tissue, fluids, neoplastic progession and infiltration; and effectively restore physiological function throughout the course of disease.

Case Study #8: South Korea's Popular "Vegetarian Liver Cancer-Fighting Diet"

Q: Some food therapy advocates in South Korea have made bold claims into the efficacy of a "vegetarian liver cancer-fighting diet," declaring that if you eat vegetables (often raw) and grains like ashitaba (immortal grass), kale, dandelion, thistle, tomato, lotus root, Brewer's yeast, wheat germ, enzymes, red beans, and pearl barley your liver cancer will shrink.

In their books and publications, they list dozens of cases supposedly verifying its effectiveness. This line of reasoning doesn't mesh with modern medicine rationale. Is this just a fad or is it for real? What's your opinion?

A: I do *not* agree at all that liver cancer patients should rely solely on food to treat their condition, and eating vegetarian (particularly a strict vegan diet) is an even worse idea. No matter what type of cancer it is, the body needs adequate nutrients to put up a defense. This is evident in studies that have been done about cancer patients losing their appetites, becoming severely malnourished following radiotherapy and chemotherapy and developing anorexia and cachexia (a hypercatabolic state that causes body tissue to break down). These patients simply waste away and die, but not from the cancer itself!

Eating a strict vegan diet over extended periods makes a person susceptible to low T-Pro and Hb levels, irreversible ascites, and pleural effusion. This is a particularly precarious situation for liver cancer patients who are already susceptible to hemolysis and may lead to hepatorenal syndrome (high BUN/Cr levels) and/or hepatic encephalopathy (cerebral edema and increased intracranial pressure

(ICP)), which may lead to death. This is why it is unequivocably inadvisable for liver cancer patients to eat a strict vegetarian diet.

The best diet for these patients includes grains and legumes like brown rice, pearl barley, and soybeans as staples; lots of nuts (all kinds); Si Shen Tang (Huai Shan, Qian Shi, Lian Zi, Yi Ren, and Fu Ling); fresh vegetables; and fish, meat, and eggs. For patients who are very weak, eating small amounts of Ren Shen (decocting pieces) is also a good idea.

The TCM approach to treating liver cancer is as follows: As long as there is *not* an accumulation of fluid or stasis obstruction in the peripheral tissue around the tumor, typically the cancer will not rapidly progress and metastasize. If the patient still has a decent appetite without signs of wasting (cachexia)—and abstains from making the often hasty and rash decision recommended by their Western medical doctor of immediately receiving chemotherapy and radiotherapy— then simply prescribe water-disinhibiting by bland percolation, heat-clearing toxin-resolving, and blood-quickening stasis-transforming TCM medicinals.

My personal preference for the treatment of liver cancer is Chai Ling Tang variant. Over the years, it has been the most effective formula I have prescribed for treating this pathocondition.

Section 7: Breast Cancer

Breast cancer is the most common type of cancer in women. However, the advancement of health education and advocacy has highlighted the importance of performing self-examinations and going for periodic screening examinations. This has resulted in early detection and initiation of treatment with more favorable outcomes. Typically, after a lump is discovered and a tumor suspected, most patients follow Western medicine protocol, having the lesion resected and then receiving adjuvant radiotherapy and chemotherapy.

That is when most patients seek TCM treatment. At this stage, TCM can provide effective relief of adverse effects and complications from Western medicine drug, surgical, and radiation therapies, inhibit proliferation of cancer cells, prevent metastatic spread, and offer adjuvant and palliative treatment for late stage disease that improves quality of life.

Case Study #1: Frequent Massage for Postoperative Arm Lymphedema

Q: I have a breast cancer patient with arm lymphedema (non-pitting). How would you treat this patient?

A: Postoperative lymphedema can be identified as qi vacuity with water amassment pattern. In addition to prescribing TCM medicinals for the treatment of this condition, it is imperative for the patient to perform massage techniques on the limb as well. Of course, having good posture and maintaining a healthy lifestyle is also important.

First, you should remind the patient that when lying down for sleep to position the arm either horizontally (perpendicular from body) or bend the elbow at a 90° angle with the palm facing upwards resting on a pillow or bedside table. Second, you should advise the patient to regularly perform massage, initially having a tui na (massage) therapist or physiotherapist conduct the procedure, and then once the patient understands the process, either have the patient do self-message or seek assistance from a close friend or family member.

Lymphedema massage should start at the back and shoulder near the region of Gao Huang (UB43) acupoint (where a myofascial "knot" will almost inevitably be found), manipulating until the hard, knotted lump has softened. Massage gently with the fingertips from the elbow up towards the back, from the wrist up to the elbow, and from the fingers up to the wrist, with each repetition ultimtely directing the flow back up towards the centrally located healthy lymphatic vessels. Do this everyday, starting from the back and shoulder, all the way down to the tips of each finger and back up again. Continue performing this daily massage until the swelling has resided and the limbs can function freely and unimpeded as normal.

As for TCM medicinals, you can prescribe a kidney yang-warming qi transformation-promoting and bland-percolating dampness- and water-disinhibiting formula such as Wu Ling San (Nephritis Formula) (including a large dose of Huang Qi, starting out at 2 liang and gradually increasing up to a maximum of 4 liang) adding Yin Xin Ye (8 qian from the onset) and Ren Shen/Chuan Qi Powder. Or you could prescribe a qi-supplementing center-fortifying blood-supplementing formula such as Gui Qi Jian Zhong Tang adding The Four Lings, Gan Jiang, and Fu Zi.

After administering this formula for a period, you can determine the effectiveness of treatment by observing if there is a reduction in hardness and tautness and the presence of wrinkles appearing in the skin of the affected arm. If so, then that is a good sign, and you should continue administering this formula. The condition will continue to improve.

Case Study #2: Intermittent Upper Limb Lymphedema

Q: Following a lumpectomy (breast-conserving surgery), the patient developed lymphedema in the upper limb (same side as surgery). After performing massage, the condition resolved, but a few days later the swelling returned? How should I approach this condition?

A: For treating lymphedema following lumpectomy you can consider prescribing either Wu Ling San (Nephritis Formula) including large doses of Huang Qi; or Bu Zhong Yi Qi Tang (including large doses of Huang Qi) adding Fu Ling, Ze Xie, Gan Jiang, Fu Zi, and Huang Qin. If after administering this formula for 1–2 weeks the edema persists and becomes even tauter, advise the patient to elevate the arm perpendicular to the body when lying down to rest or sleep. This simple measure is very helpful in improving the condition; in the great majority of patients, the swelling will gradually go down. Don't worry!

Case Study #3: Acupuncture and Moxibustion – Adjuvant & Palliative Therapy

Q: Nowadays, it is common for many cancer patients and their families to seek TCM consultation and treatment to regulate the constitution following Western medical treatment (i.e., anticancer agents, radiotherapy, surgery, and other drugs). However, oncologists at most major hospitals are not supportive of this approach, and some categorically contraindicate the use of TCM medicinals.

In recent years, there have been growing numbers of successful cases applying an integrative TCM and Western medicine approach for the treatment of cancer. These successes are making headway, turning the tides from objections and biases into acceptance. Recently, the dean of a major South Korean university contacted me about collaborating on a paper entitled "Efficacy of acupunture therapy on cancer patients."

The purpose of this paper focuses on determining the efficacy of administering acupuncture treatment to prevent and improve adverse effects following resection, radiotherapy, and chemotherapy in breast cancer patients. I am particularly interested in the adverse effects resulting from radiotherapy and chemotherapy, but I don't have enough experience in this area. I was hoping you could share your experiences and insights with me.

A: The efficacy of acupuncture treatment following radiotherapy and chemotherapy for malignant tumors is not very extensive or comprehensive. I view acupuncture as a type of complementary therapy to the administration of TCM medicinal decoctions. Acupuncture certainly plays a role in relieving symptoms, but not as important as medicinals.

One specific adverse effect that I have found acupuncture particularly effective at treating is phlebitis and damage to the vein of the limb at the site of the intravenous (IV) catheter in patients who have received chemotherapy infusions for extended periods. Acupuncture can relieve postoperative pain and reduce the amount of time it takes for the swelling to go down following removal of the IV, improve hematopoietic function following chemotherapy and radiotherapy, and boost the immune system.

If there is lymphedema on the affected side, it is best to apply warm needling Warm needling (applying moxa cubes on the handles of the needles); and after you remove the needle make sure to *press firmly* on the point of insertion. Again, it is important to *press firmly* in order to mitigate the potential for hematoma arising!

Useful acupoints to select are He Gu (LI4), Nei Guan (P6), Chi Ze (LU5), San Yin Jiao (SP6), Yin Lin Quan (SP9), Shou San Li (LI10), Zu San Li (ST36), Fei Shu (UB13), Pi Shu (UB20), Shen Shu (UB23), Tai Chong (LV3), Shen Men (HT7), Feng Chi (GB20), and Hou Xi (SI3).

During the acupunture treatment regimen, patients should *not* concomitantly receive Western medicine drug infusions; instead, they should be administered TCM medicinals. This will ensure the best results.

Case Study #4: Postoperative Ileal and Lung Metastases

Q: A 40 y/o female patient was diagnosed with left-sided breast cancer. Three years after undergoing mastectomy, follow-up examination revealed metastatic spread to the right ilium, and 1 year later metastatic spread to the lung was discovered. Over the past 3 years, the patient has been receiving infusions of Taxol and Docetaxel in an attempt to keep her condition under control.

Originally, the treatment showed effectiveness, but these results have waned. Now, she has a cough with white foamy sputum, but after being administered expectorant medication, her symptoms improved a bit.

Caught up in her other health concerns and daily life, the patient recently realized that it had been 3 months since her last menstruation. Based on the patient's history, what is the best way to treat this patient going forward?

A: For breast cancer patients with metastatic spread to the iliac and lung who receive long-term and repeated radiotherapy and chemotherapy, cancer cells will tend to develop drug resistance. Once fibrosis, induration, and stasis of the lymph nodes, lymph ducts, and microvascular circulation occur, there is *no* available Western medicine drug that offers efficacy. This is especially true for Taxol and Docetaxel, which can only reach the periphery of the tumor and incapable of penetrating the cancerous tissue, so of course they are patently inneffective.

Chemotherapy also causes endometrial inflammation that leads to atrophy and adhesions, and in more severe cases, even the ovaries become inflamed and atrophy. Sometimes the toxicity of chemotherapy and radiotherapy will damage the liver, kidney, PNS, and CNS, which disrupts the gonadal axis and inhibits its natural feedback mechanism. I suspect these two factors could play a role in your patient's amenorrhea. The patient is only 40 y/o so I anticipate that following a TCM therapeutic regimen for a period of time her menstral cycle will regain normal function.

The metastatic spread to the lung presenting with white foamy sputum can be identified as water-cold shooting into the lung with water amassment pattern and suggests the patient most likely has pleural or pericardial effusion. First, you should check to see if the patient has edema on the wrists and shins; if so, this is a sign that there is fluid build-up in the thoracic cavity and your initial prescription should be to disinhibit water in the thoracic cavity. Once the water has been disinhibited, the tumor will become inactive.

As for TCM medicinals, I would prescribe Chai Ling Tang (including large doses of Fu Ling and Ze Xie) adding Ma Huang, Xing Ren, Ting Li Zi (large dose), Fang Ji, Ren Shen/Chuan Qi Powder, and Da Huang (small dose). Remember! At the onset, you should *not* add The Three Great Yang-Supplementers, only after most of the water (fluid) has been cleared should you gradually add these yang-supplementing medicinals.

For bone metastasis, Cu Lu Rong still offers the best effectiveness at improving the patient's condition. If pleural effusion presents along with low levels of Hb, WBC, PLT, and T-Pro, then of course, you should immediately add large doses of Ren Shen (best to gradually add up to 5–7 qian), Cu Lu Rong, and The Three Great Yang-Supplementers. If there is metastatic spread to the bone of the lower extremities, then add Chuan Qi, Niu Xi, and Di Long.

If it is only *mild* pleural effusion, then you can prescribe qi- and yang-supplementing and blood-quickening stasis-transforming medicinals, along with small doses of bland-percolating water-disinhibiting medicinals. These medicinals will soften the tissue surrounding the tumor and substantially enhance efficacy if the patient decides to go ahead with chemotherapy and/or radiotherapy at that time.

If pleural effusion does *not* present, you could consider prescribing variants of either You Gui Yin, Shen Qi Wan, Zhen Wu Tang, or Shi

Quan Da Bu Tang adding Ren Shen/Chuan Qi Powder, The Three Yellows, and Lu Jiao. And if Hb is low and CR high, then add Xi Lu Rong (powder).

Note: The Four Lings (disinhibit water by bland percolation, fortify the spleen and disinhibit dampness, and discharge heat), Ting Li Zi (drains the lung and calms panting and disinhibits water and disperses swelling), and Fang Ji (dispels wind-damp, disinhibits water and disperses swelling) are exceptional medicinals for the treatment of pleural effusion.

Case Study #5: Hormonal Therapy

Q: The patient is a 62 y/o female who began hormone replacement therapy (HRT) 11 years ago to treat what her doctors suspected were menopausal transition related symptoms (hot flashes and profuse sweating).

Several years later, a malignant tumor was discoverd in her left breast. Following surgical resection, her doctor advised her to take Fareston and an aromatase inhibitor. After taking the medication, the hot flashes increased in frequency to over 20 times per day; profuse sweating occurred at intervals throughout the day; and prior to attacks, she would feel a prickly sensation in the skin all over her body.

In hopes of relieving these symptoms, I recently prescribed Bu Zhong Yi Qi Tang adding Qing Hao, Di Gu Pi, and Zhi Mu, but it wasn't helpful at all. Do you think I have failed to accurately identify the pattern? Would Jian Ling Tang variant be a better formula for her pathocondition?

A: The patient's menopausal transition type symptoms of hot flashes and profuse sweating worsened after taking Fareston (a selective estrogen receptor modulator (SERM) class drug like Tamoxifen). The underlying pattern here is clearly yin vacuity, but I have provided a more detailed pattern identification analysis below. This condition can be identified as one of the following three patterns and treated accordingly:

1) Emotionally-derived: Chai Hu Long Gu Mu Li Tang adding Qing Hao, Zhi Mu, and Di Gu Pi.

2) Kidney and liver yin vacuity and hyperactive yang pattern: Variants of either Zhi Bo Di Huang Tang or Dang Gui Liu Huang Tang; or Ba Xian Chang Shou Wan adding Zhi Mu, Huang Bo,

Qing Hao, Di Gu Pi, Long Gu, Mu Li, Dai Zhe Shi, Gan Cao, and Long Yan Gan.

3) Yang straying outward pattern: Jian Ling Tang (including Gan Cao) adding Long Yan Gan, Qing Hao, Zhi Mu, Di Gu Pi, and Huang Bo (in cases of severe heat, consider adding The Three Yellows).

Based on your description, I would identify this patient as yang straying outward pattern, thus I would go with the Jian Ling Tang (Gan Cao) variant.

Case Study #6: Lung, Liver, and Lymphatic Metastases

Q: The patient is a 62 y/o female who was diagnosed with left-sided breast cancer and had a lumpectomy performed 3 years ago. This year she began having shortness of breath and heaviness in the chest, so she went to have it checked out. Examination confirmed the cancer had spread to the lungs, liver, and lymphatics. At this stage, what is the best treatment approach?

A: If the patient has *already* started chemotherapy, then I would prescribe a heat-clearing phlegm-damp-transforming water-disinhibiting formula such as Chai Ling Tang adding large doses of Fu Ling, Ze Xie, Ting Li Zi, Ma Huang, Xing Ren, Fang Ji, Da Huang, and Ren Shen/Chuan Qi Powder. And if hematopoietic dysfunction presents, then add The Three Great Yang-Supplementers and Xi Lu Rong.

If the patient has *not* received chemotherapy, then you can still prescribe the above prescription, subtracting The Three Great Yang-Supplementers and adding Tong Jing Fang (breaks blood and frees the channels) instead. If there is metastasis to the lymphatics presenting with swollen lymph nodes and tidal fever, then add Qing Hao, Zhi Mu, and Di Gu Pi. Shortness of breath suggests pleural effusion for which Chai Ling Tang variant can be prescribed to relieve symptoms and allow the patient to live in harmony with this condition.

Remember! If chemotherapy and/or corticosteroids have *not* been administered, then this condition can be identified as stasis heat pattern, and thus, you should *not* add The Three Great Yang-Supplementers!

Case Study #7: Vegetarian Diet – Devastating for CT & RT Patients

Q: A 58 y/o female patient received treatment for breast cancer 7 years ago and a recent examination revealed multiple metastatic bone lesions. At the time of discovery, lab test results showed a CA15-3 36 (0–83) and WBC 4,000 (4.5 to 11.0 × 10^9/L). She decided to receive treatment with infusions of anticancer agents and oral aromatase inhibitors (already on her third different one).

The most recent lab test results show WBC 2,100 and CA15-3 28.4, and a computed tomography scan (CT scan) revealed metastatic spread to the skull. Other signs, symptoms, and history are as follows: reflux gastritis; Ca, P, and K levels are *normal*; and the patient has now begun a vegetarian diet.

I prescribed Xiang Sha Liu Jun Zi Tang adding Gan Jiang, Fu Zi, Mu Dan Pi, Chi Shao, Cu Lu Rong, and Chuan Qi. Do you think this approach will be effective?

A: Cancer patients must maintain healthy and balanced nutritional intake in order to overcome the side effects of chemotherapy (CT) and radiotherapy (RT), and prevent T-Pro and Hb levels from falling too low, which could lead to hemolysis and death. It really is *not* good for cancer patients to maintain a strict vegeterian diet or suddenly changing to a vegetarian diet just because of cancer diagnosis.

This is especially the case for vegetarians who receive chemotherapy. Chemotherapy inhibits a broad spectrum of metabolic and endocrine mechanisms, causing severe bone marrow suppression (hematopoietic stem cell dysfunction), while the inhibition of the kidneys' capacity to secrete hormones such as granulocyte-colony stimulating factor (G-CSF) and erythropoietin (EPO) further leads to a poor blood picture. Once these physiological mechanisms have been disrupted, the process of returning the body to homeostasis is very difficult.

Thus, you should actively encourage your patient to at the very least eat plenty of eggs and milk along with a variety of nuts and grains (including brown rice, pearl barley, and soybeans), which are all high in vitamin B complex. You should also prescribe starchy TCM medicinals to promote appetite (e.g., Si Shen Tang); Dan Shen, Dang Shen, and Ren Shen to improve hematopoiesis; and large amounts of The Three Great Yang-Supplementers and Cu Lu Rong to "boost" the metabolism and immune system and strengthen bone. Administration of these medicinals follows the key treatment principle of supplementing to benefit attacking and supplementing as a substitute for attacking (補助攻,補替攻 bǔ zhù g□ng, bǔ tì gong).

For breast cancer patients who have received chemotherapy, if the CA15-3 levels are high, this suggests potential for relapse. At this time, you can prescribe Xiang Sha Liu Jun Zi Tang variant; and if Gan Jiang and Fu Zi are added, you must remember to include appropriate amounts of The Three Yellows (to counterbalance the heat) along with Mu Dan Pi and Di Gu Pi.

Remember! Monitoring and attempting to maintain CA15-3 within the normal range is the guiding principle in my therapeutic approach. If CA15-3 levels increase again, then this suggests that bone metastases have occurred and you can add medicinals such as Cu Lu Rong, Yin Xing Ye, Chuan Qi, Sheng Du Zhong, Di Long, Gou Ji, and Xu Duan. Bone belongs to the kidney and Cu Lu Rong can inhibit the tumor vasculature from generating hormones that promote angiogenesis and tumerogenesis, thus ensuring the tumor remains stalled in the G1 to G0 phase and unable to rapidly proliferate. In fact, the actions of other TCM medicinals such as The Three Yellows, Mu Dan Pi, and Di Gu Pi function in the same way.

Case Study #8: HPV Following CT & RT – Xiao Chai Hu Tang Is Effective!

Q: A 41 y/o female breast cancer patient contracted human papillomavirus (HPV) following radiotherapy (RT) and chemotherapy (CT). I followed your advice by prescribing Xiao Chai Hu Tang adding large doses of Huang Qin (8 qian), Mu Dan Pi, Zhi Zi, Long Dan Cao, and Pu Gong Ying. After taking the formula for 1 month, the HPV completely resolved. Thanks for your guidance!

A: Ah! Yes, administering a Shao Yang-harmonizing and -resolving formula such as Xiao Chai Hu Tang adding Mu Dan Pi, Zhi Zi, Long Dan Cao, and Pu Gong Ying to successfully treat HPV in a breast cancer patient following radiotherapy and chemotherapy.

Congratulations! This is a good case study. You should organize the material and submit it to a professional medical journal in South Korea, or even an international publication.

Case Study #9: Acupuncture Treats HPV

Q: I followed your advice prescribing Xiao Chai Hu Tang adding Long Dan Cao along with acupuncture to treat a breast cancer patient presenting with flushing, hot flashes, and HPV infection following radiotherapy and chemotherapy. The treatment was very effective as the HPV tested negative.

The most noteworthy aspect of this case for me was the selection of acupoints for the treatment regimen—Feng Chi (GB20), Shen Men (HT7), Shao Fu (HT8), and San Yin Jiao (SP6)—needling 1x/week. After just four treatments (4 weeks), the condition had improved by over 70%. I intend to present these results at a TCM conference in the U.S.

A: Congratulations on your successful treatment of HPV. I wish your presentation the best of success!

Case Study #10: Intermittent Plueral Effusion

Q: A 58 y/o female patient was first diagnosed with left-sided breast cancer, surgical resection was peformed, and then 2 years later a 6 cm tumor was discovered in the right lung. After receiving radiotherapy and chemotherapy, the tumor shrank to 2 cm. The patient's condition stabilized for the most part, but she was still hindered by the pleural effusion of the right lung.

Examination did *not* reveal metastatic spread to the pleura, and the patient did *not* have the classic symptoms of intermittent fever, shortness of breath, or difficulty breathing when lying down. However, this pleural effusion problem persisted with intermittent symptoms presenting at times and then resolving. How would you treat this patient?

A: There are many potential causes of right lung pleural effusion, including spontaneous occurrence, infection, inflammation, trauma, cardiopulmonary disorder, uremia, cirrhotic sequela of ascites, immune system abnormalities, and cancer. If the patient has undergone treatment, the condition may become chronic with a small quantity of pleural effusion that typically does not produce pronounced symptoms.

I have come across something like this before with a patient having an air-filled cyst located between the lower lobe of the right lung and the diagphram, which was so large it had compressed the right lung down to the size of a fist. Despite the extent of this distortion, the patient did *not* have any noticeable symptoms, and it was only upon routine physical examination that this abnormality was discovered.

In any case, the best formula for treating right lung pleural effusion is still a heat-clearing phlegm-damp-transforming water-disinhibiting formula such as Chai Ling Tang adding large doses of Fu Ling, Ze Xie, Ting Li Zi, Fang Ji, Qing Hao, Zhi Mu, Di Gu Pi, and Ren Shen/Chuan Qi Powder. Treatment should be administered for 3–6 months and then gradually discontinued.

Case Study #11: Leukopenia Following Radiotherapy

Q: A 43 y/o breast cancer patient presented with leukopenia following radiotherapy. How should I treat this?

A: One of the potential adverse effects of radiotherapy is hematopoietic suppression. Fortunately, radiotherapy to the chest area in breast cancer patients is typically not as severe as irradiation to the bone marrow of the long bones!

The cardiopulmonary system plays an integral role in hematopoiesis with the lungs secreting "precursors" to erythropoietin (EPO), whereas the majority of "functional" EPO is secreted by the kidneys (with small portions secreted by the lungs, liver, fat, and marrow.)

Lung and myocardium damage may occur when breast cancer patients undergo radiotherapy, which can result in anemia and leukopenia. These adverse effects can be effectively treated through an integrative TCM and Western medicine approach.

Case Study #12: Is Pregnancy Safe for Breast Cancer Patients Following Western Medical Treatment?

Q: A 34 y/o breast cancer patient underwent mastectomy on her left breast followed up by radiotherapy, chemotherapy, and hormonal therapy. Now, she wants to get pregnant, but her oncologist strongly opposes this idea. What is your opinion?

A: Indeed, it is not advisable for breast cancer patients who have been administered Tamoxifen following radiotherapy and/or chemotherapy to get pregnant right away. The reason for this is that fetal cells differentiate rapidly in a very similar to cancer cells.

Once a woman becomes pregnant, the high nutrient diet required provides ample sources of fuel for cancer cells to exploit, which can differentiate faster than fetal cells. This opens up the possibility for relapse and multiple metastases during gestation, putting everyone involved in a difficult position. The best thing to do is temporarily hold off on pregnancy.

That does *not* mean she should never become pregnant. It is best for patients to wait until their breast cancer condition has stabilized. Once stabilized, discontinue the use of Tamoxifen and take a formula such as Ru Mo Si Wu Tang adding The Three Yellows; Di Gu Pi Yin variant; or Zhi Bo Di Huang Tang adding The Three Yellows, Qing Hao, and Di Gu Pi. These types of TCM medicinals have the capacity to lower the sensitivity of estrogen and progesterone hormone receptors on cell surfaces.

After a period of time, have lab tests performed to determine if the patient is hormone receptor-negative, and if so, continue administering TCM medicinals for 6 more months. At that time, the patient will be ready to prepare for pregnancy!

Case Study #13: Adverse Effects of Long-Term Administration of Tamoxifen

Q: Why is it that over 70% of breast cancer patients who take Tamoxifen for 1–2 years develop fatty liver, but their AST and ALT levels are normal? What is the best way to approach this?

A: Long-term administration of Tamoxifen (a selective estrogen receptor modulator (SERM)) may cause a number of side effects, including hepatitis, fatty liver, cirrhosis, neuropathy, edema, blood clots, and sometimes even endometrial cancer. These can all be identified as stasis heat with water amassment pattern that can be treated as follows:

1) Prescribe Ru Mo Si Wu Tang adding The Three Yellows, Mu Dan Pi, Fu Ling, and Ze Xie. This therapeutic approach inhibits the hormone receptor-positive response and reverts it to negative, while also lowering the CA12-5 and CA15-3 levels. Administration of this formula will eventually enable the patient to discontinue Tamoxifen.

2) Includes various approaches each with distinct advantages and disadvantages that can be selected based on the individual patient's constitution and condition: a) Continue taking Tamoxifen while gradually reducing the dose; b) Administer TCM medicinals and discontinue Tamoxifen; or c) Wait until CA12-5 and CA15-3 levels return to normal before discontinuing Tamoxifen.

Case Study #14: TCM Medicinal Prescriptions Must Flexibly Respond to Patient's Condition

Q: I have a 62 y/o female patient with breast cancer that has already metastasized to the lung and left femur. She *has* received various regimens of radiotherapy and chemotherapy and is currently taking Tamoxifen.

Now, her WBC remains at low levels of 2,000–2,800 (4,500 to 11,000), so I prescribed Xiang Sha Jun Zi Tang adding The Three Great Yang-Supplementers, Ren Shen/Chuan Qi Powder, and Dai Zhe Shi. I added Dai Zhe Shi because of her reflux esophagitis. After taking this formula, her WBC level increased from 3,000 to 6,000 and the patient now wants to stop taking the TCM medicinals. What is your opinion on this case?

A: Congratulations on your patient's WBC increasing! If your patient wants to stop taking the medicinals now, that would be fine. In the future, if she wants to continue with TCM treatment you must pay close attention to increases in the tumor markers CA12-5, CA19-9, CA15-3, and CEA.

If levels do *rise* above normal, then you should either *reduce* the dose of The Three Great Yang-Supplementers or *subtract* them altogether. Administration of The Three Great Yang-Supplementers may cause CA12-5, CA15-3, CEA, LDH, and CPK levels to rise; increase blood concentrations of calcium, potassium, and magnesium; and prompt peripheral blood stem cells to differentiate, thus inducing tumor relapse.

The best thing to do if the aforementioned scenario of relapse does occur is to change the prescription to include blood-cooling, blood-quickening stasis-transforming, and heat-clearing toxin-resolving medicinals such as Ru Mo Si Wu Tang adding The Three Yellows, Bai Zhu, Fu Ling, Ze Xie, Mu Dan Pi, Yu Sheng Wan, and Wan Ling Dan. If tidal heat presents, then consider adding medicinals such as Qing Hao, Zhi Mu, and Di Gu Pi; or Chai Hu, Qin Jiao, Tian Men Dong, and Mai Men Dong.

The manifestations of pathoconditions are continuously changing and new Western medicine drugs are being developed every passing day. TCM prescriptions must also continuously evolve and adapt to the conditions, just as it is written in the *Book of Changes* (易經 *Yi Jing*): "If you can one day renovate yourself, do so from day to day, and let there be daily renovation." Another verse that resonates in a similar spirit is "Be diligent and alert from morning till night," which is also a core philosophical principle of traditional Korean medicine (TKM).

But remember! You must always be discerning. Do not adjust the TCM formula contents too quickly or dramatically and always carefully consider the results of biomedical lab tests (e.g., CBC, liver enzymes, tumor markers) and other diagnostic tools. After all, these are the fundamental principles of an integrative TCM and Western medicine therapeutic approach, and combined with pattern identification, provide the basis for which to fine-tune your prescriptions.

Case Study #15: Increased CA15-3 and Thrombocytopenia

Q: I have a 60 y/o female breast cancer patient with metastatic spread to the lung and femur. After taking Tamoxifen, lab tests showed CA15-3 1869 (normal range is lower than 83) and WBC 2,400 (4,500 to 11,000).

I prescribed Ru Mo Si Wu Tang adding Huang Qin (1 liang); Huang Lian, Huang Bo, and Dai Zhe Shi (5 qian), Mu Dan Pi and Chi Shao (8 qian), and Wan Ling Dan (5 pills/3x/pay). However, after 2 months of treatment, the most recent lab test results did *not* show much improvement. Shouldn't I be seeing some positive results by now? Please offer your invaluable advice and guidance.

A: For breast cancer patients with lung and skeletal (femur) metastases who have taken Tamoxifen but still are hormone receptor-positive, it isn't necessarily appropriate to prescribe Ru Mo Si Wu Tang variant. Bone belongs to the kidneys, so Ru Xiang and Mo Yao are *not* the best choices.

You should consider changing to an yin-enriching fire-downbearing steaming bone-eliminating formula such as Zhi Bo Di Huang Tang or a blood-breaking channel-freeing and sinew- and bone-strengthening formula such as Tong Jing Fang. Just make sure to include The Three Yellows, Qing Hao, Zhi Mu, Di Gu Pi, Cu Lu Rong, and large doses of Wan Ling Dan.

Additionally, regardless of the formula you choose, make sure to include combinations of blood-quickening stasis-transforming medicinals such as Du Zhong, Sang Ji Sheng, Liu Ji Nu, Du Niu Xi (or Huai Niu Xi). If water amassment presents, then add The Four Lings, Ting Li Zi, and Fang Ji.

Case Study #16: Lung Metastases – Focus on Increasing WBCs

Q: I have a 61 y/o female breast cancer patient with lung metastases (right lung tumor 5.5 cm) and vertebral metastases (discovered during TomoTherapy). Her lab test results showed WBC 2,500 (4,500 to 11,000) and monocyte 13% (9–11%). The patient has *no* presenting symptoms. What treatment approach would you consider for this patient?

A: Typically, for breast cancer patients with lung metastases and lab test results showing WBC 2,500 and monocyte 13% following chemotherapy, you can simply focus on increasing the levels of ANC (absolute neutrophil count) and LYM (lymphocytes) to normal range. Monocyte levels will naturally follow suit, so you do *not* need to worry about them. Your focus should be on *increasing* the WBC count!

For malignancy of the lung, I generally prescribe the heat-clearing phlegm-damp-transforming water-disinhibiting formula Chai Ling Tang adding Ren Shen/Chuan Qi Powder. If chemotherapy has *not* been administered, WBC levels should quickly rebound.

If the patient takes Chai Ling Tang variant concomitantly with chemotherapy, and the WBC drops once again, then it is tyically very difficult for TCM medicinals to restore normal WBC levels. At this time, it is necessary to add small doses of The Three Great Yang-Supplementers to your main formula.

Case Study #17: Bone Metastases – Add Cu Lu Rong

Q: A breast cancer patient with bone metastases presented with elevated $Ca2^{+}$ after being administered Fareston (a selective estrogen receptor modulator (SERM)).

I have been prescribing this patient Ru Mo Si Wu Tang, and after adding Cu Lu Rong to the formula, the hypercalcemia and related symptoms have resolved. Do you think the CT/PET imaging will reveal that the bone tumor has disappeared as well?

A: Prescribing Ru Mo Si Wu Tang adding Cu Lu Rong can prevent breast cancer from spreading to the bone, but if Hb, PLT, WBC, and T-Pro levels are low, you must also nourish kidney yin and abate steaming bone heat by adding Ma Huang, Di Long, Niu Xi, and Du Zhong (or Jin Mao Gou Ji).

If the patient has poor appetite and T-Pro and A/G levels are low, then you should consider changing to a qi-boosting spleen-fortifying and qi-moving phlegm-transforming formula such as Xiang Sha Liu Jun Zi Tang or a spleen-fortifying qi-supplementing yang-upbearing formula such as Bu Zhong Yi Qi. Make sure to include Mu Dan Pi and Huang Qin in your formula selection.

If BUN/Cr levels are high, then first add The Three Great Yang-Supplementers; if the condition does *not* improve, then add Ren Shen/Chuan Qi Powder and Xi Lu Rong (powder); and if there is *still* no improvement, then treat this condition as renal failure and add other anticancer medicinals.

Case Study #18: Colorectal Metastases – Nausea and Vomiting Following CT & RT

Q: Colorectal metastasis was discovered in a 55 y/o female breast cancer patient following radiotherapy (RT) and chemotherapy (CT). After receiving 5 infusions of chemotherapy, she experienced vomiting and retching.

The patient is a very sensitive person to begin with. She has a poor appetite, cannot tolerate foods with peculiar smells or flavors, and virtually everyting she eats makes her feel nauseous (even plain white rice makes her want to retch!).

She has sought treatment from numerous TCM and Western medicine doctors, but nothing has been effective. Her bowel movements vary, sometimes 1 stool/1–2 day(s) and others 3–4 stools/day. How would you approach this case?

A: This patient sounds like she fits the classic description of "cancer neurosis." Some people will have *extreme* reactions in response to the stimulus of radiotherapy and chemotherapy. In this situation, to stop vomiting and retching, I like to prescribe Ban Xia and Fu Ling (powdered medicinals, 2g each/3–4x/day); and once the vomiting and retching subsides, then I would prescribe either Ban Xia Hou Po Tang alone or Gan Mai Da Zao Tang Combining Ban Xia Hou Po Tang.

Ban Xia and Fu Ling are virtually flavorless, but if the patient still thinks Fu Ling has an unappealing flavor, then just prescribe Ban Xia by itself: it is "absolutely" flavorless. Once the patient's symptoms improve, then you can gradually add in antiemetic medicinals (formulas) that are sweet in flavor. And once the patient is able to tolerate the sweet-flavored antiemetic medicinals, then proceed gradually, changing the formula to the slightly more robust flavors of Xiang Sha Liu Jun Zi Tang. This formula is ideal because it functions as an antiemetic, improves appetite, promotes the absorption of nutrients and medicinals, supplements the kidney, and disperses swelling.

Prescribing Xiang Sha Liu Jun Zi Tang variant at this time will prove effective in remedying the adverse effects of radiotherapy and chemotherapy, helping the patient to overcome the discomforts and enabling her to complete the scheduled radiotherapy and chemotherapy regimens. During the Xiang Sha Liu Jun Zi Tang phase of treatment, if hematopoietic dysfunction presents and this formula proves ineffective at remedying the condition, then you can add Ren Shen, Dan Shen, and Dang Shen; and if this is still ineffective, then you can go ahead and add small doses of The Three Great Yang-Supplementers

Section 8: Other Cancers & Treatment Risks

Case Study #1: Tonsillar Cancer – Salivary Gland Hypofunction, Xerostomia, and Aguesia Following RT & CT

Q: Ten years ago, this patient was diagnosed with tonsillar cancer. Following surgical dissection, radiotherapy (RT), and chemotherapy (CT), the patient experienced salivary gland hypofunction, dry mouth (xerostomia), loss of taste (aguesia), and right-sided neck pain and stiffness. My idea is to prescribe Blood Desiccation Formula variant. Do you think this is a good choice?

A: Virtually all patients receiving chemotherapy and radiotherapy for cancers of the head, neck, and mouth will experience the adverse effects of losing the sense of taste (aguesia), dry mouth (xerostomia), and salivary gland hypofunction (or complete loss of secretion). The presentation of these symptoms requires the inclusion of great yang-supplementing medicinals.

Yes, you can prescribe Blood Desiccation Formula, but you should also add The Three Great Yang-Supplementers, Huang Qin, Tian Ma, and Ge Gen. For patients currently *receiving* radiotherapy and chemotherapy, you can prescribe a lung-clearing stomach-nourishing and liquid-engendering dryness-moistening formula such as Sha Shen Mai Men Dong Tang adding Jie Geng and Ke Zi; and if salivary secretions have dried up, then add The Three Great Yang-Supplementers, Huang Qin, and Ren Shen/Chuan Qi Powder.

Both of these formulas are effective at improving the patient's condition. You can reassure the patient that positive results will be noticeable after taking these medicinals for about 3–5 weeks. However, it will take at least 6 months of ongoing administration to completely remedy this condition.

Case Study #2: Gastrointestinal Cancer – Pancreatic and Lymph Node Metastases

Q: A 58 y/o male patient was diagnosed with gastric cancer and colorectal cancer, requiring immediate partial gastrectomy and colectomy. Not too long after surgery, pancreatic and lymph node metastases were discovered, and the patient received 3 targeted therapy treatments.

Recently, follow-up examination revealed metastatic spread to the abdominal cavity and the patient is currently being administered polysaccharide K (PSK). He is still able to go on hikes in the hills and does *not* have ascites or lymphedema.

How would you treat this condition? Please offer your guidance and instruction on this case.

A: In general, the most important concern for advanced cancer patients is to maintain a good appetite. With a good appetite and positive attitude, nutrients will be efficiently absorbed and the patient will be able to continue maintaining a relatively good quality of life.

With this in mind, if the patient can still take food, then you can consider prescribing a phlegm-damp-transforming and qi-boosting spleen-fortifying formula variant such as Ban Xia Tian Ma Bai Zhu San, Bu Zhong Yi Qi Tang, Xiang Sha Liu Jun Zi Tang, or Chai Ling Tang. You can add combinations of medicinals such as Shan Dou Gen and Liang Jiang; Gan Cao, Da Zao, and Long Yan Rou; and Shan Zha and Ji Nie Jin. Remember! Regardless of which formula you choose, make sure to include Chuan Qi, Yu Sheng Wan, and Wan Ling Dan.

Ban Xia Tian Ma Bai Zhu San can remedy stomach cold and poor appetite induced by anticancer agents. If necessary, you can add Gan Cao, Da Zao, and Long Yan Gan. Formulas such as Shen Ling Bai Zhu San, Si Shen Tang, and Shui Lu Er Xian Dan are all moderate in nature (neither hot nor cold) and are appropriate for maintaining health, increasing appetite, promoting the absorption of nutrients, and boosting the body's natural capacity to fight cancer. If levels of the tumor markers CEA, CA72-4, and CA19-9 are *increased*, then you should *subtract* Gan Jiang and Fu Zi and instead *add* large doses of The Three Yellows.

Case Study #3: Cervical Cancer – Colorectal Metastases

Q: Today a female patient visited my clinic explaining that she had been diagnosed with cervical cancer. After surgical resection, follow-up examinations revealed colorectal metastases. She received chemotherapy without effective results, and then became infected with pulmonary tuberculosis. Right now, her symptoms are as follows: constipation, poor appetite, dry mouth, numbness in the upper and lower limbs, and insomnia. Lab tests show tumor markers SCC antigen (SCC-Ag) at 48.1 (22–78) and CYFRA 21 at 9.7 (0.6–126).

I prescribed Sheng Yu Tang adding Chuan Qi, Da Huang, and Yu Sheng Wan (2 pills/day). Originally, I was thinking about prescribing Ru Mo Si Wu Tang variant, but decided not to because of problems with digestion. I think the most difficult aspect of colorectal cancer is trying to get the tumor to shrink. Please offer your guidance and instruction on this case.

A: SCC and CYFRA 21 are lung cancer tumor markers and do *not* correlate with colorectal metastases. Typically, CEA and NSE are also referenced for lung metastases, but it would appear that her doctors suspect more than just infection with pulmonary tuberculosis.

As for TCM medicinals, I would prescribe Chai Ling Tang adding Qing Hao, Zhi Mu, Di Gu Pi, The Three Great Yang-Supplementers, Shan Zha, Ren Shen/Chuan Qi Powder, and Wan Ling Dan. Remember! Start out with small doses of The Three Great Yang-Supplementers (2–3 qian each), waiting until tidal fever and night sweats subside, and then increase to 5 qian or even higher.

Case Study #4: Prostate Cancer

Q: Is PSA a useful indicator for diagnosing and monitoring patients for prostate cancer?

A: Right now PSA (prostate specific antigen) offers the highest specificity of any tumor marker. The problem with accuracy is that patients with prostatitis will also test high PSA levels (false-positive test result) and sometimes PSA levels are normal in people who really do have prostate cancer (false-negative test result). But overall, I would say PSA is accurate at least 70%–80% of the time.

In TCM, prostate cancer can be identified as liver channel damp-heat pouring downward pattern, requiring the administration of a formula variant such as Long Dan Xie Gan Tang, Zhi Bo Di Huang Tang, Zhi Zi Bo Pi Tang, or Huang Lian Jie Du Tang. All of these formula variants are effective. Just make sure that the formula includes Long Dan Cao (5–8 qian), Huang Bo (5–8 qian), and Chuan

Qi; and if the patient has endured this condition for a long period of time, then add Long Yan He and Chuan Lian Zi.

Remember! Patients with chronic constipation often have blood amassment passing into the blood chamber (蓄血傳於血室之中 xù xuè chuán yú xuè shì zh□ zh□ng), which refers to static blood impairing circulation and physiological mechanisms in the pelvic cavity. This results constipation and bilateral pain in the pelvis, requiring the administration of either Tao Ren Cheng Qi Tang, Di Dang Tang (pulverized powder), or simply Ma Zi Ren and Da Huang, making sure to incrementally increase the dose of Da Huang up until the patient maintains 3–5 stools per day.

Case Study #5: Swollen Neck Lymph Nodes

Q: A 37 y/o female patient explained that she has had swollen lymph nodes in her neck since she was 20 y/o. After taking TCM medicinals for 6 months, the swellings disappeared. Is it possible for this condition to be completely cured in such a short period of time?

A: If the lymph node swelling disappeared, then it is most likely not of malignant origin. Benign cervical lymph node swelling (simple goiter) is typically caused by infection (e.g., cervical lymph nodes, ears, nose, mouth, teeth, lungs) and can be identified as Shao Yang heat pattern.

If you accurately prescribe TCM medicinals based on assessment of the signs, symptoms, and pattern identification, then you most certainly can expect to see rapid results.

Case Study #6: Non-Hodgkin's Lymphoma

Q: A 70 y/o female patient was diagnosed with non-Hodgkin's lymphoma (NHL) and she presented with swelling on the left side of her nose. She is currently receiving chemotherapy and her WBC count is slightly low, but she has a good appetite. Is it necessary for NHL patients to receive chemotherapy?

A: If the diagnosis of non-Hodgkin's lymphoma is indeed accurate, then you can follow the Shao Yang heat pattern therapeutic approach. You can prescribe Shao Yang-harmonizing and -resolving and blood-nourishing yin-enriching formulas such as Xiao Chai Hu Tang, Di Gu Pi Yin, or Xi Niu Di Huang Tang, making sure to include Qing Hao, Zhi Mu, Di Gu Pi, Huang Qin (and/or Huang Lian and Huang Bo), Chuan Qi, Yu Sheng Wan, and Wan Ling Dan. If soft, diffuse swelling of lymph nodes present, then add The Four Lings (disinhibit water by bland percolation and fortify the spleen and disinhibit dampness), or change the formula to Wu Ling San adding Huang Qin (large doses), Mu Dan Pi, and Di Gu Pi.

If chemotherapy induces leukopenia, then you should add Ren Shen/Chuan Qi Powder, which will promote a rapid increase in the WBC count. If the WBC count does *not* increase, then add The Three Great Yang-Supplementers. Remember! Once chemotherapy has been discontinued, then you must *subtract* The Three Great Yang-Supplementers; otherwise, the lymph node enlargement may return.

Case Study #7: Multiple Spinal Cord Tumors

Q: I have a 38 y/o male patient with a 2 cm x 1 cm coccygeal vertebral tumor that was discovered 5 years ago. Recently, he had experienced back pain and difficulty rotating his torso. An MRI was performed revealing the presence of 5 variably sized tumors in other parts of his sacral and lumbar vertebrae. This is a classic case of multiple spinal cord tumors. What's the best way to treat this condition?

A: If the patient does not undergo surgery, then simply prescribe a formula variant such as Ru Mo Si Wu Tang or Di Gu Pi Yin. If the patient undergoes surgery, then after the operation administer either Paralysis #2 Formula (Shi Quan Da Bu Tang Variant) or Paralysis #3 Formula (You Gui Yin Variant). Depending on the patients presenting symptoms and stage of progress, you can also consider adding Di Long, Ma Huang, Lu Jiao, and Wan Ling Dan.

Case Study #8: Cervical Artery Aneurysm

Q: An MRI revealed the presence of a cervical carotid artery aneurysm that appeared to be on the verge of rupturing. Do you think the patient should undergo bypass surgery, or should he just take Aspirin and glycerin? Please offer your guidance and instruction on this case.

A: Among cervical segments consisting of the external carotid, internal carotid, and vertebral arteries, the vertebral artery is the most important. Once occlusion or rupture of the vertebral artery occurs, virtually every case leads to severe disability with high mortality rates.

Right now, the only Western medicine drug option a patient with a cervical artery aneurysm has is to take antihypertensive medication to control blood pressure. As far as the options you provided in your letter, I think that a surgical procedure offers the best potential outcome, whether it's with coil embolization, titanium clips, or CyberKnife (though they all have potential risks!).

The use of anticoagulants like Aspirin is absolutely contraindicated. Not only are they ineffective; worse, they can induce hemolysis and rupture of aneurysms in other parts of the body. Bypass surgery is also not advisable because the cervical artery would need to withstand enormous pressure, and adequate extracorporeal circulation would be a challenge during the operation. Also, the materials used for the bypass surgery would not last for much more than 10–20 years, becoming either damaged or dislodged and likely causing sudden death.

As for TCM treatment, I would prescribe long-term administration of blood-quickening qi-supplementing and stasis-dispelling network vessel-freeing formula variants such as Ru Mo Si Wu Tang, Sheng Yu Tang, or Bu Yang Huan Wu Tang, which focus on preventing rupture by maintaining low blood pressure and vascular wall elasticity and patency.

Case Study #9: TCM Treatment for Syringoma

Q: A 48 y/o female patient explained that since about the age of 30 y/o syringomas began appearing on both of her lower eyelids. She underwent laser surgery to remove them, but the growths reappeared. Now, she has numerous growths appearing on her forehead and cheeks and wants to try treating this condition with TCM medicinals.

Would Ma Xing Yi Gan Tang variant be effective at preventing the spread of these growths? Why do these growths continue proliferating in her sweat glands? Some reports from TCM doctors in

China advocate using large doses of Xia Ku Hua. Do you think this is an effective approach?

A: Most patients with syringomas do *not* have the patience for TCM treatment. If the patient is compliant in taking Ma Xing Yi Gan Tang variant for long durations, this formula can definitely improve this condition. You can talk with your patient and suss out the situation.

Regarding reports from China advocating the efficacy of Xia Ku Hua, I don't oppose giving it a try, but you must remember that Xia Ku Hua will lower T3 and T4, so it should not be prescribed for patients with low thyroid hormone levels (hypothyroidism).

Instead of Xia Ku Hua, I would consider including combinations of the following medicinals for more effective and quicker results: Zao Jiao Ci, Ci Ji Li, Ye She Mei (*Duchesnea indica* (Andr.) Focke), Que Bu Ta (*Aralia decaisneana* Hance), Lu Lu Tong, and Yao Ren Gou (*Dendrocnide meyeniana* (Walp.) Chew). You can also consider selecting combinations of Mu Dan Pi, Bai Xian Pi, Zhi Ke, Chen Pi, Cang Bai Pi, and the leaves of citrus fruit plants such as oranges, tangerines, Buddha's hand (Fo Shou), pomelo, and grapefruit.

Case Study #10: Radiotherapy-Induced Salivary Gland and Gustatory Nerve Damage

Q: I provided acupuncture treatment (Tian Chuang (SI16), Tian You (SJ16), Yi Feng (SJ17), He Gu (LI4), and Xia Guan (ST7)) to a patient presenting with dry mouth (xerostomia) following radiotherapy.

After four treatments (1 per week), the patient had noticeably increased salivary flow, but the patient's sense of taste (hypoguesia) was still impaired (everything tastes bitter). The patient has a very poor appetite, and oddly, the only dish he likes to eat is fried saucy noodles, anything else is hard to swallow. Why would this be?

A: For patients incurring dry mouth and loss of taste following radiotherapy, as long as they can still discern some flavor (e.g., bitter), then this indicates gustatory nerve damage is mild and gradual recovery eminent. Continue with the acupuncture treatment, but I recommend adding moxa for quicker results. I would also recommend prescribing an orally administered dual supplementation of qi and blood TCM formula adding yang-supplementing medicinals such as Shi Quan Da Bu Tang (including a large dose of Huang Qi (2–4 liang)) adding Tian Men Dong and Mai Men Dong; large doses of The Three Great Yang-Supplementers (5–8 qian each); and Ren Shen/Chuan Qi Powder.

This approach should facilitate quick recovery of gustatory sense for spicy and sweet flavors and promote increased salivary flow rate. At the onset, the patient may experience profuse salivary secretions, and then the patient will gradually regain capacity to draw in and swallow the saliva normally. Additionally, your patient may have incurred damage to the cranial nerves in the brainstem that control swallowing. That is why the patient probably likes to eat fried saucy noodles because this dish is moist, so all the patient has to do is lift up his head and let the noodle covered in sauce flow down his esophagus.

Remember! You still need to prescribe TCM medicinals to ensure complete recovery of nerve function, and this will require continuous administration over a long period. If the patient takes TCM medicinals for short interval, shows improvement, and then decides to discontinue treatment, at some point the incompletely healed nerves will likely begin regressing into a progressive atrophy.

I have a classmate whom had difficulty swallowing (dysphagia) food nearly 20 years after receiving radiotherapy to the neck, and he refused to have an NG tube inserted. In the end, he suffered from severe depression and died of starvation—basically, committing suicide. Inserting an NG tube or undergoing a percutaneous endoscopic gastronomy (PEG) procedure would have enabled the patient to continue taking TCM medicinals through the feeding tube, which would have allowed at least partial recovery and extended his life. I advise you to continue striving to help this patient by providing the best care possible.

Case Study #11: Chemotherapy-Induced Peripheral Neuropathy of the Upper and Lower Limbs

Q: Many of the cancer patients I have treated who have received chemotherapy have experienced peripheral neuropathies of the upper and lower limbs and urticaria that sometimes is so severe the entire body is swollen. How would you treat these side effects?

A: Peripheral neuropathy following chemotherapy can be identified as qi vacuity pattern. Simply add large doses of qi-supplementing medicinals (e.g., up to 2 liang of Huang Qi) into your main formula and you will quickly see positive results. Naturally, you could also needle acupoints along the corresponding channels of the affected limbs.

For drug-induced urticaria (wind papules), you can first bleed (above, on, and below) Da Zhui (DU14) and the well points of the three yang channels (hands and feet) and then needle Feng Chi (GB20), Tian Zhu (UB10), Shou San Li (LI10), Zu San Li (ST36), Tai Chong (LV3), and He Gu (LI4). I would also add Lu Lu Tong, Ma Huang, and Gui Zhi, along with large doses of Huang Qin and Sheng Shi Gao to your main formula.

These therapeutic approaches will provide quick and effective relief for those drug-induced side effects.

Case Study #12: Immunotherapy (Biologic Therapy)

Q: Immunotherapy (biologic therapy) involves drawing blood from a patient, cultivating the immune system components (e.g., monoclonal antibodies, interferon, interleukin-2 (IL-2), several types of colony-stimulating factors (CSF, GM- CSF, G-CSF)), and then transfusing them back into the patient. Is this an effective treatment solution? Thanks for sharing your knowledge and advice!

A: For some patients this method can be very effective, but it does come with the risk of causing an allergic reaction, and in severe cases, cerebrovascular, CNS, cardiovascular, and peripheral nerve disorders.

Types of immunotherapy include monoclonal antibodies (e.g., Avastin, Erbitux, Herceptin), non-specific immunotherapies (e.g., interferons, interleukins), and cancer vaccines. Some Western medicine physicians will also concomitantly administer immunosuppressants (e.g., corticosteroids, Methotrexate, cyclosporine) as anticancer agents.

The key for TCM physicians is the same—focus on the signs, symptoms and pattern identification, which naturally involves assessing the blood work up and other lab test results.

II. AUTOIMMUNE DISEASES

Section 1: Rheumatoid Arthritis

Case Study #1: Five Approaches to Treating Rheumatoid Arthritis

Q: A 35 y/o female patient explained that 5 years ago she began feeling aches and soreness in joints all over her body, with the symptoms worse at night. Finally, it got to the point where she really couldn't stand it anymore and went to see a rheumatologist.

She was diagnosed with rheumatoid arthritis and immediately began taking medication to treat this condition. After 4 years of continuous administration, she doesn't feel that the treatment has been very effective overall, so she decided to try TCM treatment.

Right now, the patient's condition is as follows: mild symptoms of aching, red, and swollen joints during the daytime that increase in severity at nighttime, occasional indigestion and incontinence at nighttime, stringlike and fine pulse, and normal stool.

I prescribed Feng Shi Fang increasing the dose of Ma Huang to 3 qian. After two weeks of administration, the effects have not been noticeable. Please share your experiences and advice about treating this condition. Thank you!

A: In classical TCM pathologic terminology, rheumatoid arthritis (RA) correlates with wind-damp traveling influx (moving impediment) (**走注** zǒu zhù) or joint-running wind (**歷節風** lì jié f□ng). For the majority of cases, this pathocondition is not that difficult to effectively treat—it just takes some time!

Critical factors that will affect the outcome of treatment are the following:

1) Whether the patient is willing to accept the long-term TCM therapeutic regimen and encounter slight discomfort along the way.

2) Whether the patient has already been administered Western medicine RA drug treatment for a long duration.

It's been my experience that patients who do *not* receive Western medicine RA drugs, and instead solely receive TCM treatment, were more likely to show marked improvements in their symptoms and get this condition under control at the soonest in about 3 months. If the patient *has* been administered various types of potent anti-inflammatory and analgesic Western medicine pharmaceutical agents, then it will take at least 6 months before seeing effective results. For those who are very sensitive to pain and unwilling to accept a bit of discomfort, the therapeutic regimen will take longer for results to appear.

Five approaches I most often use in the treatment of RA:

1) Administer bleeding at the site of swollen and painful joints and also Da Zhui (DU14) (above, at, and below the acupoint); and needle He Gu (LI4), Feng Chi (GB20), Tian Zhu (UB10), Zu San Li (ST36), Yang Ling Quan (GB34), and Jue Gu (GB39).

2) For acute flare-ups presenting with severely swollen and painful joints that the patient finds unbearable, prescribe Huang Lian Jie Du Tang with Wu Ling San adding Ma Huang.

3) If the patient's RA condition has already entered the chronic stage, then prescribe (Yu Sheng) Hyperactive Immune Formula.

4) If the patient has been receiving TCM treatment for a long duration with effective results (no longer has red and swollen joints), the patient still must continue taking the formula for 2–3 more months until the aching and pain resolves to the point the patient only feels slight tightness during work or other activity.

At this point, you can change the formula to variants of Zhi Bo Di Huang Tang or Zuo Gui Yin, and administer it for about 2 weeks, assessing to make sure there is *no* joint swelling. If there is *not*, then gradually add incremental doses of The Three Great Yang-Supplementers.

5) If you are treating the patient during the initial flare-up *prior to* receiving treatment with Western medicine RA drugs, or if the patient has *never* received treatment with Western medicine RA drugs (which tend to mask the symptoms), then this condition can be identified as being in its "essential state" and is easier to treat.

In the absence of Western medicine RA drug intervention, advise the patient to perform lab tests on rheumatoid factor (RF), ESR, and C-reactive protein (CRP). If ESR and CRP levels are *elevated*, then the condition can be identified as yang hyperactivity pattern, requiring administration of heat-clearing toxin-resolving medicinals adding exterior effusion medicinals (e.g., Hyperactive Immune Formula adding Ge Gen and Ma Huang, or Ge Gen Tang adding The Three Yellows, Qing Hao, Zhi Mu, and Di Gu Pi). If ESR and CRP levels are *normal*, but rheumatoid factor (RF) *is* (+), then prescribe Ma Gui Wen Dan Tang or Gui Zhi Jia Ling Zhu Fu Tang adding Huang Qin and Shi Gao. This should resolve the patient's symptoms and effectively control the condition.

Case Study #2: Scan Image Reveals Joint Inflammation

Q: Six months ago, a 44 y/o female patient came to my clinic for an initial consultation, complaining of morning stiffness, tenderness, and swelling in the joints of every finger. I prescribed Huang Lian Jie Du Tang with Wu Ling San variant and her symptoms completely resolved. However, the patient was worried that she might have inherited "intractable" [her description!] rheumatoid arthritis (RA), since a relative of hers had been afflicted with RA for over 15 years without any improvement.

With this in mind, the next time she had an episode of joint stiffness, tenderness and swelling, she made an appointment with a rheumatologist, had a blood test, and performed an MRI. Results revealed hypointensity in the wrist joint and glenohumeral joint (sites where she had experienced tenderness and pain). Her doctors suspected RA and administered drug treatment, but after 3 months of treatment, the patient did *not* feel there was any noticeable improvement, so she returned for another TCM consultation.

I started her out with a Zhi Bo Di Huang Tang variant and 2 weeks later her joint pain resolved. She had a blood test performed with results showing RF, CRP, and ESR normal, but she hasn't had another MRI performed. I am still uncertain if she really has RA or not.

I think this patient may have avascular necrosis caused by insufficient blood supply to the joints, and not RA. Please offer your respected advice and opinion on this case. How would you treat this patient?

A: Strictly speaking, RA is not a hereditary condition, though there is a genetic presdisposition making certain people's immune systems more susceptible to external contraction (e.g., microbial infections). In TCM, RA can be identified as heat with mild exterior pattern, and it is a relatively easy pathocondition to remedy. If severe swelling and heat present, then add large doses of The Three Yellows, Qing Hao, Zhi Mu, and Di Gu Pi. Administer this formula until the symptoms resolve and both rheumatoid factor (RF) and ESR levels are normal. At this time, the patient can discontinue Western medicine RA drugs as well. Remember! For patients who have *never* been administered Western medicine RA drugs, effective results from TCM treatment will appear even faster!

The hypointensity appearing on the CT scan and MRI images is most likely a result of arthritic degeneration and *not* ischemic necrosis. You can look at it like "the sediment and mud that deposits between architectural structures following a severe flood." Don't worry about this "sediment," just continue prescribing the heat-clearing toxin-resolving and blood-quickening stasis-resolving medicinals (possibly adding yin-supplementing medicinals in some cases).

This approach will successfully prevent inflammation from recurring, while the body will naturally do the rest by gradually reabsorbing the metabolic waste ("sediment") from previous inflammatory episodes, putting the body back on the track of recovery.

Case Study #3: Differential Diagnosis – Periodic Paralysis, Subacute Combined Degeneration, Ankylosing Spondylitis, and Rheumatoid Arthritis

Q: A 24 y/o female patient came to my clinic complaining of left-sided hemilateral pain. In her childhood, she experienced severe abdominal pain on numerous occasions, and in high school, she experienced left ankle pain following a fever. Later in life, left-sided joint pain gradually developed in her upper limb, lower limb and jaw. At that time, lab test results showed rheumatoid factor (RF) 735, HLA-B27 (+), and low K+.

Despite being administered various Western medicine drugs, her condition has continued to deteriorate. Over the past several years, she has felt generalized weakness and lack of strength, especially in her legs. The patient has seen numerous TCM and Western medicine doctors, but no one has been able to diagnose her condition.

Do you think this could be rheumatoid arthritis (RA), periodic paralysis (PP), or subacute combined degeneration (SCG)? I want to prescribe Gui Qi Jian Zhong Tang with Chai Hu Jia Long Gu Mu Li Tang adding Yu Sheng Wan and Huo Luo Dan. Please offer your perspectives and advice on this perplexing case. Thank you!

A: Ah! The presentations and treatment approaches of these conditions are all significantly different. These conditions are clearly distinguishable based on evaluation of lab tests, diagnostic tools, and clinical presentation.

RA can typically be identified as yang hyperactivity, exterior-interior triple burner repletion heat with exterior, and steaming bone heat pattern. For the treatment of this condition, you can prescribe Hyperactive Immune Formula (including large doses of The Three Yellows, Qing Hao, Zhi Mu, and Di Gu Pi) adding Mu Dan Pi, Shan Zhu Yu, and Ma Huang. This formula should be administered continuously up until the ESR, CRP, and RF levels test (-). At that time, you can advise the patient to gradually reduce and eventually discontinue Western medicine drugs altogether.

A definitive diagnosis of PP is contingent upon blood test results showing *normal* levels of K, T3, and T4, with TSH levels either *elevated* or *decreased.* If the patient tests HLA-B27 (+), then this strongly suggests ankylosing spondylitis (AS). For AS patients whose condition has progressed to the stage of vertebrae fusions (aka "bamboo spine") and hunchback, then you can consider prescribing a formula such as Shi Quan Da Bu Tang or You Gui Yin adding Ma Huang, Du Zhong, Niu Xi, Di Long, Gan Jiang, and Rou Gui. Long-term administration of this formula will prevent further deterioration and gradually improve the patient's condition.

During the administration of TCM medicinals, all of the key blood test levels will be *elevated.* Don't worry about this! Just continue administering the formula. The patient's agonizing symptoms of stiffness, aching, and pain in the torso, shoulders, upper back, and lumbar region will quickly be relieved and strength and flexibility improved. At this time, it's fine if the patient wants to continue taking Western medicine drugs (e.g., NSAIDs, TNF, corticosteroids, interferon, Methotrexate). Of course, the optimal scenario is for the patient to gradually reduce the drug dosage until complete discontinuation is achieved, though this process will take a long period of time.

If *increased* ESR, RF, and HLA-B27 levels persist after administering yang-supplementing medicinals for a period of time, then this can be identified as true heat pattern, requiring the addition of large doses of Huang Qin (or Huang Lian) and Huang Bo to the main formula above, or changing the formula to (Yu Sheng) Hyperactive Immune Formula adding Ma Huang, Gui Zhi, Niu Xi, and Sheng Du Zhong.

If the patient has *not* been administered Methotrexate, and increased ESR, RF, and HLA-B27 levels persist, then this can be identified as exterior-interior triple burner repletion heat with exterior wind heat pattern. For this pattern, you should consider prescribring a formula such as (Yu Sheng) Hyperactive Immune Formula, Huang Lian Jie Du Tang, or Ge Gen Qin Lian Tang adding Ma Huang (or Ge Gen), Qing Hao, Zhi Mu, Di Gu Pi, Du Zhong, Niu Xi, Huo Luo Dan, and in some cases Wan Ling Dan. Administer this formula up until the blood test results are normal.

If K and T4 levels are *low*, then you must supplement yang, qi, and blood; conversely, if K and T4 levels are *high*, then you must prescribe heavy settling and heat-abating medicinals; and if K and T4 levels are normal, then you must carefully consider the possibility of damp heat, qi vacuity, or dryness pattern, adjusting your formula accordingly. For instance, if damp heat pattern presents, then prescribe a formula such as Er Miao San, San Miao Wan, Si Miao Wan, or Jia Wei Er Miao San; and if dry pattern presents, then prescribe a formula such as Qing Zao Jiu Fei Tang, Bai He Gu Jin Tang, or Ba Xian Chang Shou Wan.

SCD is a rare disorder of the spine, brain, and nerves, which is caused by vitamin B12 deficiency. Symptoms involve weakness, abnormal sensations, cognitive dysfunction, and vision difficulties. For details about this disorder you can reference *Neuropathy: Traditional Chinese Herbal Treatment in a Modern Medical Environment* (中西醫結合中醫腦神經治療學) pp. 620–625. My personal approach is to prescribe Gui Qi Jian Zhong Tang, Shi Quan Da Bu Tang, or You Gui Yin adding Huang Qi, Ma Huang, and Di Long. Or, for certain cases, you can prescribe Blood Desiccation Formula with Si Ni Tang adding Huang Bo (or Huang Qin) and Huang Qi. From a dietary perspective, advise the patient to eat plenty of liver and garlic and supplement with B-complex vitamins. Also, Dang Gui contains an abundance of B-complex vitamins, including B12, vitamin A, and vitamin E among other nutrients.

Case Study #4: Ankylosing Spondylitis

Q: A 34 y/o female patient began experiencing lower back pain in her teens, but subsequent medical tests and examinations were unable to pinpoint a cause. After her second child was born, the pain became even more severe. Two years ago, she went for another evaluation and was diagnosed with ankylosing spondylitis (AS). She does *not* take regular medication for this condition, but when symptoms become unbearable, she *does* occasionally take corticosteroids.

Two months ago, she once again began experiencing left-sided lower limb and finger numbness, right-sided neck pain, and lower back pain. The last time she took corticosteroids she was initially reluctant because it made her gain weight, but the pain was too much to endure, so she went ahead with the treatment. However, this time it wasn't nearly as effective at relieving her pain, so she decided to seek TCM treatment. Do you have any suggestions or advice about treating AS?

A: That sounds like the typical history and presentation of an AS patient. In recent years, this condition has become much more prevalent in Taiwan. A key determinant for pattern identification and treatment of this condition is whether HLA-B27 is positive (+) or negative (-).

If HLA-B27 is (-) and the patient complains of soreness and backache after sleeping in cold weather or even air conditioning, then the condition could simply be identified as cold impediment of the urinary bladder channel. If HLA-B27 is (-), but the history and presentation of symptoms and elevation of inflammatory markers suggest AS, then Western medical doctors will typically administer corticosteroids, Methotrexate (a disease-modifying antirheumatic drug), quinine, or potent analgesics.

If HLA-B27 is (-) and *no* other inflammatory markers are elevated, simply prescribe You Gui Yin variant, administer acupuncture (warm needling), and advise the patient to get enough sleep (at least 8–10 hours per day), dress warmly, and exercise regularly (e.g., swimming, walking). Also, tell the patient to eat sensibly (no dietary restrictions) and lead a normal sex life (just don't overindulge!). If the patient also presents with tearing on exposure to wind, then add large doses of Ma Huang and Bai Zhi. Continue long-term administration of TCM medicinals and acupuncture, and when the pain subsides the patient may gradually discontinue the use of corticosteriods.

If the vertebral joints feel hot and swollen upon palpation, the patient has night sweats, HLA-B27 (+), and CRP, ESR, and RF are all *elevated*, then this condition can be identified as yang hyperactivity pattern, indicating that the immune system is in the midst of a hyperactive episode, overreacting and "attacking" the vertebral joints. For this condition, you can prescribe formula variants such as Hyperactive Immune Formula, Huang Lian Jie Du Tang, Ge Gen Qin Lian Tang, Da Qing Long Tang, or Yang Dan Tang. Just make sure your formula includes Sheng Du Zhong, Niu Xi, Ma Huang (or Ge Gen), Qing Hao, Zhi Mu, Di Gu Pi, Mu Dan Pi, and Chi Shao. You can also bleed Da Zhui (DU14) (above, at, and below) and administer acupuncture on the acupoints Feng Chi (GB20), Tian Zhu (UB10), Wei Zhong (UB40), Hou Xi (SI3), and Guan Yuan Shu (UB26).

If HLA-B27 is (+) and chronic symptoms have aleady set in, then the condition can be identified as cold impediment of the urinary bladder channel with exterior pattern. In these patients, stiffness of the spine extends all the way up to C1 and C2; and in severe cases fusion ("bamboo spine"), dislocation, and fracture will occur, resulting in upper limb weakness, limp paralysis, limp wilting back and legs, and hunchback. Pain in the sternum and ribs can become so unbearable that it may cause breathing difficulties. This condition can be identified as cold strike with exterior and qi vacuity pattern for which you can prescribe a formula such as Shi Quan Da Bu Tang, You Gui Yin, Du Huo Ji Sheng Tang, or San Bi Tang, making sure to include Ma Huang, Di Long, Lu Jiao, The Three Great Yang-Supplementers, and Huo Luo Dan. Also, perform acupuncture (warm needling) on acupoints such as Feng Chi (GB20), Hua Tuo Jia Ji Xue (EX-B2), Shen Shu (UB23), Guan Yuan Shu (UB26), Huan Tiao (GB30), Ba Liao (UB31–34), Yang Ling Quan (GB34), and Jue Gu (GB39).

Case Study #5: Zygomatic Bone Swelling – Don't Prescribe Feng Shi Fang

Q: A 28 y/o male patient was diagnosed with rheumatoid arthritis (RA) at the age of 13. Over the past two years, he has felt aches and pain in the muscles of his entire body. Western medical doctors diagnosed him with polymyalgia rheumatica, and he has been on medication to control this condition since then.

Three months ago, the right side of his face below the zygomatic (cheek) bone suddenly swelled up. His doctors recommended surgery, but the patient was concerned his face may become disfigured, so he came to me seeking TCM treatment instead. I prescribed Huang Lian Jie Du Tang adding Qing Hao, Zhi Mu, Di Gu Pi, Mu Li, and Tao Ren. Please offer your invaluable advice on this case.

A: RA can be identified as hyperactivity yang pattern. Unless the patient has been (or is currently being) administered corticosteroids or high dosages of Methotrexate (both have immunosuppressive effects), then do *not* prescribe Feng Shi Fang. The reason is that it derives from Huang Lian Jie Du Tang and thus contains Zhi Zi. Long-term administration of Zhi Zi will tint the skin of some people a greenish color, especially the face and torso.

A student of mine, Dr. Cheng, Shu-mei (鄭淑鎂) first discovered this phenomenon during clinical treatment and research. She observed that patients with overactive immune systems (e.g., Sjogren's, rheumatoid arthritis) had heightened pigment absorption sensitivity. When these patients were adminstered TCM formulas containing Zhi Zi, their skin gradually acquired a noticeable greenish tint. However, quite the opposite, when TCM formulas containing Zhi Zi are administered for hepatitis patients (e.g., hyperbilirubinemia) their jaundice (yellowish skin coloration) is effectively abated.

This greenish skin discoloration can be reversed by simply discontinuing use of the Zhi Zi containing formula for a period of time, or subtracting Zhi Zi from the formula altogether. For your patient, I would stay on the safe side; you don't want to give him any more challenges to overcome. Prescribe Huang Lian Jie Du Tang (subtracting Zhi Zi) adding Qing Hao, Zhi Mu, and Di Gu Pi. This is essentially the composition of a signature formula that I have recently designed called (Yu Sheng) Hyperactive Immune Formula, offering excellent efficacy without the potential for "unsightly" side effects.

For those patients who *have* been administered corticosteroids without effectiveness, I have had great results prescribing Zhi Bo Di Huang Tang adding Ma Huang, Sheng Shi Gao, and Wan Ling Dan, which will keep RF, ESR, and CRP in check. Once ESR and CRP return to normal levels, even though RF may still be elevated, you can advise the patient to gradually reduce the dosage of analgesics, antiinflammatories, Methotrexate, and corticosteroids. If the patient incurs a mild relapse along the way, then simply add large doses of The Three Yellows; and bleed Da Zhui (DU14) (above, at, and below) and the well points of the corresponding channels presenting with pain or discomfort.

Section 2: Systemic Lupus Erythematosus (SLE)

Case Study #1: Three Keys to Treating SLE

Q: This 22 y/o female is my first systemic lupus erythematosus (SLE) patient. Two months ago, a butterfly rash appeared on her face, along with generalized joint pain. Lab tests showed RF 120 (0-20 u/ml). Currently, she is taking prednisolone (2 pills/day).

What is the best approach for treating SLE? How long will it take before the symptoms (e.g., joints, skin) start to improve?

A: According to the Western medical perspective, SLE is an autoimmune disease similar to rheumatoid arthritis (RA). Determining a diagnosis requires performing basic tests on ANA, C3 and C4, and RF levels. If SLE has been accurately diagnosed, the TCM treatment approach involves long-term administration of TCM medicinals, healthy lifestyle and nutritional intake, and making sure the body is warm (e.g., thermal underwear, ambient heating).

In my clinical experience, administration of approximately 185 packets (the fastest 75 packets and the slowest 615 packets) will effectively remedy this condition to the point where the patient can discontinue use of Western medicine drugs. Administration of approximately 320 packets (the fastest 82 packets and the slowest 795 packets) will effectively cure this condition to the point where the patient can discontinue use of TCM medicinals. The patient will be able to lead a normal life without having to take drugs or medicinals.

It is commonly known that the long-term administration of Western medicine drugs (mainly corticosteroids) in the treatment of SLE can lead to ischemic necrosis of the joints, retinal detachment, Raynaud syndrome, nerve atrophy, and renal failure. Based on my clinical experience, TCM effectively treats SLE and its complications. It just takes some time and a lot of patience!

These are the three formulas I most commonly administer for the treatment of SLE patients:

1) Xiang Sha Liu Jun Zi Tang adding The Three Great Yang-Supplementers, Huang Qin, Huang Qi, Tu Si Zi, and Ren Shen/Chuan Qi Powder.

2) You Gui Yin adding large doses of Gan Jiang, Rou Gui, Ren Shen/Chuan Qi Powder, and Huang Qi.

3) If autoimmune hemolytic anemia presents, then subtract Chuan Qi and add Zhu Qi and Xi Lu Rong (powder); or change the formula to Sheng Yu Tang adding Gan Jiang, Fu Zi, Huang Qin, Tu Si Zi, Ren Shen, Xi Lu Rong (powder), and Zhu Qi.

Remember! Make sure to add stomach-opening (appetite promoting) medicinals, Yu Sheng Wan, and also Huo Luo Dan to remedy pain. If uremia presents, then add large doses of Fu Ling, Ze Xie, and Ting Li Zi. If pleural, pericardial, or mediastinal effusion presents, then change the formula to Wu Ling San (Nephritis Formula) (including large doses of Fu Ling and Ze Xie) adding large doses of Ting Li Zi and Fang Ji along with Ren Shen/Chuan Qi Powder. If anemia presents, then add Xi Lu Rong (powder). Administer this formula up until the C3/C4 levels return to 100/15—that's when you can begin discontinuing administration of prednisolone.

During cold weather months, the patient may feel discomfort in the fingers (Raynaud phenomenon). Raynaud phenomenon requires the administration of Wu Zhu Yu Tang, but this formula is very bitter, pungent, and spicy, and some patients cannot tolerate the flavor. This is why I have Wu Zhu Yu Tang processed into pills, so the patient can simply add it into a decocted TCM formula, thus ameliorating the unpalatable flavor. South Koreans generally like to eat spicy foods and drink alcoholic beverages, so during cold weather months, decocted Wu Zhu Yu Tang would probably provide a palatable solution!

Note: One packet denotes a single prescription of decocting pieces, which are decocted into 600 ml of decoction and taken orally typically 3 times per day in 200 ml dosages.

Case Study #2: SLE – Mediastinal Effusion Indicates Chronic Renal and Brain Damage Stage

Q: A 38 y/o female patient of mine has been living with systemic lupus erythematosus (SLE) for many years. After being diagnosed 10 years ago, she received inpatient care at a hospital for 3 months until her condition stabilized, and then was administered 20 mg of predinsolone daily to keep the disease in check.

Five years ago, she experienced a sudden onset of palpitations along with swollen extremities, right-sided jugular veinous distention, shortness of breath, and dry cough. Examination results revealed costal and pericardial effusion for which she was administered high dose intravenous corticosteroid therapy daily on an outpatient basis, along with oral diuretics.

The patient's relatives couldn't stand seeing her in this condition and came to me wondering if TCM treatment could get her back to normal.

A: When SLE presents with pleural effusion it usually indicates the disease has already entered the renal (e.g., interstitial nephritis, nephrotic syndrome, membranous GN, renal failure) and brain (e.g., CNS, behavioral, memory) damage stage. At this time, you must keep an eye out for elevated BUN/Cr levels, cerebrovascular disease, and CNS disorders.

My treatment approach is to prescribe a qi-boosting spleen-fortifying and qi-moving phlegm-transforming formula such as Xiang Sha Liu Jun Zi Tang or Ban Xia Tian Ma Bai Zhu San, making sure to include large doses of Fu Ling, Ze Xie, Ting Li Zi, and Fang Ji. And if uremia presents, then add Ding Shu Xiu and Ren Dong Teng, along with Tu Si Zi, Huang Qi, The Three Great Yang-Supplementers, Ren Shen/Chuan Qi Powder, Xi Lu Rong (powder), Da Huang, and Ma Huang.

Remember! For Da Huang, add incremental doses of 5 fen up until the patient maintains 2–3 stools/day; and for Ma Huang, I typically add a maximum dose of 3 qian, but in cold climates like South Korea, you may need to add more.

Case Study #3: SLE – Acupuncture and TCM Medicinals

Q: A 33 y/o female SLE patient has decreased C3/C4 levels. Since receiving a definitive diagnosis, she has been taking prednisolone and quinine to control her condition (3 pills (5mg)/day). Despite this treatment, her condition has been getting worse, and now she wants to try TCM treatment. Her symptoms are as follows: cold, painful knees, and since she stopped taking her Western medicine drugs, the generalized joint pain worsens during menses, but she does *not* have swelling.

While administering acupuncture treatment, it was difficult inserting the needles into Xi Yan (EX-LE5) and Du Bi (ST35); it felt like something was blocking the way. Could this be synovial adhesion? I prescribed (Yu Sheng) Hyperactive Immune Formula adding Gan Jiang, Fu Zi (Tian Xiong), and Rou Gui (starting out with small doses and incrementally increasing). Do you think this is the right approach?

A: Once an SLE patient is administered prednisolone, the condition can be identified as either yang vacuity pattern or true cold false heat pattern; and at this time, the patient can discontinue administration of quinine, but not prednisolone.

First, prescribe kidney yang-supplementing medicinals to dispel cold stasis and cold-damp, along with swelling-dispersing, heat-abating, and dampness-disinhibiting medicinals. Then, advise the patient to try discontinuing prednisolone. If after a period of 1–2 weeks, the patient does *not* present with any significant discomfort, then continue this approach of administering only TCM medicinals.

Remember! As a general rule, I would *not* needle directly into the joints of SLE patients, because it could result in rupture of a synovial cyst or cause infection. Depending on the presenting signs, symptoms and pattern, for this type of joint pain and swelling, I would typically prescribe large doses of The Three Yellows and The Four Lings; Qing Hao, Zhi Mu, and Di Gu Pi; and if necessary, small doses of The Three Great Yang-Supplementers.

However, based on your description of this patient, she has decreased C3/C4 and Hb levels. Thus, you should *not* increase the dose of The Three Yellows and The Four Lings for this patient; instead, simply add larger doses of The Three Great Yang-Supplementers and a small dose of Ma Huang.

Case Study #4: SLE and Idiopathic Thrombocytopenic Purpura

Q: A 22 y/o female SLE patient experienced malaise and went to the hospital for an examination. Results of lab tests revealed a PLT count of only 30,000 and her doctors diagnosed her with idiopathic thrombocytopenic purpura (ITP).

Three months later, she suffered from enteritis and diarrhea and her PLT count continued to spiral downward, prompting admission to the hospital for treatment. Despite being administered intravenous immunoglobulin (IVIG) and intravenous corticosteroids, her PLT continued falling down to 5,000 before her diarrhea symptoms began showing improvement.

The patient has been in the hospital for 3 weeks now, receiving PLT infusions 2x/day, but her body has been disposing of the PLTs as fast as they can be administered, making the treatment ultimately ineffective. She has been plagued by a persistent cough, nausea, and fever, and it looks like she may be about to pass away. Please offer your guidance and advice on the best approach for this patient going forward.

A: SLE patients are susceptible to hemolytic disorders. The presence of severely low PLT count (thrombocytopenia) resulting from immune system malfunctions and causing the body to errantly destroy platelets is called idiopathic thrombocytopenic purpura (ITP).

As for TCM medicinal treatment, you can consider prescribing Sheng Yu Tang variant. If the patient has been administered corticosteroids, then this pathocondition requires the prescription of medicinals that treat either spleen yang vacuity with cold stasis pattern (e.g., Xiang Sha Liu Jun Zi Tang) or kidney yang vacuity with cold stasis pattern (e.g., You Gui Yin). At this time, advise the patient to reduce the dose of corticosteroids (do *not* completely discontinue administration!) and as the PLT count returns to normal levels, then gradually reduce the corticosteroid dose further until it is eventually discontinued. If after discontinuing corticosteroids, the PLT count again gradually decreases, then simply prescribe Sheng Yu Tang variant to bring the PLT back up and maintain normal levels.

During the onset of idiopathic thrombocytopenic purpura (ITP), when the immune system is attacking renegade antibodies that have attached to platelets throughout the entire body, or during the acute heat stage of external contraction (i.e., microbial infection), you can add yin-enriching fire-downbearing and vacuity heat-clearing steaming bone-eliminating medicinals (e.g., Qing Hao, Zhi Mu, and Di Gu Pi) and blood-cooling heat-clearing and blood-quickening stasis-dispersing medicinals (e.g., Mu Dan Pi and Chi Shao). However, if the pathocondition evolves into the chronic stage, you must stop administering these medicinals, because they should only be prescribed for pathoconditions presenting with Shao Yang heat, steaming bone, taxation heat, late afternoon tidal heat (fever), night sweats, or meningitis.

Case Study #5: Rheumatoid Arthritis and Systemic Lupus Erythematosus

Q: I have a 34 y/o female patient diagnosed with rheumatoid arthritis (RA) and systemic lupus erythematosus (SLE). Her chief complaint is generalized aches and redness, heat, and swelling of both deltoid muscles (near Bi Nao (LI14)). Her lab results were as follows:

RF 28 (0–20 u/ml), C3 54 (80–160 mg/dL), C4 9 (16–48 mg/dL), and WBC normal.

What are the distinguishing diagnostic features of these two conditions and should different treatment approaches be applied?

A: First of all, they are both autoimmune diseases, and you can assess blood tests to make a diagnostic distinction between RA and SLE. A distinguishing diagnostic feature of SLE patients is low complement C3 and C4 levels, whereas the rheumatoid factor (RF) level *may* or may *not* be high, and if high, it will *not* be as high as in RA patients.

Also, in SLE patients, ANA and anti-dsDNA will be positive; CRP and ESR levels may be normal, high or low; and LDH and CPK levels may be high. In RA patients, during the initial onset and flare-ups, ESR and CRP will be increased, and only when the disease has spread to the heart and vasculature wall changes in PT and APTT occur. For details about these autoimmune diseases and more, you can reference *Harrison's Principles of Internal Medicine.*

If you determine that the diagnosis of SLE is indeed correct, and the patient has *not* taken corticosteroids or Methotrexate, then prescribe (Yu Sheng) Hyperactive Immune Formula (including large doses of at least 8 qian for each medicinal); and if joint swelling and pain present, then add Ma Huang (and/or Ge Gen). The redness, heat, and swelling near Bi Nao (LI14) sounds like it might be vasculitis, and if so, then add Chuan Qi and Dan Shen, which will gradually resolve the inflammation.

Remember! Any type of massage or manipulation, and even local bleeding is *contraindicated* for this pathocondition; and if you do decide to bleed, then bleed the well points of the fingers.

Section 3: Idiopathic Thrombocytopenic Purpura

Case Study #1: It's Probably Purpura!

Q: A 26 y/o female patient explained that "her face broke out into a pimply mess" (which was actually seborrheic dermatitis), so she decocted some San Bai Cao (*Saururus chinensis* (Lour.) Baill., Asian lizard's tail) at her own discretion. Not long after taking this decoction, she experienced hematuria and bleeding gums, prompting her to get examined at a hospital. The doctors diagnosed idiopathic thrombocytopenic purpura (ITP) and simply prescribed corticosteroids to maintain a stable PLT count.

Eight months passed without elevation of the PLT count. Her doctors thought the condition was severe enough to warrant splenectomy, but the patient didn't want to have this done and instead continued corticosteroid administration. Follow-up examination 1 year later showed a PLT count of about 5,000. The patient has occasionally experienced bleeding gums, hematuria, nosebleeds (epistaxis), and excessive bruising (purpura) on the medial side of the elbow joint.

I prescribed Xiang Sha Liu Jun Zi Tang adding Gan Jiang, Fu Zi, Rou Gui, Huang Qin, Zhi Zi, and Han Lian Cao. Please share your views and advice about this case. Do you think San Bai Cao could cause idiopathic thrombocytopenia purpura (ITP)?

A: No, I do *not* think San Bai Cao had anything to do with your patient's condition. San Bai Cao is a heat-clearing toxin-resolving and bone- and sinew-consolidating medicinal. The only scenario I could imagine this medicinal having any possibility of inhibiting PLT production is if the patient took enormous doses (up to 500g–1,000g of the dried raw herb) over a long period of time. Based on your description of the patient's symptoms, it clearly indicates she has purpura.

A characteristic feature of purpura is spontaneous external bleeding, which involves mild spontaneous bleeding from the gums, nasal cavity, skin, etc. In Western medicine, this condition is classifed as resulting from either low platelet count (thrombocytopenic purpura), which is more commonly seen in young women, or normal platelet count (nonthrombocytopenic purpura), which is more commonly seen in the elderly with fragile blood vessels (senile purpura).

As for TCM treatment, I would prescribe (Yu Sheng) Sheng Yu Tang adding The Three Great Yang-Supplementers, Huang Qin, Ren Shen, Niu Xi, Xi Lu Rong (powder), and Zhu Jie Qi. For Xi Lu Rong and Zhu Jie Qi, start out with 1 qian and gradually increase the dose, and since Zhu Jie Qi tends to cause diarrhea add Cang Zhu and Ze Xie to counteract this potential side effect. Remember! You should *not* prescribe Chuan Qi (anticoagulant action) for this condition, but Han Lian Cao is fine.

If the patient is being administered Western medicine drugs, such as Methotrexate and corticosteroids, once the patient begins taking the TCM formula you can advise her to first discontinue Methotrexate. And when PLT levels increase up to the 10,000–20,000 level, then advise her to gradually discontinue corticosteroids.

Case Study #2: What Is Idiopathic Thrombocytopenic Purpura?

Q: It seems that the prevalence of idiopathic thrombocytopenic purpura (ITP) is increasing, especially among children. Incidences of ITP cases are being reported all over the Internet, but the only available Western medical treatment is intravenous immunoglobulin (IVIG) or IV Rho immunoglobulin (RhIG), corticosteroids, other immunosuppresants, and vitamin supplements. A lot of parents have been contacting me for advice and consultation wondering if TCM could provide effective treatment.

Please share your experiences in treating ITP. Why are increased incidences of this disease occurring? What types of patterns does this condition manifest? Aside from blood stasis type patterns that require (Yu Sheng) Sheng Yu Tang for treatment, are there any yang vacuity type patterns that I should be aware of? What is the best treatment approach?

A: Idiopathic thrombocytopenic purpura (ITP) is also known as immune thrombocytopenic purpura or simply purpura. This condition manifests when the immune system errantly manufactures antibodies that attack and destroy platelets. This decrease in PLT (blood platelet) count and/or the inability of PLT to return to functionally adequate levels produces the classic array of thrombocytopenic symptoms (e.g., easy bruising, bleeding gums, nosebleeds (epistaxis), petechiae, hematuria, tarry stools (melena)).

Western medicine classifies this pathocondition into two types: primary ITP—triggered by a viral infection that causes an autoimmune reaction; and secondary ITP—associated with the presence of another chronic disease or viral infection such as lymphoma, leukemia, SLE, RA, HIV, and hepatitis C virus (HCV) that causes an autoimmune reaction. It is a rather common disorder with the prevalence much higher in children (e.g., mumps, measles, respiratory infection) and in women (e.g., develops gradually, incidental finding).

Typically, Western medicine treatment will begin before the platelet count drops down to a lower limit threshold of 20,000–30,000/mm3 (normal range > 150,000/mm3), because that is when the chances for spontaneous bleeding increases. You mentioned the Western medicine first-line treatment already, and for cases of refractory thrombocytopenia and severe bleeding, the second-line treatment is splenectomy.

As for TCM treatment, yes, based on my experience Sheng Yu Tang adding The Three Great Yang-Supplementers, Huang Qin, Ren Shen, Zhu Qi, Xi Lu Rong (powder), and Tu Si Zi provides the best therapeutic efficacy.

Thrombocytopenic patients may develop splenomegaly caused by increased destruction and sequestration of platelets, which can also result in severe hepatosplenomegaly. This is very difficult to treat, which is why some Western medical doctors will then recommend splenectomy. In TCM, hepatosplenomegaly can be identified as heart and spleen qi and blood vacuity with heat pattern or spleen failing to control the blood with heat pattern, requiring administration of a qi- and blood-supplementing and boosting and spleen-fortifying heart-nourishing formula variant such as Gui Pi Tang or Jia Wei Gui Pi Tang.

On the general topic of thrombocytopenia, here are some additional thoughts and clinical experiences. The high living standards and medical advancements of modern civilization have made it possible to control or cure many previously intractable diseases with drugs. However, many of these "wonder drugs" also happen to be toxins that may harm the body if administered in high doses or over long periods of time. One such complication is damage to platelets that causes drug-induced hemolysis. Chemotherapeutic agents that kill cancer cells (and healthy cells too!) wreak the most havoc, followed by analgesics (e.g., NSAIDS, anti-inflammatories, quinine, aspirin, acetaminophen, anticonvulsants). Of course, prolonged and serious illnesses such as cancer, severe hemorrhage, malaria, or hemolytic liver diseases (e.g., cirrhosis, hepatic carcinoma, fulminant hepatitis) and excessive weight loss or a long-term strict vegan diet that results in malnutrition and bone marrow suppression will also lead to thrombocytopenia. Severe cases of dengue fever (i.e., dengue hemorrhagic fever), which more likely occur upon contraction a second time, can also cause severe thrombocytic purpura.

The following are TCM therapeutic approaches for conditions associated with the manifestation of thrombocytopenia from varying etiologies:

1. Chronic exposure to malaria may lead to hepatosplenomegaly. The classical TCM pathologic term for this disease is mother-of-malaria (瘧母 nüè mǔ). In the early stage, prescribe a formula variant such as Xiao Chai Hu Tang, Chai Hu Gui Zhi Tang, or Chang Shan Wan; and for interupt malaria (截瘧 jié nüè) prescribe large doses of vacuity heat-clearing, summerheat clearing, and malaria-treating medicinals (e.g., Qing Hao).

2. Insufficient production of thrombopoietin by the kidneys, long-term administration of chemotherapeutic agents, losing excessive weight (e.g., anorexia, cachexia), or long-term strict vegan diet resulting in malnutrition and bone marrow suppression can all be identified as kidney yang vacuity pattern. For treating this condition, you can prescribe either You Gui Yin, Shen Qi Wan, Shi Quan Da Bu Tang, or Ren Shen Yang Rong Tang, making sure to include Ren Shen, Xi Lu Rong (powder), Zhu Qi, The Three Great Yang-Supplementers, and Huang Bo.

3. Insufficient production of thrombopoietin by the liver can be identified as liver blood vacuity pattern. For treating this condition, you can prescribe (Yu Sheng) Sheng Yu Tang adding The Three Great Yang-Supplementers, Ren Shen, Zhu Qi, Xi Lu Rong (powder), and Huang Qin (or Huang Bo).

4. Dengue hemorrhagic fever can be identified as exterior blood heat pattern. For treating this pathocondition, you can prescribe formula variants such as Di Gu Pi Yin, Xiao Chai Hu Tang, or Yin Qiao San adding Qing Hao, Zhi Mu, Di Gu Pi, Yin Hua, Lian Qiao, Ou Jie, and Ce Bo Ye. Or, possibly consider adding combinations of medicinals such as Mu Dan Pi, Zhi Zi, Shi Shang Bo (aka Selaginella, Herba Selaginellae Doederleinii), Ji Xue Teng, and Luo Shi Teng.

5. The most difficult of these pathoconditions to treat are the hemolytic type that present in cirrhosis, hepatic carcinoma, and fulminant hepatitis. Treatment of acute hepatitis is less demanding

and easier to control and stablize. Patients with cirrhosis must be administered TCM medicinals for a long duration before the condition resolves, and then continue taking medicinals for at least another 6 months to 1 year to ensure the condition remains stabilized and completely cured. Hepatocellular carcinoma (HCC) requires long-term administration of TCM medicinals and follow-up evaluation.

6. For patients with drug-induced hemolytic pathoconditions (e.g., thrombotic thrombocytopenic purpura (TTP), hemolytic uremic syndrome (HUS)), you can prescribe a formula variant such as (Yu Sheng) Sheng Yu Tang or You Gui Yin. For patients with leukemia, renal cancer, and myeloma in the acute stage, you should prescribe formula variants such as Tong Jing Fang adding Huang Bo, Qing Hao, Zhi Mu, and Di Gu Pi; or Zhi Bo Di Huang Tang variant. And in the chronic stage, you should prescribe a formula variant such as Zhi Bo Di Huang Tang, Dang Gui Liu Huang Tang, or Zuo Gui Yin. For patients presenting with thrombocytopenia resulting from repeated administration of radiotherapy and chemotherapy, if immature cells are *not* found in the blood and abnormal cells are *not* found in bone marrow aspiration, then prescribe a You Gui Yin variant.

Case Study #3: Gong Zhen Dan – It's Not Sheng Yu Tang!

Q: I have an idiopathic thrombocytopenic purpura (ITP) patient with the following history:

The patient originally presented with PLT 7,000/mm3 (normal range > 150,000/mm3). After taking the TCM formula Gong Zhen Dan, which the patient took on his own discretion, it increased to 27,000. Then, 2 weeks later, PLT fell to 5,000, and the patient took more Gong Zhen Dan; after another 2 weeks, the PLT jumped back up to 65,000 and 87,000; and just as before, 2 weeks later, PLT dropped back down to 5,000 again.

This patient has an inexorable superstition about the "elixir" Gong Zhen Dan. I have told the patient over and over again that Gong Zhen Dan will only provide "ephemeral" efficacy, but he just doesn't believe me. As you advised, the last time the patient visited I prescribed (Yu Sheng) Sheng Yu Tang adding The Three Great Yang-Supplementers, Ren Shen, and Xi Lu Rong (powder). Do you have any further advice on this patient?

A: Unfortunately, for this type of obstinant patient, sometimes the only "medicine" that seems to work is having the patient find out for themselves what can happen when they do not listen to the doctor's advice. Why would the PLT go up and down like a roller coaster ride? Gong Zhen Dan contains Xi Lu Rong (powder), Dang Gui, Shan Zhu Yu, and She Xiang, which all promote an increase in hematopoietic function. However, once corticosteroids are discontinued, then PLT levels will gradually fall back down again. Also, the dose of each medicinal is small, with the effects relatively slow to appear; and nowadays She Xiang is usually synthetically manufactured, which has reduced its efficacy in the treatment of hematological disorders.

In the past, many TCM doctors have advocated prescribing Shi Quan Da Bu Tang, You Gui Yin, or Xiang Sha Liu Jun Zi Tang adding The Three Great Yang-Supplementers, Huang Qin, Ren Shen, Xi Lu Rong (powder), Tu Si Zi, Huang Qi, and Zhu Qi. I have tried some of these approaches, but none has provided the effectiveness of (Yu Sheng) Sheng Yu Tang. One of my patients has gone into a "permanent" remission using this formula, going nearly 20 years now without a relapse.

Despite the patient's obstinance, my advice is to try again, firmly iterating your case and assuring him that Sheng Yu Tang variant provides the best treatment for quick and sustained results. For even faster results, try adding wine-soaked Zhu Qi (1 qian/day). Remember! For Xi Lu Rong (powder), start at 1 qian and gradually increase the dose (not too quickly!). First, wait for the PLT to increase up until it plateaus; once the PLT remains at that plateaued level for about 3–5 weeks without rising, then you can begin adding large doses of The Three Great Yang-Supplementers. If at that point PLT levels do not rise, then you can gradually add 5 fen incremental doses of Xi Lu Rong (powder). These small incremental increases will alleviate the potential for loose stools and overstimulation causing insomnia.

Case Study #4: Sheng Yu Tang – It's the Best!

Q: I have a patient who was diagnosed with idiopathic thrombocytopenic purpura (ITP). Both the patient and the family members are very concerned and want to know specifics about the integrative TCM and Western medicine treatment approach, asking me questions such as: What Western medicine drugs should I take? When is the best time to discontinue taking the drug(s)? What is the plan if the PLT count falls again and the condition worsens? What is the role of TCM treatment if splenectomy is performed? I am curious myself about just this medicinal Zhu Jie Qi is anyways? If I don't have access to Zhu Jie Qi, can I use Han Lian Cao instead?

A: Normally, all you need to do for positive results is prescribe (Yu Sheng) Sheng Yu Tang adding The Three Great Yang-Supplementers, Huang Qin, Ren Shen, Zhu Qi, Xi Lu Rong (powder), and Tu Si Zi. If the patient *has* been administered corticosteroids or testosterone and *has* had blood transfusions, then the above formula will increase PLT up to around 200,000 within 1–3 weeks; and after 2–3 more weeks of administering this formula, then you should advise the patient to begin gradually reducing the doses of Western medicine drugs.

If these drugs are discontinued too quickly, then the TCM medicinals will *not* have enough time to rejuvenate the hematopoietic function of the bone marrow and compensate for the natural release of thrombopoietin by the kidneys. This will result in an initial decline followed by a subsequent rebound. In the great majority of cases, once you bring the PLT count back up to normal levels, the PLT count will remain sustained with relapse only rarely occurring.

As for splenectomy patients, if the PLT count is still low, then continue prescribing Sheng Yu Tang variant. If splenitis or splenomegaly present and result in excessive platelet destruction, this is when you should prescribe Gui Pi Tang variant adding combinations of medicinals such as Mu Dan Pi, Zhi Zi, The Three Great Yang-Supplementers, Huang Qin, Ren Shen, Zhu Qi, and Xi Lu Rong (powder). You could also consider changing the formula to You Gui Yin variant instead, depending on the patient's presenting signs, symptoms, and pattern identification.

Note: Zhu Jie Qi (竹節七/*Tupistra ensifolia* Wang et Tang/aka Zhu Qi) appears in the book *Selected Medicinal Plants of Yunnan* (雲南中草藥選 *Yunnan Zhong Cao Yao Xuan*). It is bitter, slightly sweet in flavor and cold in nature and has heat-clearing toxin-resolving, blood-quickening pain-relieving, and water-disinhibiting swelling-dispersing actions.

Case Study #5: ITP in Menopausal Patient with Vaginal Bleeding

Q: I have been treating a 55 y/o female idiopathic thrombocytopenic purpura patient for several months now, prescribing (Yu Sheng) Sheng Yu Tang adding Gan Jiang, Fu Zi, Rou Gui, Huang Qin, and Xi Lu Rong (each 6 g); Ren Shen (3 g); Han Lian Cao (6 g); and Tu Si Zi (10 g). I have been following up and evaluating her PLT count every 2 weeks with the results listed below:

1st month: 5,000 □ 67,000 □ 3,000
2nd month: 3,000 □ 85,000 □ 5,000
3rd month: 5,000 □ 110,000 □ 10,000

Her last menses was 3 years ago, so it was presumed that she had entered menopause; but unexpectedly her menstrual cycles started up again (after taking (Yu Sheng) Sheng Yu Tang, the patient felt mild fullness in her lower abdomen). Please share your views and advice about this patient's condition.

A: The dramatic fluctuations in platelet count are likely due to excessive vaginal bleeding (menorrhagia) caused by endometrial hypertrophy. All you need to do is add Fu Ling, Ze Xie, Ou Jie, and Ce Bo Ye, or consider adding a small dose of Zhu Sha to the mix. Technically, you can prescribe up to 12 g per day of Zhu Sha (powder), because this mineral medicinal is very dense by weight. Your plan should be to first reduce and check menstrual bleeding since this will enable PLTs to sustain high levels.

Your treatment appears to be very effective; many patients would have dropped down to a low of 3,000–5,000, but your patient has leveled off at a minimum of 10,000. Good work! Actually, it is *not* that uncommon for a 55 y/o woman who has been menopausal for 3 years to have menses again. Adding Zhu Sha and large doses of Huang Qin and Huang Bo should stop the menstrual cycle (and bleeding) and ensure that the PLT count does not drop back down again.

Case Study #6: Why Such Extreme Fluctuation in PLT Count?

Q: I am treating a 35 y/o female idiopathic thrombocytopenic purpura (ITP) patient with infertility that has undergone intrauterine insemination (IUI) on two occasions. Last October, she experienced sudden onset of high fever, prompting her doctor to prescribe drug treatment that proved ineffective. She still had a fever after 10 days of drug administration, prompting admission into the hospital and low PLT discovered. In the hospital, she was administered 10 mg/day of corticosteroids and eventually her PLT rose back up to 170,000/mm3 (normal range > 150,000/mm3), after which she was released.

However, her concerns over side effects of long-term corticosteroid administration prompted her to stop taking this medication, instead, substituting it with another type. After switching medications, her PLT suddenly dropped to 3,000 and due to persistent, severe nosebleeds she was admitted into the hospital again where corticosteroids and immunoglobin were administered. Her condition stablized once again, but after being released from the hospital she developed mild hepatosplenomegaly and continued taking oral corticosteroids, giving her the classic "moonface" appearance. Please offer your advice and guidance on this case?

A: Idiopathic thrombocytopenic purpura (ITP) patients who rely on corticosteroids to increase PLT above 100,000 must *not* immediately stop taking corticosteroids. These patients must wait at least 3–5 months with PLT levels reaching between 150,000–400,000 before gradually reducing the dose by small incremental amounts.

Remember! Hematopoietic function may be severely suppressed and result in a dramatic drop in PLT levels unless a gradual approach to reducing and eventually discontinuing corticosteroid administration is employed.

Case Study #7: Splenectomy – Eliminates Platelet Destruction and Sequestration

Q: Right now, I am treating five different idiopathic thrombocytopenic purpura (ITP) patients; all are taking cortiscosteroids and some have received splenectomies. An increasing number of potential patients are contacting me inquiring about TCM treatment for this condition. Among these patients, some are antinuclear antibody (ANA) (+) and/or anti-dsDNA antibody (+) and another has Von Willebrand's disease. These patients either have received or are currently being administered therapies such as corticosteroids, immunoglobulins (IVIG), and IV Rho immunoglobulin (RhIG).

Are there any potential side effects or complications from these therapies? Is it necessary to suppress the immune system in ANA (+) and anti-dsDNA antibody (+) patients? When should I suppress (drain)? When should I supplement? What factors should I consider in conducting pattern identification as the basis for determining treatment?

A: In my opinion, for idiopathic thrombocytopenic purpura (ITP) patients it is better to evaluate the complement levels. If antibodies are positive (+), then complement levels will typically be decreased. Common clinal pictures are as follows:

1) For patients in the *chronic stage* that *have* been administered corticosteroids in the past, but still present with antibodies (+) and decreased complement levels, this can be identified as qi and blood vacuity with heat and mild yang vacuity pattern, requiring administration of qi and blood-supplementing and yang-supplementing medicinals adding small doses of heat-abating medicinals as a counterbalance.

2) For patients *currently* being administered corticosteroids (during administration, antibodies and complement levels may or may not be maintained in the normal range), this pathocondition can be identified as spleen, kidney, and liver yang vacuity pattern, requiring great spleen and yang-supplementing medicinals such as Xiang Sha Liu Jun Zi Tang, Sheng Yu Tang, You Gui Wan, Shen Qi Wan, or Shi Quan Da Bu Tang adding The Three Great Yang-Supplementers, Ren Shen, Xi Lu Rong (powder), Tu Si Zi, Huang Qi, and Huang Qin.

3) If antibodies (+) and C3 and C4 are normal, and the patient has *not* been administered corticosteroids, then this can be identified as blood heat with yin vacuity pattern or Shao Yang heat with yin vacuity pattern, requiring administration of formulas such as (Yu Sheng) Hyperactive Immune Formula, Xiao Chai Hu Tang, Di Gu Pi Yin, or Qin Lian Ru Mo Si Wu Tang adding Qin Hao, Zhi Mu, and Di Gu Pi, along with Ce Bo Ye, Ou Jie, Qian Cao, Niu Xi, and Chuan Qi.

4) If antibodies are (+), but C3 and C4 are normal, and the patient is *currently* being administered corticosteroids, then this can be identified as yin vacuity with residual heat pattern, for which you should prescribe (Yu Sheng) Hyperactive Immune Formula variant to induce a rapid increase in PLT levels and a decrease in antibody levels.

Remember! For patients receiving long-term administration of corticosteroids, once corticosteroids have been discontinued (or the effect wears off), PLT levels will inevitably drop, but the antibody levels will slightly increase, and C3 and C4 will remain normal or only moderately decreased: it is for these types of patients with fluctuating levels due to stoppage and continuation of corticosteroid treatment who *should* have The Three Great Yang-Supplementers added to (Yu Sheng) Hyperactive Immune Formula.

If you apply the yang-supplementing approach to decreasing antibody levels for ITP patients, while gradually discontinuing administration of Westerm medicine drugs, there is no need to worry about the yang-supplmenting medicinals inducing a relapse. However, for rheumatoid arthritis (RA) patients, the situation is different, as you must immediately *subtract* the yang-supplementing medicinals if any were added to the (Yu Sheng) Hyperactive Immune Formula.

The purpose of receiving a splenectomy is to eliminate platelet destruction (and antibody production to some extent). If the procedure is performed and PLT levels remain low, then this indicates that the source of the problem was in fact *not* the spleen, but another mechanism (e.g., liver). In this situation, you can prescribe Xiang Sha Liu Jun Zi Tang, Gui Pi Tang, Bu Zhong Yi Qi Tang, Shi Quan Da Bu Tang, Ren Shen Yang Rong Tang, or Sheng Yu Tang adding The Three Great Yang-Supplementers, Huang Qin, Huang Qi, and Tu Si Zi. This approach will be effective in increasing and sustaining PLT levels.

Case Study #8: Familial (Inherited) ITP – It's Worth Following Up!

Q: I have an idiopathic thrombocytopenic purpura (ITP) patient who has already *discontinued* corticosteroids. Previously, I had prescribed (Yu Sheng) Sheng Yu Tang for 3 1/2 months and observed his PLT count increase from 3,000 up to 168,000/mm3 (normal range > 150,000/mm3). This patient's younger brother also has ITP and has been battling the disease for more than 20 years. He has tried corticosteroids in the past without successful results and has suffered cerebral hemorrhage on 3 occasions (*no* subsequent physical or cognitive sequelae).

He has received treatment regimens prescribed by one of South Korea's most renowned traditional Korean medicine (TKM) physicians for over 2 years. Now his PLT is 3,000, and he said that the treatment was not at all effective (the patient just remembers the formula contained Lu Rong among other medicinals). What's your opinion on this case?

A: This case of familial (inherited) ITP is worth following up. I recommend you contact the chairperson of the hematological oncology foundation to see if you can collaborate in an effort to investigate the blood or marrow of these two patients (brothers) with familial (inherited) ITP and compare the results with their parents to determine if any genetic precursors exist. This is really a fascinating case!

Case Study #9: ITP Prevalence Increasing in South Korea – Patients Seek TCM Treatment

Q: I never imagined there were so many idiopathic thrombocytopenic purpura (ITP) patients. In the past, the public did not believe TCM could effectively treat ITP.

Right now, I am treating two ITP patients. One of them has already had PLT levels increase to 160,000, and the other took my TCM prescription for 1 week with PLT increasing from 5,000 to 22,000, and then up to 25,000 after the second week. (I prescribed relatively large doses of Gan Jiang, Fu Zi, and Rou Gui (4 qian each)).

Can you offer more insights from your experiences treating this pathocondition?

A: Ah! It is obvious you are gaining more confidence and experience treating ITP patients.

Remember! (Yu Sheng) Sheng Yu Tang variant is only suitable for liver blood vacuity pattern. If increased PLT destruction occurs in the spleen or splenomegaly (platelet sequestration) presents, then you can prescribe a formula such as Gui Pi Tang or Jia Wei Gui Pi Tang; and if mother-of-malaria (**瘧母** nüè mǔ) presents, then prescribe a formula such as Bie Jia Jian Wan. If liver damage presents from chemotherapy or poisoning (Western medicine drugs or food) resulting in spontaneous bleeding of the flesh (petechiae or purpura), then prescribe a formula such as Sheng Yu Tang, Xiang Sha Liu Jun Zi Tang, Blood Desiccation Formula, Qi Bao Mei Ran Dan, You Gui Wan, Shen Qi Wan, Shi Bu Da Quan Tang, or Ren Shen Yang Rong

Tang.

Liver damage induced by poisoning can be identified as stasis heat pattern, requiring the administration of heat-clearing toxin-resolving medicinals. However, if high-dose platelet transfusions and corticosteroids have been administered, but the PLT count still does *not* increase, then Sheng Yu Tang variant is more suitable for this condition. External contraction (e.g., dengue hemorrhagic fever) can be identified as vacuity heat with frenetic movement of hot blood pattern and Shao Yang heat pattern, requiring the administration of a formula such as Di Gu Pi Yin, Xi Jiao Di Huang Tang, or Xiao Chai Hu Tang adding Mu Dan Pi, Zhi Zi, Qing Hao, Zhi Mu, and Di Gu Pi.

When renal production of thrombopoietin is insufficient, then this can be identified as kidney yang vacuity with cold stasis pattern, requiring the administration of a formula such as You Gui Wan or Shen Qi Wan adding Ren Shen, Xi Lu Rong (powder), and Zhu Qi (wine-soaked). If the patient presents with a histology of hypoplasia and fibrosis inducing suppression of hematopoietic function in the bone marrow, then you should prescribe a formula such as You Gui Wan or Shen Qi Wan adding Ren Shen, Chuan Qi, Xi Lu Rong (powder), and Er Xian Miao.

Acute myelogenous leukemia patients with hematopoietic disorders can be identified as steaming bone taxation heat (fever) pattern, requiring administration of a formula such as Zhi Bo Di Huang Tang, Xiao Chai Hu Tang, Di Gu Pi Yin, or Xi Jiao Di Huang Tang adding Qing Hao, Zhi Mu, Di Gu Pi, Ce Bo Ye, and Ou Jie.

Remember! You must carefully differentiate each individual case. From my experience, the most difficult patients to treat are those incurring graft failures following allogeneic bone marrow transplant (aka stem cell transplant) who have the resulting insufficiency of platelet, RBC, and WBC production. This condition demands a lot of patience. You must first verify whether or not there are abnormal cells in the marrow aspiration and biopsy; if there *are*, then it can be identified as steaming bone pattern; and if *not*, then it can be identified as kidney yang vacuity with cold stasis pattern.

Multiple myeloma patients can be identified as steaming bone with stasis heat pattern, requiring administration of (Yu Sheng) Tong Jing Fang or (Yu Sheng) Ru Mo Si Wu Tang adding Qing Hao, Zhi Mu, and Di Gu Pi.

Case Study #10: Other Heat Pattern Conditions Complicated By ITP

Q: I have a 42 y/o female idiopathic thrombocytopenic purpura (ITP) patient. One week ago, she discovered tiny pinpoint lesions (petechiae) spread over the medial aspect of both lower legs and the medial aspect of both elbows. These spots varied in color from red, purple and brown, did not itch, and were not painful.

I prescribed Gui Pi Tang variant. Please offer you advice and guidance on this patient's condition.

A: Has the patient been definitively diagnosed with ITP? What are the lab test results (e.g., PLT count)? Was bone marrow aspiration performed? What are the presenting signs, symptoms, and history?

If a definitive diagnosis has not been verified, you must consider the possibility of this being a febrile disease complicated by wind heat rash (macules and papules), requiring the administration of Yin Qiao San or Di Gu Pi Yin variants, and *not* Gui Pi Tang.

Remember! Gui Pi Tang and Sheng Yu Tang are administered for patients with low PLT counts, while blood heat and wind heat rash (macules and papules) *may* or may *not* be associated with low PLT count. As you know, external contraction (i.e., microbial infection) can also cause platelet destruction, which at the onset can be identified as Shao Yang heat, exterior wind, and blood heat pattern. If the administration of these types of medicinals *fails* to increase PLT levels, then you can switch to Gui Pi Tang or Sheng Yu Tang; and if the patient has *not* been administered high doses of corticosteroids and/or received platelet transfusions, then you should add Mu Dan Pi and Zhi Zi, which forms Jia Wei Gui Pi Tang. If you know for sure that high doses of corticosteroids *have* been administered, then add The Three Great Yang-Supplementers, Ren Shen, Xi Lu Rong (powder), and Zhu Jie Qi.

ITP is relatively rare in Taiwan and I didn't realize there were so many patients with this condition in South Korea. It is possible that patients' patterns (e.g., cold, heat, vacuity, repletion) are not being accurately identified, as Western medicine doctors are repeatedly administering corticosteroids whose actions may suppress and disguise the underlying condition. Thus, I think the more likely scenario is that many of these cases are simply maculopapular eruptions and not actually ITP. It is just that accurate pattern identification is not being made over and over again, resulting in one errant diagnosis after another!

Case Study #11: ITP and Evans Syndrome

Q: I have a 38 y/o female patient who experienced postpartum hemorrhage (epistaxis and menorrhagia) and went to the hospital for examination, during which a PLT count below 10,000/mm3 (normal range>150,000/mm3) was revealed. She was diagnosed with idiopathic thrombocytopenic purpura (ITP) and since the hemorrhage was intractable her doctors recommended uterectomy.

Following treatment the patient's PLT levels remained between 20,000–30,000, and after administration of intravenous immune globulin (IVIG), PLT levels dropped further down to 5,000, resulting in spontaneous bleeding (epistaxis (nosebleeds) and bleeding gums). Current lab test results are as follows: Hb 7 (12–16 g/dl) and PLT 38,000. Her doctors have diagnosed her with Evans syndrome. What is the best treatment approach for patients with this pathocondition?

A: In my opinion, you can consider prescribing a formula such as Sheng Yu Tang, You Gui Yin, or Shen Qi Wan adding yang-supplementing medicinals, Ren Shen, Zhu Qi, Xi Lu Rong (powder), and Ai Cao (or Ce Bo Ye). If symptoms of hyperactive immune system present, manifesting in steaming bone taxation heat and yin vacuity blood heat pattern, then add Qing Hao, Zhi Mu, Di Gu Pi, and Mu Dan Pi.

Additionally, you can advise the patient to eat plenty of raw lotus root and drink fresh lotus root juice, or also add Lian Ou Jie into your formula. This approach will provide effective treatment for remedying the patient's condition.

Section 4: Behcet's Disease

Case Study #1: My First Behcet's Disease Patient

Q: I consulted and provided treatment for my first Behcet's disease (BD) patient recently. The patient explained that 10 years ago she began having recurrent oral ulcers (aphthous stomatitis) in her mouth and frequently caught common colds. These symptoms endured for a long duration with treatment efforts proving ineffective and prompting her to undergo thorough examination at a hospital.

Doctors diagnosed her with Behcet's disease and she began receiving treatment with Western medicine drugs. The medication did *not* offer any noticeable improvement in her condition, so she decided to seek TCM consultation and treatment.

Since her only presenting symptoms were recurring oral ulcers and susceptibility to catching common colds (external contraction), typically aversion to cold with heat pattern type, I prescribed Da Qing Long Tang adding Huang Qin and Sheng Pu Huang. Do you think this is a good approach? What about long-term treatment?

A: Behcet's disease (aka fox-creeper (狐惑 hú huò) in classical TCM pathologic terminology) patients simply presenting with oral ulcers and susceptibility to external contraction can be identified as exterior pattern with residual damp-heat. So in this case, yes, Da Qing Long Tang adding Huang Qin and Sheng Pu Huang is a good choice, and you can also consider adding Huang Bo and Huang Lian. This formula can be prescribed long-term. TCM physicians in Japan commonly prescribe Wen Qing Yin, comprised of Si Wu Tang combining Huang Lian Jie Du Tang.

If it has really been that long since the patient received Western medicine drug treatment, then the physiological side effects should have already spontaneously metabolized by now, so you do *not* need to consider adding yang-supplementing medicinals to Da Qing Long Tang variant.

In periods of remission, you can prescribe Xie Xin Tang (drains fire and resolves toxin and dries dampness and drains heat) adding Pu Huang or just simply prescribe Pu Huang, instructing the patient to decoct these medicinals and drink the solution like a beverage.

Case Study #2: Behcet's Requires Long-Term Administration of TCM Medicinals

Q: I have a 43 y/o female patient presenting as follows: painful sores (ulcerations) on the tongue and mouth cavity and swollen, inflamed sores on external genitalia that flare up and then spontaneously resolve, and mild pain in both knee joints. The patient explained that she has been suffering from this condition for 11 years and had been on long-term administration of Western medicine drugs *without* effectiveness.

She decided to try TCM and came to see me for consultation. Upon inspection, I observed she had white thick tongue fir, aphthous ulcerations on her tongue and mouth cavity, and mild pain in both her knee joints without swelling. Her appetite, urine, and stool were all normal, and she did *not* have a fever.

Suspecting this is Behcet's disease (fox-creeper), I thus prescribed Wen Qing Yin adding Sheng Pu Huang. Do you think this was the correct diagnosis and treatment approach? Please offer your advice about the treatment course and prognosis.

A: References to Behcet's disease can be found in *On Cold Damage and Miscellaneous Diseases* (**傷寒雜病論** *Shang Han Za Bing Lun*) under Fox-Creeper (**狐或** hú huò). Actually, for most patients this condition is not particularly difficult to treat.

The key for treatment is long-term administration of a formula that contains The Three Yellows and Pu Huang (large doses of each), Mu Dan Pi, Qing Hao, Di Gu Pi, and Zhi Mu. And if joint pain presents, then add Huo Luo Dan; if erosions of the genitals present, then add Long Dan Cao; if erosion of the anus presents, then add Bai Zhi, Huai Hua, Di Yu, Fang Feng, and Bai Zhi; and if red and inflamed eyes present, then add Ru Xiang, Mo Yao, and Chuan Qi (or Hong Hua).

The formula you prescribed will provide effective treatment for heat toxin with yin and blood vacuity pattern of your patient. But remember! TCM treatment of this disease requires long-term administration of medicinals. The patient should have lab tests periodically performed so you can assess ESR and CRP levels. Once these levels are normal, you should change to a formula such as Xian

Fang Huo Ming Yin (clears heat and resolves toxin, disperses swelling and breaks hardness, and quickens the blood and relieves pain), Sheng Yu Tang (supplements qi and nourishes the blood), or Bu Yang Huan Wu Tang (quickens the blood and supplements qi) adding The Three Yellows.

Case Study #3: Once Western Medicine Drugs Have Been Discontinued – (Yu Sheng) Hyperactive Immune Formula

Q1: A 38 y/o female patient has suffered from oral cavity aphthous ulcerations (tongue and mouth) for more than 20 years. She explained that at the age of 9 she began having pain in both knees, prompting her to undergo examination, which revealed rheumatoid factor (RF) (+). She was administered Western medicine drugs at the time and her symptoms were partially relieved, but ever since then she has felt malaise and tidal heat (潮熱 cháo rè).

Recently, a severe flare up in both wrist joints forced her to spend 5 months in the hospital until the pain resolved, and she worried that her illness would relapse again. Past administration of immunosuppressant medication caused allergic reactions so she does *not* want to take them anymore.

Now, she wants to try TCM treatment. After assessing the patient's history and carefully examining her, despite the fact that she does *not* have the telltale genital ulcerations, I suspect she *has* Behcet's disease (BD). Please offer your advice and guidance.

A1: BD commonly presents in women and your description indeed suggests she has fox-creeper (aka Behcet's disease). Remember! If your patient has simply been administered analgesics, colchicine, and/or topical corticosteroids, and *not* immunosuppressants (e.g., corticosteroids) or chemotherapeutic agents, then this can be identified as yin vacuity heat with steaming bone pattern.

Blood test results will *not* necessarily reveal abnormalities in C3/C4, ANA, and anti-ds DNA, but *abnormal* levels of Ig, ESR, CRP, and RF can all be identified as heat pattern, requiring the administration of Hyperactive Immune Formula (including large doses of The Three Yellows) adding Sheng Pu Huang. If swollen and painful joints present, then add Ma Huang, Niu Xi, and Sheng Du

Zhong (specifically for the lower extremities); and if loose stools present, then add Cang Zhu, Fu Ling, and Ze Xie.

The administration of TCM medicinals in patients who have *not* been administered Western medicine drugs is the optimal scenario that provides the most effective treatment. For patients who *have* already received long-term administration of Western medicine immunosuppressants and chemotherapeutic agents (e.g., corticosteroids, Methotrexate), you should evaluate Hb and C3 and C4 as the basis for pattern identification and determining treatment. If *decreased* levels Hb and complement present, then prescribe a formula that supplements qi, blood, and yang. If complement levels are *normal*, then advise the patient to begin gradually discontinuing Western medicine drugs.

Once these drugs have been completely discontinued and an extended period goes by without any flare-ups occurring, then you can change the formula to (Yu Sheng) Hyperactive Immune Formula variant. Administration of this formula will ensure that the patient's condition remains symptom free, and eventually, the administration of this formula can be gradually reduced and discontinued altogether.

Q2: Sorry to trouble you again! Since she began taking (Yu Sheng) Hyperactive Immune Formula adding Sheng Pu Huang and Lian Qiao, the patient has had loose stools (5–10 times/day), cold hands and feet, chest distention and heaviness, and her oral ulcers have worsened.

I want to change formulas to Xiang Sha Liu Jun Zi Tang adding Huang Lian Jie Du Tang, Lian Qiao, Pu Gong Ying, Wu Zhu Yu, Dang Gui, and Xi Xin. Do you think this is a good approach?

A2: If you are sure she has BD, the original formula is still the best. Again, if the patient presents with loose stools, then either add Cang Zhu and Ze Xie to your formula and reduce the doses of the other medicinals, or change the formula to Huang Lian Jie Du Tang (subtracting Zhi Zi) adding Sheng Pu Huang and The Four Lings.

Cold hands and feet is a typical psychosomatic symptom of the autonomic nervous system, thus it is *not* necessary to add Dang Gui, Xi Xin, and Wu Zhu Yu. If necessary, you can consider prescribing Xiang Sha Liu Jun Zi Tang (boosts qi and fortifies the spleen and moves qi and transforms phlegm), Sheng Yang Yi Wei Tang (supplements the spleen and stomach and drains yin fire), Ping Wei San (dries dampness and fortifies the spleen and moves qi and harmonizes the stomach), or even Qing Zao Jiu Fei Tang (clears dryness and moistens the lung). Just make sure to include The Three Yellows (clear heat and resolve toxin) and Sheng Pu Huang (transforms stasis and stanches bleeding).

Though I rarely prescribe these types of formulas, for some people's body constitutions it may be necessary. For instance, it sounds like I have a similar type of body consitition as this patient, because whenever I take The Three Yellows it causes me to have loose stools as well; and when I get a common cold (external contraction), I must apply Li Dong-Yuan's approach by adding spleen and stomach-supplementing medicinals to the formula.

Q3: Thanks for your advice and guidance.

After changing the formula to Xiang Sha Liu Jun Zi Tang adding Qing Hao and Zhi Mu (8 qian each), Lian Qiao, Pu Gong Ying, and Dang Shen (5 qian each), Jin Yin Hua, and Huo Luo Dan, the patient's condition has improved dramatically.

Not only have her bowel movements, cold hands and feet, and chest heaviness normalized, but also the oral ulcers, joint pain, and eye inflammation are getting much better.

A3: BD can be identified as true heat with yin vacuity and vacuity fire pattern. This is a good example of how different people's body constitutions require the physician to modify the formula and customize the approach to meet the therapeutic needs of each patient. Congratulations on the accurate pattern identification and treatment. This makes both the patient and doctor happy!

Case Study #4: Painful Oral Ulcerations on the Tongue and Mouth – It Could Be Behcet's Disease

Q: Three years ago, a female patient (now 6 y/o) went for a medical examination to get the oral (aphthous) ulcers on the side of her tongue and mouth (so painful she couldn't eat or drink hot or spicy foods) and excessive tearing (epiphora) checked out. At the time, blood tests were *normal*; and neither the medication (for oral ulcers), nor the surgical procedure (for epiphora) were effective. To this day, she is still troubled with recurring painful tongue and mouth ulcerations, prompting her mother to bring her in for consultation.

Despite the aphthous ulcers on her tongue and oral cavity suggesting the patient has Behcet's disease (BD), I think her condition looks more like Sjogren's syndrome (SS). Thus, I prescribed Hyperactive Immune Formula adding Sheng Pu Huang and Mai Men Dong. Administration of this formula resulted in rapid improvement in the patient's symptoms. Do you think I have accurately identified the pattern and provided an appropriate treatment?

A: According to TCM theory, a painful tongue can be identified as effulgent heart fire pattern and ulcerations on the side of the tongue and mouth cavity can be idenfitied as stomach heat pattern.

The diagnosis of fox-creeper (aka Behcet's disease) is correct; it is *not* Sjogren's syndrome (SS). However, your prescription of Hyperactive Immune Formula adding Sheng Pu Huang and Mai Men Dong accurately treats the pattern identified, so naturally you will have effective results!

Section 5: Other Autoimmune Disorders

Case Study #1: Sjogren's Syndrome – It's More Than Sicca Syndrome!

Q: I have a 62 y/o female patient who presented with dry mouth (xerostomia), painful gums, dry-fissured tongue, and swollen parotid glands. She explained that 1 year ago, the same symptoms occurred, but test results couldn't isolate a definitive diagnosis. She takes Western medicine drugs, which are sometimes effective in remedying symptoms, but eventually recur in 2–3 days.

Recently, her dry mouth has been so severe that when eating food she has a "burning" sensation, so she decided to visit my clinic. What are your thoughts on the diagnosis and treatment of this pathocondition?

A: Your description of this patient's sicca syndrome symptoms strongly suggests the diagnosis of Sjogren's syndrome (SS), but technically this diagnosis is *not* made unless there is laboratory evidence of autoimmune disease.

Regardless of the Western medicine diagnosis, for this condition you can consider prescribing formulas such as Hyperactive Immune Formula variant; Huang Lian Jie Du Tang (subtracting Zhi Zi) combining Si Wu Tang (aka Wen Qing Yin); or Wen Dan Tang. Just make sure to include Huang Bo, Huang Lian, and combinations of yin-enriching fire-downbearing, vacuity heat-clearing, and dryness-moistening medicinals such as Qing Hao, Zhi Mu, Di Gu Pi, Tian Men Dong, Mai Men Dong, Tian Hua, Yuan Shen, and Sheng Pu Huang.

The "burning" sensation your patient feels when she eats is likely phantom pain or phantom heat, and for this you can add Quan Xie, Bai Jiang Can, Wu Gong, and Yu Sheng Wan.

Case Study #2: Viscous Saliva May Indicate Sjogren's Syndrome

Q: A 70 y/o female patient began experiencing severely dry mouth (salivary gland hypofunction) with viscous saliva. In the past, she had taken Western medicine drugs, but treatment attempts were *not* effective; and now, she has sought my consultation to treat this condition. What is the best approach for treating this patient?

A: Dry mouth (xerostomia), viscous saliva (sicca syndrome), and dry eyes (xerophthalmia) are the most commonly presenting symptoms in patients with the autoimmune disorder Sjogren's syndrome (SS). You should prescribe Hyperactive Immune Formula (including large doses of each medicinal, especially The Three Yellows) adding Sheng Pu Huang. This formula should effectively remedy this patient's condition.

Case Study #3: Exposure to Water Induces Skin Rash (Papules)

Q: A 49 y/o female patient complained of a skin rash presenting with reddish, slightly raised papules on her arms and legs. She said that this condition began 3 days ago, explaining, "every time my arms and legs touched water, a rash would appear on my skin."

During her clinic visit, I saw this rash (tiny papules) appear myself when I sprinkled water on her arm as a test. Have you ever heard of this type of reaction before?

A: Exposure to water inducing skin rash with red papules can be identified as reversal cold (厥冷 jué leng) and strongly suggests Raynaud's disease, which occurs when the amount of cryoglobulin in the blood is too high (cryoglobulinemia).

TCM treatment of reversal cold typically calls for a formula such as Dang Gui Si Ni Tang or Dang Gui Si Ni Tang combining Wu Zhu Yu Gan Jiang Tang adding Huang Qin, Fu Zi, and Huang Qi.

Case Study #4: Reversal Cold Inducing Red Rash – Raynaud's Disease

Q: I have a 48 y/o female patient who is allergic to cold. Exposure to cold objects (e.g., cold water, ice) will initially induce itchiness (urticaria) and reddish painful swelling (angioedema), and then progress to a generalized rash (papules) over the entire body. She is so sensitive to cold that even air conditioning and raindrops will cause a rash (papules) to present. Her latest allergic reaction began about 3 weeks ago. How would you treat this condition?

A: Allergic reaction upon exposure to cold indicates the reversal cold (厥冷 jué leng) of Raynaud's disease (RD), which is caused by increased levels of cryoglobulin (CR) in the blood (cryoglobulinemia) and results in cutaneous ischemia. Remember! This condition must *not* be identified as exterior wind-cold pattern.

In the winter, these patients are susceptible to sloughing flat-abscess (脫疽 tuo ju) (gangrene) in which severe peripheral vasculature ischemia leads to necrosis. In Taiwan, we call this black-hand disease and black-foot disease. In the past, frostbite inducing gangrene was much more prevalent among people who worked outdoors (e.g., farmers, laborers) during the cold weather months. Nowadays, with the development of effective cold weather gear, improvement of labor conditions, and healthier nutritional intake, this condition is much less common. In your mother and father's (definitely grandmother and grandfather) generation, the cracked skin and purulent erosions of sloughing flat-abscess (gangrene) were a much more common (though unpleasant!) sight.

To treat this condition, if a "painful" rash (papules) presents, then prescribe a blood-nourishing yin-enriching dryness-moistening formula such as Blood Desiccation Formula adding The Three Great Yang-Supplementers, Wu Zhu Yu, and Huang Qin; or Dang Gui Si Ni Tang combining Wu Zhu Yu Gan Jiang Tang adding Fu Zi, Huang Qin, and Ren Shen/Chuan Qi Powder.

Case Study #5: Irritable Bowel Disease – Ulcerative Colitis and Crohn's Disease

Q: I have a 40 y/o female patient whom has endured 10–20 stools (often with small amounts of fresh blood) per day for the past 30 years. Recently, her condition has worsened, prompting her to go to the hospital for an examination. Colonoscopy revealed continuous areas of inflammation and ulcerations in the lining of the colon and rectum. Her doctors prescribed corticosteroids, which have proven to be very *effective*. However, she can only take this medication for 2 months and thus is worried about the condition recurring, so she decided to try TCM treatment.

I diagnosed her condition as irritable bowel disease (IBD), and specifically chronic ulcerative colitis (UC), based on the location, distribution, and depth of the lesions. Please offer your advice and guidance on this patient's condition.

A: Colorectal ulcerations and Behcet's disease (BD) both correlate with the classical TCM pathologic term fox-creeper (狐或 hú huò). In the early days of Western medicine, morphine was prescribed to treat this condition and now corticosteroids are administered. Ulcerative colitis (UC) and Crohn's disease (CD) are the two main types of irritable bowel disease (IBD) in which the immune system attacks the mucous membrane lining of the intestinal walls (CD and UC) and other parts of the digestic tract and body (only CD).

In TCM, *regardless* if immunosuppressants (e.g., glucocorticoids, Methotrexate) or immunotherapies *have* been administered, this pathocondition can still be identified as great heat vacuity fire pattern or possibly vacuity fire with Shao Yang heat pattern. To treat this condition, I typically prescribe (Yu Sheng) Hyperactive Immune Formula adding The Four Lings.

Case Study #6: Aphthous Tongue Ulcers – Heat Pattern of "Fox-Creeper"

Q: A 52 y/o male patient suddenly began having raised lesions and painful ulcers on his tongue. He was administered treatment with Western medicine drugs, which were *not* effective. Do you think this could be Sjogren's syndrome (SS)?

A: Raised lesions and painful ulcers on the tongue can be identified as heat pattern and can be classified as fox-creeper (狐或 hú huò); it's not Sjogren's syndrome (SS).

You can prescribe Hyperactive Immune Formula (including large doses of The Three Yellows, Qing Hao, Zhi Mu, and Di Gu Pi) adding Sheng Pu Huang. Instruct the patient to drink this decocted formula as follows: make sure it has cooled to at least room temperature, drink it like a beverage in small amounts over a 24-hour period, and thoroughly rinse the entire mouth slowly, letting the liquid soak into the mucous membrane of the oral cavity prior to swallowing.

SS typically presents with the sicca syndrome symptoms of dry eyes (xerophthalmia) and dry mouth (xerostomia) caused by the immune system errantly attacking the salivary and lacrimal glands, but may affect other areas (i.e., mucous membranes) of the body as well. It's possible for patients with SS to also have Behcet's disease (BD) and thus present with aphthous ulcerations, but up to now, I have not witnessed this type of case in my clinical practice. If the sores and ulcerations appear *bright red* colored, then you can consider adding Pu Gong Ying, Yu Sheng Wan, and Wan Ling Dan.

Remember! Both BD and SS can be idenfitied as great heat vacuity fire pattern, thus the approach for treating this pathoconditions is similar. Typically, I will prescribe (Yu Sheng) Hyperactive Immune Formula, making modifications to this formula and possibly changing to another formula as the condition evolves and completely resolves.

Case Study #7: Autoimmune Diseases – Amyloidosis Predisposition

Q: Two years ago in June, a 50 y/o female patient began suffering symptoms of diarrhea with blood, cramping, and rectal pain, prompting a hospital examination and a diagnosis of ulcerative colitis (UC). The patient was treated with hydrocortisone rectal suspension for 3 months, which produced *effective* results.

One year later in early July, she began experiencing difficulty breathing (when walking upstairs) and dry cough, for which she took Western medicine drugs *without* effective results. After hospital examination, she was diagnosed with bronchiolitis obliterans organizing pneumonia (BOOP) and was treated with large doses of corticosteroids. Blood oxygen levels were normal and aside from the breathing difficulty, dry cough, and loose stools, all other test results were normal and the symptoms were not severe.

The patient's husband is the editor-in-chief of South Korea's largest newspaper. They have several Western medicine doctors in their family and don't have much faith in TCM. However, after ineffective Western medicine treatment, the director of the radiology oncology department (also my academic advisor) at my university's hospital personally introduced me to this patient. I have a lot of pressure on this case. Please offer your invaluable advice and guidance.

A: UC and Crohn's disease (CD) are two closely related types of irritable bowel disease (IBD) caused by the immune system attacking the lining of the GI tract and other mucous membranes (only in the case of CD). Both UC and CD can be classified under the TCM pathocondition called fox-creeper.

If large doses of methylprednisolone pulse therapy, chemotherapeutic agents (e.g., large dosages of Methotrexate), or immunotherapy *have* been administered, which suppress hematopoiesis, hormone, and immune functions, this can be identified as kidney yang vacuity pattern. In all other cases, these pathoconditions can be identified as in the "essential state" of great heat vacuity fire pattern or possibly vacuity fire with Shao Yang heat pattern.

For kidney yang vacuity pattern, once the patient has discontinued Western medicine drugs for 3–6 months, then the pathocondition has returned to its "essential state." This is when you should prescribe Hyperactive Immune Formula variant.

People with autoimmune disease are predisposed to amyloid deposits forming in the tissues and capillary membranes of organs (e.g., heart, lungs, eyes, and brain), thus interfering with normal function. The presentation of difficulty breathing and dry cough suggests this type of secondary amyloidosis.

For this condition you should prescribe Hyperactive Immune Formula variant adding medicinal combinations such as Ma Huang, Xing Ren, Ting Li Zi, Fu Ling, and Ze Xie; Chuan Xiong, Chi Shao, Dan Shen, Yin Xing Ye, Ma Huang, and Xing Ren; Tian Men Dong, Mai Men Dong, Sha Shen, and Yuan Shen (lung yin-nourishing action); and Ci Yuan, Kuan Dong Hua, Wu Wei Zi, and Bai Bu (dispels watery phlegm). These medicinals will effectively treat pathoconditions involving water amassment, stasis heat, lung yin vacuity, and lung cold-phlegm shooting into the lung. Carefully assess the patient's condition to identify the pattern and determine the best medicinals for treatment.

Remember! The key factors during diagnosis are to differentiate between dry cough and watery phlegm, the presence of pleural effusion, edema of the upper and lower limbs, and night cough. Some telltale signs of pleural effusion are the following: the patient will begin to cough after sitting for a while, but when lying down they won't cough; or possibly cough for a brief period of time after lying down and then stop coughing; or cough upon turning over.

Case Study #8: Adult-Onset Still's Disease

Q: A 30 y/o female patient began experiencing symptoms of generalized joint pain and swelling about 3 years ago, prompting her to undergo hospital examination. Doctors suspected rheumatoid arthritis (RA) and did a workup only to find RF (-), ESR normal, and CRP slightly elevated. Based on these results, her doctors suspected adult-onset Still's disease (AOSD).

Ever since then she has been receiving corticosteroids (her distinctive "moonface" will attest to that) to relieve the symptoms, but this approach has *not* offered lasting results. What is your opinion about this patient's condition?

A: AOSD is an immune hyperactivity pathocondition that causes an inflammatory type of arthritis similar to RA. Does the patient have any other symptoms such as tidal fever or sore throat? Additionally, you should advise the patient to have the following lab tests performed: C3/C4, ANA, anti-dsDNA, BUN, and Cr. Rheumatologists will typically administer prednisone, other immunosuppressants, and immunotherapy (aka biologic response modifiers (BMR)) for the treatment of this pathocondition.

Regardless of the Western medicine drugs prescribed, in TCM this pathocondition can be identified as yin vacuity heat pattern and treatment is the same as for dermatomyositis or RA.

Thus, I would prescribe Hyperactive Immune Formula adding combinations of the following medicinals: Ci Shi, Sheng Long Gu, and Dai Zhe Shi (quiet the spirit with heavy settlers), Chi Shao and Sheng Di Huang (clear heat, cool the blood, and nourish yin), and Wan Ling Dan. I would also bleed Da Zhui (DU14) (above, at, below), Wei Zhong (UB40), Tai Yuan (LU9), and the well points of the pericardium, liver, spleen, and stomach channels; and perform acupuncture on the acupoints of the Shao Yang channel (applying the draining technique). This approach should provide effective results in a relatively short period of time.

III. NEUROLOGICAL DISORDERS

Section 1: Stroke

Case Study #1: Hemiparesis Resulting from Cerebral Infarction

Q: I have a male patient who suffers from hemiparesis resulting from cerebral infarction and has a history of chronic bleeding hemorrhoids. One day last year, he overstrained while on the toilet leading to a stroke that caused left-sided hemiparesis, manifesting as stiffness in the left arm and leg. The patient's doctor diagnosed him with cerebral infarction.

How do you treat cerebral infarction? Using TCM medicinals, how long do you think it will take to recover function of the stiff appendages so that he will able to move about freely and autonomously carry out basic daily activities? I am estimating at least 1 year, does that sound about right?

A: Overstraining while on the toilet (e.g., holding the breath and straining at the same time) in people with constipation, bleeding hemorrhoids, or anal prolapse can most certainly cause cerebral ischemia (hypoxia), cerebral infarction, and cerebral hemorrhage, resulting in hemiparesis (sensory and motor deficits) and in severe cases hemiplegia. In fact, overstraining while on the toilet is the most common cause of anal prolapsed, with incidence rates on the rise.

There are increasing numbers of people with anal prolapse and anal fissures. People of today eat a lot of rich foods, not enough fruits and vegetables, and don't get enough exercise—dietary and lifestyle habits that lead to constipation problems. Additionally, sit-down toilets are now in virtually every modern household. These toilets offer the benefit of convenience for those physically unable to squat; alleviate the discomfort of soreness, numbness, and pain for those who have to wait for their bowels to move; and even provide a leisurely gettaway for those in the habit of reading periodicals or browsing on their smartphone while "doing their business."

The problem is that these toilets were invented by people of European descent, with designs standardized to accommodate the physical stature of Europeans and Americans, and *not* the relatively smaller statures of Asians whose legs are often left hanging in the air or straining in flexion to reach the floor below. People with constipation sit on the toilet for long periods, exerting themselves unsuccessfully and not getting everything evacuated. Since sitting there is a relatively comfortable endeavor, constipated people tend to spend excessive amounts of time straining away. This puts too much pressure on the anal orifice, constricting the canal instead of opening it, and making it difficult to defecate and more likely to induce anal fissures and anal prolapse. In severe cases, this overstraining may lead to cerebral hypoxia and ischemia (especially for those with anal fissures or anal prolapse who sit on the toilet and bleed) and possibly may even induce cerebral infarction (ischemic stroke) that results in hemiparesis or hemiplegia.

For cerebral infarction patients, it is best to administer both TCM medicinals and acupuncture (warm needle).

As for medicinals, you can prescribe a blood-quickening qi-supplementing formula such as Bu Yang Huan Wu Tang adding The Three Great Yang-Supplementers, Huang Qin, and Ren Shen/Chuan Qi Powder. You can start out by prescribing 2 liang of the sovereign medicinal Huang Qi, and incrementally increase the dose up to 2.5 liang and then 3 liang to enhance the qi-supplementing action. This approach will be effective in treating hemiparesis and hemiplegia caused by cerebral infarction (ischemic stroke), improving motor function and strengthening the limbs.

As for acupuncture, to treat hemiparesis (or hemiplegia) you can consider warm needling the following acupoints: He Gu (LI4), Shou San Li (LI10), Wai Guan (SJ5), Zhong Zhu (SJ3), Zu San Li (ST36), Yang Ling Quan (GB34), Xuan Zhong (GB39), San Yin Jiao (SP6), Tai Chong (LV3), Di Wu Hui (GB42), Feng Chi (GB20), Tian Zhu (UB10), Bai Hui (DU20), Guan Yuan Shu (UB26), Wei Zhong (UB40), and Kun Lun (UB60). Naturally, if the patient actively engages in rehabilitation, the outlook for functional recovery (especially the arms) is even better. For remedying hemorrhoids, anal fissures, and anal prolapse, you can needle He Gu (LI4), Shou San Li (LI10), Chi Ze (LU5), Xia Bai (LU4), Bai Hui (DU20), and the Four Anal Perimeter Acupoints; and bleed Shang Yang (LI1), Er Jian (LI2), and San Jian (LI3).

Remember! The duration of treatment for hemiparesis and hemiplegia varies greatly with each patient. Sometimes it is a quick process and other times it can be very slow. It depends on the extent of brain damage (both the size and location of the lesion), the duration of time elapsed prior to beginning TCM treatment, the age of the patient, and also on how motivated the patient is to achieve recovery along with the level of family support. Patients with mild hemiparesis who retain motor function capacity and cognitive clarity should stay actively involved in hobbies and engage in social interactions. For example, getting together with friends for therapeutic mahjong sessions is a great way to combine an interest that stimulates the brain, encourages social interaction, and provides rehabilitation for upper limb motor function.

Note: The Four Anal Perimeter Acupoints (**肛門口四周** g□ng mén kǒu sì zh□u) are four acupoints roughly corresponding with Hui Yin (CV1) and Chang Qiang (DU1) longitudinally, along with two accompanying latitudinal acupoints at each side of the anus, which together form symmetrical x-y axis coordinates. Needle at a distance of approx. 0.5 cun from the external anal sphincter and insert at a depth of approx. 1.5–1.8 cun parallel to the anal canal.

Case Study #2: Cerebral Infarction (Stroke) Complicated by Hemorrhage and Hydrocephalus – Is There Cerebral Atrophy?

Q: A 62 y/o male patient suffered from cerebral infarction and received treatment. Then, 6 months later, hydrocephalus presented with secondary cerebrovascular infarct and mild hemorrhage.

I prescribed Bu Yang Huan Wu Tang variant. After taking this formula for 3 months, the symptoms of heaviness of the entire body and mental fogginess dramatically improved, helping him make close to a full recovery.

Yesterday, his daughter called notifying me that her father has been lethargic and clumsy over the past month, prompting another MRI that showed signs of hydrocephalus, but without increased ICP and without fever. Do you think this could be cerebral atrophy? How should I treat this?

A: In patients with cerebral infarction, a loss of cerebral tissue occurs and the ventricular system enlarges to compensate for this loss, resulting in a secondary (normal-pressure or communicating) hydrocephalus. For this condition, you can consider prescribing a kidney yang-warming qi transformation-promoting and bland-percolating dampness- and water-disinhibiting formula such as Wu Ling San (Nephritis Formula) adding Da Huang, and Ren Shen/Chuan Qi Powder; or s spleen- and stomach-supplementing, phlegm-damp-transforming, and wind-stabilizing formula such as Ban Xia Tian Ma Bai Zhu San variant.

If constipation presents, incrementally increase the dose of Da Huang (drains heat and frees the intestines) up to 8 qian, and if this still does *not* prove ineffective, then add Mang Xiao (drains heat and frees the stool and moistens dryness and softens hardness), starting at 5 fen increasing incrementally up until the patient maintains at least 1 stool/day.

Remember! In cases where hydrocephalus develops from a cyst or tumor that blocks CSF circulation (i.e., obstructive noncommunicating hydrocephalus), then the patient will present with increased ICP, requiring the prescription of a different formula. You should also advise the patient to avoid rigorous activities and situations that might injure the already compromised brain tissue (cells).

Case Study #3: Dizziness Following Cerebellar Infarction

Q: This patient is a male with robust stature who likes to drink alcohol and has a history of high blood pressure. Recently, he went to the hospital to examine the cause of his severe dizziness and get treatment. An MRI revealed left-sided cerebellar infarction. The patient's urine output and stool are normal. What is the best approach for treating this patient?

A: There are many causes of dizziness, and cerebellar infarction is one of them. You must carefully identify the pattern and then decide on the right treatment. Here are three formulas you may consider prescribing:

1) Bu Yang Huan Wu Tang adding The Three Great Yang-Supplementers, Tian Ma, Huang Qin, and Ren Shen/Chuan Qi Powder.

2) Ban Xia Tian Ma Bai Zhu San adding heavy doses of Tian Ma, Huang Qi, Chuan Qi, Chi Shao, and Yin Xing Ye.

3) In cases involving visceral agitation (**臟躁** zàng zào), prescribe

Ban Xia Tian Ma Bai Zhu San adding Gan Cao and Long Yan Gan (or Da Zao).

Case Study #4: TIA – A Type of Cerebral Infarction

Q: A 65 y/o male patient suffered from stroke and sudden collapse. After this incident, he has continued experiencing temporary loss of consciousness during the nighttime while sleeping at least once a month.

What is the etiology of these blackouts (syncope)? Could they be caused by cerebral infarction?

A: Repeated bouts of passing out or collapse (syncope) following a stroke results from a type of cerebrovascular infarction, the correct medical term for this is transient ischemic attack (TIA), also called a "mini-stroke."

To treat this condition, you can prescribe a blood-quickening qi-supplementing formula such as Bu Yang Huan Wu Tang adding The Three Great Yang-Supplementers, Huang Qin, and Ren Shen/Chuan Qi Powder. If the patient experiences periodic paralysis, then you should request that he get lab tests (e.g., complete blood count (CBC), electrolyte panel) performed to determine further modifications to your formula.

Case Study #5: Retinal Vascular Occlusion (Ocular Stroke)

Q: One month ago, a 43 y/o female patient visited my clinic complaining of partial vision loss in one of her eyes. She explained that 6 months ago she was walking to her car when suddenly "half the sky turned dark" in one eye's field of vision. She rushed to the hospital, was diagnosed with retinal vascular occlusion (ocular stroke), and received treatment for 5 months *without* substantial improvement in her vision. That's when she decided to seek TCM consultation.

I prescribed Bu Yang Huan Wu Tang adding large doses of Yin Xing Ye (8 qian), The Three Great Yang-Supplementers, Huang Qin, Ren Shen/Chuan Qi Powder, Fu Ling, and Ze Xie. Unfortunately, this formula has *not* produced very effective results: she still has partial vision loss. Do you have any suggestions? Is it possible to treat this condition?

A: Retinal vascular occlusion is also known as ocular stroke. Just by the name you know the etiology and pathomechanisms are similar to a cerebrovascular attack (i.e., stroke), and so is the therapeutic approach.

In the treatment of stroke, the process is always slow, and it is even slower for ocular stroke; it will take at least 3 to 5 months before you will see any noticeable improvement. That has been my experience treating this condition…patience…patience…patience…and eventually there will be gradual improvement. Prescribing Bu Yang Huan Wu Tang variant is the right approach, just have patience!

Section 2: Other Cerebrovascular Disorders

Case Study #1: Nocturnal Cramps – Periodic Paralysis, *Not* Cerebral Infarction

Q: In recent years, a 66 y/o female patient has been experiencing frequent nighttime cramps during sleep throughout her entire body (especially in her arms and legs). She had an MRI performed and was diagnosed with a lacunar infarct (the most common type of ischemic stroke).

Following several months of Western medicine drug treatment, the cramps continued to occur, though with lesser intensity. Now, she has the sensation of ants crawling under her skin (formication). Do you think this could be a side effect of Western medicine drug treatment? How would you treat this patient's condition?

A: It sounds to me like this patient has periodic paralysis, *not* cerebral infarction, and the "ants crawling" sensation is phantom itch. I base this presumption on the fact that if it were cerebral infarction causing her symptoms, she would have these attacks the entire day and they should be even more severe during the day when she is active. These symptoms would *not* just manifest at nighttime! Also, cerebral infarction generally would involve motor function impairment of the extremities, and the absence of these symptoms indicates that your patient's condition has nothing to do with cerebral infarction.

You should advise the patient to have an electrolyte panel performed (specifically Na+ and K+ levels). In cases of *hypo*kalemic-induced attacks, the patient can take oral potassium chloride supplements and avoid carbohydrate-rich meals and strenuous exercise. In cases of *hyper*kalemic-induced attacks, the patient can eat carbohydrate-rich, low-potassium foods, and avoid strenuous exercise and fasting. Another helpful bit of dietary advice is telling her to buy salt-free soy sauce.

As for TCM medicinals, I would prescribe a formula variant such as a kidney yang-warming and -supplementing, blood-quickening stasis-dissipating, sinew- and bone-strengthening, and dampness-eliminating pain-relieving formula such as You Gui Wan or Shen Qi Wan.

Case Study #2: Hypertension and Headache During Menopausal Transition

Q: A 51 y/o female patient sought my consultation for the treatment of hypertension and headache during menopausal transition (aka climacteric period). Just as I have done in the past for similar pathoconditions, I prescribed Jian Ling Tang adding Zi He Che. Unexpectedly, the patient's blood pressure rose even higher. Why would this happen?

A: Prescribing Jian Ling Tang variant for hypertension and headache during menopausal transition is a logical formula selection for ascendant hyperactivity of liver yang pattern.

If your patient's blood pressure increased, then I would try adding Qing Hao, Zhi Mu, Di Gu Pi, Long Yan Gan, and Gan Cao to your original formula. If headache presents, then add Tian Ma, Chuan Qi, Wu Zhu Yu, and Yu Sheng Wan. You could also consider changing to a formula variant such as Di Gu Pi Yin, Zhi Bo Di Huang Tang, Bu Yang Huan Wu Tang, or Wen Dan Tang, making sure to include Long Gu, Mu Li, Tian Ma, Qing Hao, Zhi Mu, and Di Gu Pi in your selection.

Case Study #3: Sexual Headaches (Coital Cephalgia)

Q: A 48 y/o female patient came to my clinic with the chief complaint of getting headaches during sexual intercourse. She explained that recently during intercourse she felt stiffness and pain in the right side of her neck and a sharp pain in her right Tai Yang (EX-HN5), which occasionally extended up to Shuai Gu (GB8). The first time this happened the pain was so bad she even checked into the emergency room, but was too embarrassed to fully explain the circumstances. It has happened 3 times now.

She wants to know the cause, if it could be life-threatening, and what she can do, if anything, to prevent these headaches.

A: Sexual headaches most often occur in men, especially in those who are overworked and stressed out. It is relatively rare for this to occur in women. The cause similarly could be from overwork, stress, or emotionally-derived; however, the possibility of cerebral aneurysm must be ruled out, so you should advise her to have an MRI performed.

I have treated several patients with this condition and even presented one of the cases when I was invited to share my clinical experiences treating vertigo, dizziness, and headache at the International Symposium of Traditional Korean Medicine held in South Korea. I discussed the administration of formulas such as Jîan Ling Tang, Wen Dan Tang, Ru Mo Si Wu Tang, and Da Chai Hu Tang adding Tian Ma and Wu Zhu Wu to treat these conditions.

If an MRI *does* reveal a cerebral aneurysm in your patient, then surgery should be immediately performed, either undergoing open craniotomy to clip the aneurysm or endovascular repair using a titanium coil, or coil and stenting to plug up and prevent the aneurysm from rupturing. Otherwise, a life-threatening rupture could occur at any moment. You must be vigilant!

As I understand, cerebral aneurysms usually occur along a loop of arteries that run between the underside of the brain and the base of the skull. Any type of excessive tension or stimulation, not just sexual intercourse, can cause pulsating pain. A cerebral aneurysm is an extremely dangerous condition that must not be taken lightly, and when it comes to health, there is nothing to be shy about.

What you should do now is urge your patient to get a functional MRI (fMRI) and angiography performed as soon as possible, and also prescribe mild TCM medicinals to ensure her condition remains stabilized. Your formula should include The Four Lings and large doses of The Three Yellows. Remember! It is *not* advisable to prescribe blood-quickening stasis-transforming (e.g., Chuan Qi) or qi-supplementing yang-upbearing (e.g., Huang Qi) medicinals. These types of medicinals may expedite a ruptured aneurysm episode.

If you want to gain further insight into this condition, you can check out a book called *When the Air Hits Your Brain: Tales of Neurosurgery* by Frank Vertosick, Jr., MD. There is a section that presents a case involving mortality from an "accidentally ruptured aneurysm."

This is a critical condition. When you receive this letter, you should immediately contact your patient and strongly advise her to go in for a thorough examination as soon as possible; and if tests do confirm cerebral aneurysm, then seek immediate treatment.

Case Study #4: Hemilateral Edema – It's *Not* Alzheimer's Disease!

Q: A 70 y/o male patient began having symptoms of slow and slurred speech and motor function impairment. He was diagnosed with Alzheimer's disease (AD) by a neurologist, and unfortunately, has not shown any discernible improvement after taking medication for many years now.

Recently, he visited me seeking treatment for right-sided edema of the arms and legs. I prescribed Wu Ling San (Nephritis Formula) adding large doses of Huang Qi, Yin Xing Ye, Dan Shen, Ren Shen, Chuan Qi, Tian Ma, Cang Zhu, Fu Ling, and Ze Xie. Do you think this is a good approach?

A: Current research indicates that symptoms of AD arise from extracellular senile plaques formed by the deposition of beta-amyloid protein (A□ protein) and from intracellular neurofibrillary tangles formed by the accumulation of tau protein. At first, damage to the medial temporal lobe (e.g., hippocampus) results in memory loss, which becomes more noticeable over time as diffuse cortical atrophy occurs. As the disease progesses, degeneration of cholinergic neurons in the basal forebrain structure occurs, which is likely the main factor in the severe decline of cognitive abilities.

The rate AD progresses varies among individuals. Symptoms may develop slowly over a period of years, but will be very pronounced in later stages with relatively rapid degeneration. Typically, progression from the first onset of symptoms (e.g., mild memory loss (forgets where keys are placed), mood swings, mild coordination problems) to the moderate stage (e.g., difficulty planning and solving problems, decline of language recall and expression, confusion about time and place) may occur slowly over a period of years. But progression from the moderate stage to the late stage (e.g., severe memory loss (fails to recognize friends and family), severe cognitive and motor function impairment, hallucinations, weight loss, incontinence) of this pathocondition usually develops rapidly over a 6-month period.

In my opinion, if the patient really has AD, it is highly unlikely that he would remain in the same cognitive and motor function state after 10 years have elapsed. To me, this suggests that the diagnosis of AD is inacccurate. These types of symptoms (e.g., forgetfulness, memory loss, disorientation, expressive aphasia) could be more aptly diagnosed as chronic cerebrovascular disease, a chronic CNS disorder, or cerebral atrophy. Hemilateral edema has nothing to do with Alzheimer's disease; most likely it is due to nutritional imbalance, remaining in a sitting position for too long, or other systemic disease (e.g., renal disease).

I agree with the approach of "first treating the edema," but suggest you change the formula to a blood-quickening qi-supplementing formula such as Bu Yang Huan Wu Tang adding Si Ni Tang, Huang Qin, and large doses of Ren Shen/Chuan Qi Powder (best to use the raw, pulverized form of these medicinals, gradually increasing the dose up to 5–8 qian/day).

Case Study #5: Posterior Cerebral Artery "Beating Like a Drum"

Q: The patient's blood pressure is normal, and he does *not* have headaches or neck pain and stiffness. It's just that his posterior cerebral artery (PCA) pulsates forcefully and frequently, and sometimes it almost feels as if it's "beating like a drum." Why would this be? How should I treat ths condition?

A: A PCA pulsating too quickly and too strongly indicates the condition arises from yang hyperactivity of the urinary bladder channel. In severe cases, patients will be able to hear their heartbeats "beating like a drum."

There are many potential causes for this with the most common being sleep deprivation or excessive sexual activity, or both of these together, which makes this condition even more likely to arise.

Treating this condition requires quieting the spirit with heavy settling medicinals such as Jian Ling Tang adding Gan Cao and Long Yan Gan. If the pulse pounds so forcefully that it "beats like a drum," then add The Three Yellows; and if headache presents, then add Tian Ma. If it turns out that your patient does suffer from sleep deprivation and excessive sexual activity, then you could also consider adding Zhi Mu and large doses of Huang Bo, or instead prescribe an yin-enriching fire-downbearing formula such as Zhi Bo Di Huang Tang adding Sheng Mu Li and Sheng Long Gu. The most important advice you can give your patient is to get enough sleep—it's optimal to get in 8–10 hours every night!

Case Study #6: Cerebellar Atrophy and Cerebral Infarction Inducing Dizziness

Q: A heavy-set male patient with high blood pressure, who says he still "enjoys his share of alcohol," recently went in for a medical examination due to frequent dizziness. MRI results revealed cerebral infarction and cerebellar atrophy. Stool and urine are normal. Please offer your advice and guidance on treating this patient.

A: Both cerebrovascular and brain stem infarction can cause dizziness, while cerebellar atrophy will present with balance and gait disorders often manifesting in the difficulty and apprehension of walking downhill or down stairs (even if the slope is very slight!).

For the treatment of dizziness caused by cerebral infarction, I can suggest three approaches:

1) Bu Yang Huan Wu Tang adding The Three Great Yang-Supplementers, Tian Ma, Huang Qin, and Ren Shen/Chuan Qi Powder.

2) Ban Xia Tian Ma Bai Zhu San adding large doses of Tian Ma and Huang Qi along with Chuan Qi, Chi Shao, and Yin Xing Ye.

3) In cases involving visceral agitation, then prescribe Ban Xia Tian Ma Bai Zhu San adding Gan Cao, Long Yan Rou, and Da Zao.

Case Study #7: Tuberculous Meningitis

Q: I have a 61 y/o female patient with tuberculous meningitis. Two months ago, she began presenting with exterior pattern symptoms of headache, mild fever, body aches, and dry cough. One week ago, she suddenly began vomiting and suffered from a severe, splitting headache. After hospital admission, examination revealed tuberculous meningitis.

Now, after taking a regimen of antibiotics, the headache and vomiting have resolved, but the nausea remains. Her doctors told her that she needs to continue treatment for at least 1 year. What is the best way to approach this condition?

A: Tuberculous meningitis can be identified as Shao Yang heat pattern. Thus, you can prescribe Xiao Chai Hu Tang adding Qing Hao, Zhi Mu, Di Gu Pi, and Tian Ma. If increased ICP and abscesses present, but a shunt has *not* been surgically implanted, then you should add The Four Lings to promote resolution.

An integrated regimen of TCM medicinals and Western medicine drugs should be administered concomitantly. After about 3 months, ask the patient to get another blood, mucus, and CSF culture performed. If these results show no sign of the mycobacterium, then continue administering the therapeutic regimen for 3 more months changing the formula to a blood-supplementing essence-replenishing formula such as Zuo Gui Yin adding Tian Ma, Qing Hao, Zhi Mu, Di Gu Pi, Chai Hu, and Qin Jiao.

Section 3: Concussion

Case Study #1: Post-Concussion Syndrome – Double Vision

Q: On the afternoon of August 16, a 9 y/o boy accidentally fell off his bed and hit his head on the floor while playing. His parents were concerned that he may have suffered a concussion. Sure enough, that evening he developed symptoms of headache and nausea. He was rushed to ER and admitted to the hospital, where he received mannitol (osmotic diuretic) infusions. The next day he still had a severe headache. The MRI revealed a small hemorrhagic lesion in his brain and he had double vision (diplopia).

The attending physician planned to give the patient drugs to promote the absorption of the hemorrhage, but his mother came to me first to ask my opinion. To tell you the truth I am not sure myself about the prognosis of solely relying on Western medicine treatment for this condition. I hope you can give me advice and direction on this case. Your input and instruction is greatly appreciated!

A: Post-concussion diplopia can be caused by damage to the visual center at the back of the head or the oculomotor nerve and optic chiasma in the brain stem. Persistence of cerebral edema and headache despite administration of mannitol suggests that the brain injury has produced a large amount of exudate with brain tissue (cell) swelling and elevated intracranial pressure (ICP). The MRI also reveals a hemorrhagic lesion. Taking these factors into consideration, this condition can clearly be identified as stasis heat with water amassment pattern.

As for TCM treatment, you can prescribe a blood-nourishing blood-quickening, stasis-dispelling pain-relieving, and network vessel-freeing channel-regulating formula such as Ru Mo Si Wu Tang adding The Four Lings, Tian Ma, Huang Qin, Huang Lian, and Chuan Qi to expedite stabilization of ICP, minimize the area damaged, and reduce the extent and severity of the ensuing drug side effects and complications. Once ICP has *stabilized*, you can add The Three Great Yang-Supplementers (gradually increasing the dose up to 5 qian each) to the original formula.

Administer this treatment for a period of time until the symptoms have *stabilized*, then change the prescription to a blood-quickening qi-supplementing formula such as Bu Yang Huan Wu Tang or Sheng Yu

Tang, or a spleen- and stomach-supplementing, phlegm-damp-transforming, and wind-stabilizing formula such as Ban Xia Tian Ma Bai Zhu San. Just make sure to include Chuan Qi, Chuan Xiong, Chi Shao, and Yin Xing Ye. The patient should continue taking this formula for a minimum of 6 months–1 year. There will be noticeable improvement in the patient's condition. If the patient has epileptic seizures, then the formula should be adjusted based on the presenting signs and symptoms.

Presently, the treatment of cerebral hemorrhage in most hospitals involves promoting spontaneous resorption by administering the anticoagulants aspirin and warfarin (Coumadin), which merely function to lower blood viscosity. There are *not* any pharmaceuticals specifically targeted at treating this condition. TCM medicinals, on the other hand, have proven efficacy in facilitating spontaneous resorption and can prevent hemorrhaging at other sites. You can definitely prescribe TCM formulas for this patient!

Case Study #2: Head Trauma – Concussion and Hemorrhage

Q: A patient of mine suffered a concussion that caused intracranial hemorrhage and edema. The patient was admitted to the hospital for treatment and management, and his family sought my consultation for TCM treatment.

After administering TCM medicinals, an MRI revealed that 2/3 of the hemorrhagic lesion had already been resorbed. The patient's doctor prescribed antiepileptic drugs and processed the patient for discharge.

A: Naturally, in cases of concussion resulting in epidural, subdural, or subarachnoid hemorrhage, the sooner resorption occurs, the better. This will minimize the amount of brain cells damaged from compression and the ensuing swelling and lysis (necrosis), dramatically reducing the potential for causing behavioral changes, cognitive impairment, and progressive brain atrophy. You must be vigilant about these potential outcomes. Brain hemorrhage will usually resolve spontaneously within 2 weeks. If spontaneous hemorrhage does not resolve within 2 weeks, TCM identifies this as cold stasis pattern.

As is the case for many types of brain disorders, antiepileptic medication must be administered to prevent epileptic seizures. Severe (e.g., grand mal) epileptic seizures may lead to cerebral vasospasm, cerebral infarction, or cerebral infarction secondary to cerebral hemorrhage, resulting in enlargement of the necrosed area and an increased severity and frequency of epileptic attacks—a viscous cycle!

My belief is that antiepileptic medication should be concomitantly administered along with TCM medicinals that regulate the constitution. This integrative approach provides the best method of both accelerating the resorption of blood and protecting the patient's brain tissue (cells) from irreversible loss of function.

Case Study #3: Concussion – Cold Hands and Feet and Profuse Sweating Following Mannitol Administration

Q: A patient suffered a concussion and was admitted into the hospital where he was administered a mannitol (osmotic diuretic) injection. Afterwards, the patient developed cold hands and feet and profuse sweating. Why would this happen?

A: Once the condition of a patient with concussion stabilizes, the patient will be susceptible to a host of autonomic nervous system and neuropsychiatric symptoms, such as spontaneous sweating, night sweats, aversion to cold (phantom cold), aversion to heat (phantom heat), fear, fright palpitations, circadian rhythm disturbance, late afternoon tidal heat, etc. These symptoms will resolve as brain circulation improves and returns to normal.

Case Study #4: Post-Concussion Complication – Night Sweats

Q: I am treating a 41 y/o male patient who suffered a head trauma injury with intracranial hemorrhage. He never underwent a cranial decompression procedure, but stayed in the hospital for 6 months following the accident, receiving medication until recovery.

What is strange about this case is that ever since the accident occurred, every night for the past 3 years just about 5 minutes after falling asleep, he has profuse sweating "flowing like water" on the neck and upper back. The patient has received both TCM and Western medicine treatment, but none has provided any significant results for his night sweats. How would you treat this condition?

A: Patients suffering from a concussion resulting in intracranial hemorrhage and leading to the complication of night sweats can be identified as Yang Ming channel with Shao Yang enduring heat pattern. You can consider prescribing a liver-settling wind-extinguishing and yin-enriching yang-subduing formula such as Jian Ling Tang (including Gan Cao) adding Da Zao (or Long Yan), Huang Bo (up to 8 qian), Qing Hao, Zhi Mu, Di Gu Pi, Ma Huang Gen, and possibly Chuan Qi. Following the administration of these medicinals, his symptoms should rapidly improve.

Remember! In the future, if the patient catches a cold (external contraction), you should *not* prescribe Ma Huang due to its potent sweat-promoting actions. If cough presents, then you can add extra amounts of Xing Ren, Gui Zhi, and Hou Po to avoid hyperstimulation of the patient's perspiration centers. You can also administer acupuncture treatment, selecting the acupoints Feng Chi (GB20), Feng Fu (DU16), Bai Hui (DU20), San Yin Jiao (SP6), Tai Xi (KD3), Xuan Zhong (GB39), Tai Chong (LV3), and Shen Men (HT7).

Case Study #5: Post-Concussion Syndrome or Neurosis?

Q: A 50 y/o female patient suffers from post-concussion complications of blurred vision in her left eye, explaining "it feels like it's swollen" (but actually it's not!). She also has mental fogginess, limb weakness, dizziness, nausea, a sensation of heat on the vertex of the head, heaviness in the chest, and slight edema of the arms and legs.

In March of this year, she was standing at the doorway of a bank when the metal security door dropped down on her forehead. The MRI revealed nothing abnormal with her neck and head, and her blood pressure is normal, but the patient continues to worry about the concussion and insists she is suffering from post-concussion syndrome (PCS). What do you think I should do?

A: This does *not* sound like post-concussion complications to me; it sounds more like neurosis. People with neurotic disorders have an uncanny way of finding "points of attack" to blame for all of their discomforts (either real or perceived). If they have been injured, hit by something, contracted an infection, been irritated, felt pressured in some way, etc., they just cannot get over it, mired and overcome by a cascade of travails.

You can prescribe a heat-clearing phlegm-transforming formula such as Wen Dan Tang or a spleen- and stomach-supplementing, phlegm-damp-transforming, and wind-stabilizing formula such as Ban Xia Tian Ma Bai Zhu San adding Gan Cao, Da Zao, Qing Hao, Zhi Mu, Di Gu Pi, and Yu Sheng Wan.

Make sure to verify if the patient really does have edema of the arms and legs or if it just "feels" like heaviness and swelling. If there really is edema, then add large doses of Bai Zhu, Fu Ling, and Ze Xie. If there is just the "feeling" of heaviness and swelling, then simply add Yu Sheng Wan (quiets the spirit and calms the nerves) and combinations of heart- and spleen-supplementing and blood-nourishing spirit-calming medicinals such as Da Zao, Long Yan Gan, or Hei Tang (dark, unrefined, cane sugar). If pitting edema presents, then add The Three Great Yang-Supplementers.

Case Study #6: Amnesia and Dysphasia Following Car Accident

Q: I have a 35 y/o male patient who suffers from amnesia (trouble remembering complex ideas and concepts) and dysphasia (speaks like a young child) following a car accident. Motor function is normal. How would you treat this patient?

A: It is very common to suffer amnesia following a concussion. The first thing I would do is determine whether he has undergone surgery and/or been administered large amounts of corticosteroids. If *not*, then prescribe Ru Mo Si Wu Tang adding Dan Shen, Chuan Qi, Yin Xing Ye, Huang Qi, and a small dose of Da Huang. This formula will activate the blood, break stasis, and promote circulation, thus resolving the static blood (thrombosis) in the prefrontal and temporal lobes that is causing this patient's symptoms.

Section 4: Parkinson's Disease

Case Study #1: Parkinson's Disease

Q: This is the first Parkinson's disease (PD) patient I have treated. I prescribed Bu Yang Huan Wu Tang adding Gan Jiang, Fu Zi, Rou Gui, Huang Qin, Ren Shen, and Lu Rong (powder). I also needled Feng Chi (GB20), He Gu (LI4), Zu San Li (ST36), Tai Chong (LV3), and Tou Lin Qi (GB15). I added Tou Lin Qi (GB15) because I recently read that research indicates this acupoint improves blood circulation to the brain. The patient currently takes 2 dopamine pills per day.

Please share with me your experiences in treating this condition: treatment approach, formula variants, prognosis, etc. Thank you again!

A: I am thrilled that you have embarked into the fascinating realm of neurology! The prevalence of PD will continue increasing in the future, so you should keep pace with the latest discoveries and developments in this field.

For the treatment of PD, acupuncture assumes a complementary role combined with the primary treatment of TCM medicinals. Indeed, Tou Lin Qi (GB15) may also be effective, but in my experience, Feng Chi (GB20) is the essential acupoint for treating this condition.

As for TCM medicinals, a blood-quickening qi-supplementing formula such as Bu Yang Huan Wu Tang is an excellent choice. And yes, it is also a good idea to add The Three Great Yang-Supplementers, starting out with small doses and gradually increasing. However, you don't want to overdo it! Even if CNS symptoms (e.g., tremor, rigidity) are severe, with concomitant administration of Madopar (Levodopa + benserazide (a decarboxylase inhibitor)) at 6–8 times or more per day, the maximum dose of Gan Jiang, Fu Zi, and Rou Gui I would prescribe is a combined total of 7 qian. For Ren Shen (powder), you should incrementally increase the dose up to 4–5 qian/day.

By administering this integrative approach, the side effects (e.g., dyskinesia) of the Western medicine drugs can be remedied, enabling the patient to walk with greater stability and maintain more fluid functional movement.

Case Study #2: Limb Tremor – Early Sign of Parkinson's Disease?

Q: I have a 53 y/o female patient presenting with tremor in the left hand, which is more pronounced in cold weather and when fatigued. The patient had similar symptoms previously when she had frozen shoulder of her left arm, but that condition has already resolved. This winter after the first big cold front, the tremor in the fingers of her left hand intensified.

Based on my limited experience treating other Parkinson's disease (PD) patients who had this type of tremor at the onset, I suspect that this patient is also presenting with an early sign of PD. Thus, I prescribed Ban Xia Tian Ma Bai Zhu San adding Quan Xie, Wu Gong, Bai Jiang Can, Yu Sheng Wan, and Niu Huang Qing Xin Wan. After taking this formula her symptoms dramatically improved. Please share your views and advice on this case.

A: Yes, your description of this case does suggest PD, and the formula you prescribed should definitely be effective. However, Niu Huang Qing Xin Wan (clears heat and resolves toxin and frees the orifices and quiets the spirit) is very expensive, and unless the patient is financially well off, she will *not* be able to afford this for very long.

PD is not a condition that can be cured in a short period of time. It is a chronic condition that requires long-term administration of medicinals in order to reduce the severity of symptoms, slow down the rate of degeneration, and ensure a good quality of life. The long-term administration of Bu Yang Huan Wu Tang adding Gan Jiang, Fu Zi, Huang Qin, and Ren Shen offers excellent efficacy for the treatment of PD. This is the simplest and best approach I have found!

Case Study #3: Early-Onset Parkinson's Disease

Q: A 35 y/o female patient came to my clinic presenting with finger tremor and chest distention. The patient said that prior to getting married about 10 years ago, any time she felt excessive nervousness or anger the fingers of her right hand would shake. About one year after marriage, her symptoms gradually worsened.

Recently, she experiences resting tremor even in the absence of emotional swings or pressure, and she feels distention in the chest and sighs frequently. I diagnosed this condition as Parkinson's disease (PD) and prescribed Ban Xia Tian Ma Bai Zhu San adding Huang Qi (2 liang), Ban Xia, Fu Ling, Ren Shen, and Chuan Qi (large dose of 3 qian). Do you think this is a good approach?

A: Hand tremor in a 35 y/o patient does suggest early-onset Parkinson's disease. You can prescribe Bu Yang Huan Wu Tang adding The Three Great Yang-Supplementers and Ren Shen/Chuan Qi Powder. That's right, I noticed you did *not* prescribe The Three Insects this time, as we discussed before, you do *not* need to for PD.

For frequent sighing and distention in the chest, you can add large doses of Ren Shen (start out with 3 qian gradually increasing to 5 qian/day) and Huang Qi (start out with 2 liang incrementally increasing by 1/2 liang doses up to a maximum of 4 liang) to remedy these symptoms.

For Parkinson's patients suffering from depression, you can consider adding medicinals such as Yu Sheng Wan, Da Zao, Long Yan Gan, or You Gui Yin (pulverized raw powder) to your therapeutic regimen.

Case Study #4: Parkinson's Disease, CSF Hypovolemia, or Cerebral Atrophy?

Q: A 57 y/o male patient with severe neck rigidity so tight it causes extension (head tilted back), didn't feel up for making a visit to my clinic in person, so a family member sought my consultation instead.

The patient's history is as follows: Three years ago, he began having tremors in his fingers, and over the past month his neck rigidity has become so severe that his neck involuntarily remains in an extended position. Even when he uses his hands to draw his neck forward, not long after the neck will gradually slide back into extension. It is difficult for him to get around, and that's why he doesn't want to leave the house.

During the past few days, his neck has been gradually angling to the left side. I am concerned that he may be showing early signs of

Parkinson's disease (PD). What is your assessment of this patient?

A: Involuntary extension of the neck and spasms suggest CSF hypovolemia or cerebral atrophy, *not* PD. As for treating this condition with TCM medicinals, you can consider prescribing You Gui Yin (supplements kidney yang, supplements qi and blood, and eliminates dampness and pain) combining Bu Yang Huan Wu Tang (quickens the blood and supplements qi) adding Ren Shen/Chuan Qi Powder.

In the past, I have also had successful results prescribing Ban Xia Tian Ma Bai Zhu San (supplements the spleen and stomach, transforms damp-wind, and stabilizes wind) adding Huang Qi (serves as the sovereign medicinal), Ren Shen/Chuan Qi Powder, The Three Insects, and Lu Rong (powder). You can consider either of these approaches based on your patients presenting signs, symptoms, and patterns.

Case Study #5: Cerebral Atrophy, Parkinson's Disease, or Atypical Parkonsonism?

Q: Four years ago this patient first experienced symptoms of lower limb flaccidity, slow and disjointed speech (expressive aphasia), and hand tremors upon exertion, prompting him to go in for a thorough examination by a neurologist.

MRI findings resulted in the diagnosis of cerebral atrophy, and after receiving years of ineffective Western medical treatment, he lost faith in their approach. The patient has a good appetite and nutritional intake and his stool is normal.

Do you think this diagnosis could be accurate? How should I treat this condition? What is the prognosis? Even if TCM can successfully remedy his symptoms, is it possible to restore brain function back to normal?

A: Based on your description of his symptoms, it does *not* sound like he has cerebral atrophy. It seems more likely to be "atypical Parkinsonism" and specifically vascular Parkinsonism (aka multi-infarct Parkinsonism) involving progressive atherosclerosis and embolization.

You can prescribe a blood-quickening qi-supplementing formula such as Bu Yang Huan Wu Tang adding The Three Great Yang-Supplementers, Huang Qin, and Ren Shen/Chuan Qi Powder. The condition should gradually stabilize over time. If you want to gain a more in-depth understanding of this condition, I highly recommend reading the book *Neuropathy: Traditional Chinese Herbal Treatment in a Modern Medical Environment* (**中西醫結合中醫腦神經治療學**).

Case Study #6: Lower Jaw Spasms and Twitching

Q: A 73 y/o female patient began having involuntary spasms in her lower jaw 10 years ago. Recently, the condition has intensified over the past 2 weeks to the point where aside from its subsiding during sleep, her lower jaw continuously spasms and twitches. However, it does *not* affect her speech, and her blood pressure and stool are normal. Please share your views on this case. Thank you!

A: An elderly female patient presenting with lower jaw spasm and twitching clearly indicates some type of extrapyramidal involvement. The TCM classical pathologic terminology for this condition is spasm (**痙攣** jìngluán) and tugging and slackening (clonic spasm) (瘛瘲 chì zòng), which is now commonly described as Parkinsonism.

You can consider prescribing a blood-quickening qi-supplementing formula such as Bu Yang Huan Wu Tang or a qi-supplementing center-fortifying blood-supplementing formula such as Gui Qi Jian Zhong Tang. Just make sure to add The Three Great Yang-Supplementers, The Three Insects, Huang Qin, Ren Shen/Chuan Qi Powder, and Yu Sheng Wan. Remember! It is imperative to add Yu Sheng Wan for this type of condition!

You can also administer acupuncture (warm needling) selecting the acupoints Feng Chi (GB20), Tian Zhu (UB10), He Gu (LI4), and Zu San Li (ST36). Treating this condition will take a long time and a lot of patience, but eventually this approach should produce effective results.

Section 5: Essential Tremor

Case Study #1: Head Tremor – Essential Tremor and Cerebellar Atrophy

Q: A 50 y/o male patient began having head tremors about 3 years ago. When he is nervous or angry his tongue will even tremble, and the only time he does *not* experience these tremors is during sleep. The patient went through a full range of tests to rule out dopamine, blood sugar, and blood pressure abnormalities. His diet and sleep habits are healthy, but he is impatient and loses his temper easily.

I diagnosed his condition as head tremor (essential tremor) and prescribed Bu Yang Huan Wu Tang adding The Three Great Yang-Supplementers, Huang Qin, The Three Insects, and Ren Shen/Chuan Qi Powder. Is there anything in particular about this condition that I should look out for?

A: When head tremor presents (especially in males), you *cannot* overlook the possibility of Parkinson's disease (PD) or brain stem pathology. Now let's take a look at what the cause of your patient's head tremor could be.

Generally, if head tremor presents when a person is calm and at rest (e.g., sitting down talking, watching television), this is called "quiet" tremor, which is strongly suggestive of Parkinson's disease. If the head tremor is brought on by action (e.g., walking, working with hands), this is called "intention" tremor, which is suggestive of essential tremor, cerebellar atrophy, or pathologies of the nerves or vasculature in sub-cerebellar regions. One sign in particular that verifies the diagnosis of cerebellar atrophy is when the patient cannot walk down the stairs even when accompanied by someone alongside (oftentimes even the slightest degree of slope will cause reluctance and apprehension!). For all of these conditions you can prescribe a blood-quickening qi-supplementing formula such as Bu Yang Huan Wu Tang variant.

In cases of elevated intracranial pressure (ICP), the patient will present with neck flaccidity and weakness, and a gait like someone with poliomyelitis, lurching forward one step at a time. For these patients, it is best to prescribe a spleen- and stomach-supplementing, phlegm-damp-transforming, and wind-stabilizing formula such as Ban

Xia Tian Ma Bai Zhu San combining Bu Yang Huan Wu Tang adding the Three Great Yang-Supplementers and Ren Shen/Chuan Qi Powder.

Overall, for any type of brain atrophy, degeneration, or dementia caused by vascular disease, long-term administration of Bu Yang Huan Wu Tang variant will prove very effective.

Case Study #2: Essential Tremor in the Elderly

Q: A 75 y/o female patient began having tremors in her upper and lower limbs about 10 years ago. At first, these tremors only occurred when she was in stressful situations and under exertion, with the tremors on the left side much more pronounced. When she is at rest there is *no* tremor, and she does *not* have any motor, speech, or cognitive impairment. Could this be Parkinson's disease?

A: There are many potential causes of arm and leg tremor, with the most common being physiological factors, cerebrovascular and CNS disorders, cerebral atrophy, cerebellar disorders, chorea, and PD. One of the main symptoms of Parkinson's disease is hand tremor, which is usually a resting tremor that classically presents as a "pill-rolling" action of the hands, and typically tremor in the legs is rare up until the late stage when some patients also develop a shuffling gait. Conversely, the tremors presenting in chorea (dyskinesias) occur when the body is engaged in movement or action.

However, TCM treatment for all of these conditions is very similar—based on the same pattern identification and treatment principles. You can prescribe Bu Yang Huan Wu Tang (quickens the blood and supplements qi) adding The Three Great Yang-Supplementers, Ren Shen/Chuan Qi Powder, and Huang Qin as the main formula.

If the patient presents with spleen and stomach vacuity, then you can consider prescribing a spleen-fortifying qi-supplementing and phlegm-damp transforming formula such as Bu Zhong Yi Qi Tang, Shen Ling Bai Zhu San, Xiang Sha Liu Jun Zi Tang, or Ban Xia Tian Ma Bai Zhu San. Just make sure to add in the essential medicinals of the main formula—Bu Yang Huan Wu Tang.

Case Study #3: Lower Jaw and Upper Limb Tremor – Essential

Tremor in the Elderly

Q: An 83 y/o female patient began having tremor in her lower jaw and right upper limb. Generally, the tremor *only* occurs when she feels nervous or under stress and *not* when she is at rest or talking. Drinking a small amount of alcohol also tends to help remedy the condition.

I diagnosed her condition as essential tremor of the elderly and prescribed Bu Yang Huan Wu Tang adding The Three Insects, Qi Cao, Ren Shen, Long Yan Gan, and Yu Sheng Wan. The patient has taken this formula for over 2 months *without* any discernible effects. Please off your advice on this case. Thank you!

A: Yes, her symptoms do suggest essential tremor. However, it is *not* necessary to add the The Three Insects and Qi Cao; instead, I would try adding small doses of The Three Great Yang-Supplementers. Also, make sure to remind her to eat healthy (full spectrum of nutrients), keep active, and get enough sleep. Keep me updated!

IV. CARDIOVASCULAR DISEASE

There is more to the etiology of cardiovascular disease than just angina pectoris and myocardial infarction. For instance, anemia can also cause arrhythmia and sweating from the chest. The key is to be aware of these complexities and nuances in order to accurately diagnose and effectively treat pathoconditions of the cardiovascular system. This section also includes peripheral vascular disorders such as intermittent claudication and deep vein thrombosis.

Case Study #1: Wolff-Parkinson-White Syndrome

Q1: A friend of mine has had a feeling of oppression in the chest since childhood, but never underwent any special investigations or treatment. Recently, his company provided free medical examinations for employees, which resulted in the diagnosis of Wolff-Parkinson-White (WPW) syndrome, a condition that commonly causes chest pain and tightness, palpitations, and tachycardia among other symptoms. His cardiologist recommended performing a radiofrequency catheter ablation procedure; otherwise, he ran the risk of ventricular fibrillation that could rapidly lead to sudden cardiac arrest and death.

The only symptoms the patient has are occasional palpitations and these really do *not* affect his livelihood or quality of life at all. Is this condition really as severe as the Western medical doctors say it is? Considering the potential complications of surgery, what advice should I give him? Forego surgery and solely administer TCM medicinal treatment? Or go ahead with the surgery first and then administer TCM medicinal treatment to regulate his constitution?

A1: If you are *certain* about the WPW syndrome diagnosis, I am *not* opposed to performing the catheter ablation procedure. His cardiologist will have determined whether the patient has the classic or concealed type, which will determine the treatment options. For a classic type, the cardiologist may advise the patient to go ahead with the catheter ablation procedure, which offers the potential for promising results. This is a relatively minor procedure that is, in principle, very safe.

As for TCM medicinals, you can consider prescribing a formula variant such as Zhi Gan Cao Tang, Gan Mai Da Zao Tang Combining Ban Xia Hou Po Tang, Zhi Bo Di Huang Tang, or Wen Dan Tang adding Fu Ling and Hou Po (large doses each), Sheng Long Gu, and Sheng Mu Li. All of these variants should provide effective results.

Q2: A 26 y/o male patient experienced symptoms of palpitations and tachycardia, prompting him to go in for an examination. He was diagnosed with Wolff-Parkinson-White (WPW) syndrome. Two years ago, the patient had a surgical procedure done on his heart.

Since then, he has been taking Western medicine drugs continuously over the past 2 years, yet he still frequently has palpitations and tachycardia. These attacks are very painful and distressing. What would you do for this patient?

A2: WPW syndrome is a congenital condition characterized by intermittent tachycardias and described as a type of atrioventricular reentrant tachycardia in which there is an extra electrical pathway of the heart. Regardless of the Western medicine treatment administered (e.g., vagal maneuvers, radiofrequency catheter ablation, drug therapy), the TCM therapeutic approach is pretty much the same.

I would consider prescribing a formula variant such as Xiao Chai Hu Tang combining Long Gu Mu Li Tang; Jian Ling Tang adding Gan Cao, Long Yan Gan, Huang Qin, Mu Dan Pi, and Zhi Zi; Gan Mai Da Zao Tang Combining Ban Xia Hou Po Tang; or Wen Dan Tang adding Sheng Long Gu and Sheng Mu Li.

Administration of TCM treatment can effectively relieve symptoms, manage the condition, and promote a better quality of life.

Case Study #2: Coma Following Cardiac Arrest

Q: A patient is now comatose after incurring sudden cardiac arrest, but stimulus to the fingers did elicit a contraction response. What is the best approach for treating this pathocondition? How long does it usually take until the patient regains consciousness? Thank you for your ongoing guidance and advice!

A: Coma following cardiac arrest results from the cerebral hypoxia brought on by impaired cerebral perfusion. You can prescribe Bu Yang Huan Wu Tang adding The Three Great Yang-Supplementers, Huang Qin, and Ren Shen/Chuan Qi Powder. After administering this formula for a period of time, the patient will show gradual improvement and eventually regain consciousness. After regaining consciousness, the patient may feel sluggishness and weakness with limp limbs, weak neck, inability to lift eyes upwards, and drooling similar to that of a stroke patient.

Assess the patient's condition after administering the above formula for 1 month, and if there has *not* been much progress, then change the formula to You Gui Yin adding Huang Qi and Ren Shen/Chuan Qi Powder. If there is neck and lumbar weakness, start out by adding Xi Lu Rong (powder) (5 fen) and incrementally increase the dose by 5 fen each time up to as much as 3 qian/day. The patient's family must have patience. This therapeutic regimen will take time, but gradually the patient will achieve substantial recovery of functional capacity and increased quality of life.

Case Study #3: What is Marfan Syndrome?

Q: I have a 13 y/o female patient who is 178 cm tall with disproportionately long arms and legs. Recently, she has experienced shortness of breath during activity, so her mother brought her in for a visit. Ten years ago, her father suddenly died as he was eating dinner, and on his death certificate, the listed cause was ruptured aneurysm. Ever since then she has been worried about following in his fateful footsteps.

Five years ago (8 y/o), she experienced irregular heartbeats, prompting a thorough cardiac examination and subsequent diagnosis of heart valve disorder. Considering her disproportionately long arms and legs and concomitant heart condition, her doctors suspected Marfan syndrome, but since there were *no* other specific symptoms to support the diagnosis, she was advised to return for follow-up investigation every 6 months.

Please share with me your knowledge of Marfan syndrome? What kind of treatment and/or advice can TCM provide?

A: Marfan syndrome is a genetic disorder of the connective tissue caused by defective genes and commonly leads to abnormalities in the limbs, eyes, and internal organs (i.e., heart). Most patients will present with a distinguishing feature of long arms that extend down near their knees. In classical TCM texts, this condition is described as abnormal contention (異相 yì xi□ng) or "out of sync." Throughout antiquity, a number of famous leaders, both civic and military, were described as having this feature, such as the legendary character Liu Bei in *Romance of the Three Kingdoms* (三國演義 *San Guo Yan Yi*) with "arms and legs that hung beyond his knees."

As for your patient, if she does *not* present with any symptoms, then treatment is *not* necessary. If symptoms do arise, then simply identify the pattern and treat the symptoms accordingly. For instance, if cataracts present, then treat the cataracts; if cardiovascular disorders present, then treat the cardiovascular disorders, and so on. Usually, these complications will not cause mortality, but patients with this condition can expect a slightly shorter life span than average (late 60s).

There is no evidence whatsoever that her father's aneurysm had anything to do with Marfan's, so she doesn't need to worry about that at all! If taking TCM medicinals would make the patient feel at ease, then you can prescribe long-term administration of Bu Yang Huan Wu Tang variant. If edema presents, then add The Four Lings and Ren Shen/Chuan Qi Powder.

Case Study #4: Angina Pectoris (Stable Angina), Psychosomatic Disorder, or Esophageal Ulcer?

Q: A 43 y/o male patient has experienced pain and discomfort in his chest for the past 3 years. He was diagnosed with angina pectoris by Western medical doctors and administered treatment with nitroglycerin and anticoagulants.

Three months ago, while in bed at night, he incurred an attack of sudden, severe pain in his chest with pain radiating to his left-side pericardium channel. At other times following this initial attack, he would experience similar sudden episodes of pain when at rest, which forced him to check into the emergency room on numerous occasions.

Previously these episodes would only occur at night or dawn with the chest pain lasting for increasingly longer durations. A recent episode lasted 6 hours and went unremedied despite taking medication and receiving an injection.

Do you think this patient's condition would improve by having a surgical procedure performed?

A: From your description, it sounds like this patient may *not* actually be suffering from angina pectoris; instead, his symptoms may derive from psychoneurosis or psychosomatic disorder. If the patency of this patient's coronary arteries were compromised to the degree of manifesting in these types of symptoms, then his cardiologist would have either recommended a surgical procedure or he would have passed away by now.

Thus, I recommend you prescribe a spirit-calming formula and try to help him open up and resolve underlying psychological issues. By doing so, the patient's condition should improve. There are so many cases of this sort nowadays.

However, you must also rule out other possible causes of this patient's condition such as the following:

1) GERD-induced esophageal ulcer.

2) Intake of oral medication without adequate water or while eating, resulting in the pill or capsule sticking to the mucous membrane and causing erosion.

3) Eating a "bedtime snack" of spicy, scalding hot soup right before going to sleep may induce acid reflux and result in these nighttime "attacks."

For these types of conditions, you can prescribe Bu Yang Huan Wu Tang adding Ban Xia, Fu Ling, Lai Fu Zi, Hai Piao Xiao, The Three Yellows, Yuan Hu, and Mu Xiang. Remember! It is important to instruct the patient to sip and gargle the decocted liquid, and make sure it is taken either cold or at room temperature. You could also needle the acupoints Tai Chong (LV3), Zhong Feng (LV4), Zu San Li (ST36), Nei Guan (PC6), and Shen Men (HT7) as well.

Case Study #5: Arrhythmia Resulting from Anemia

Q: Last year a 38 y/o male patient suffered from acute lower limb edema, difficulty breathing, and oliguria (urine output < 500 cc). He went to the hospital for examination and was prescribed diuretics and antihypertensives, and advised to maintain a low-salt diet. After his symptoms resolved, he was then prescribed Aspirin.

Currently, the patient has *no* symptoms, but has a cardiac contractility of 15% (normal range 55–75%). He wants to take TCM medicinals to regulate his constitution. Do you have any advice or suggestions?

A: The patient's signs and symptoms suggest chronic heart failure with anemia, and the patient may also have mild lung blood depression (stasis) and obstruction (i.e., pericardial effusion, pleural effusion).

For this condition, you can prescribe a blood-quickening qi-supplementing formula such as Bu Yang Huan Wu Tang adding Gan Jiang, Fu Zi, The Four Lings, Ting Li Zi, Fang Ji, Huang Qin, Ma Huang, Xing Ren, and Ren Shen/Chuan Qi Powder. Or you could prescribe a kidney yang-warming qi transformation-promoting and bland-percolating dampness- and water-disinhibiting formula such as Wu Ling San (Nephritis Formula) (including large doses of Fu Ling and Ze Xie) combining Bu Yang Huan Wu Tang adding Ting Li Zi, Fang Ji, Ma Huang, Xing Ren, and Ren Shen/Chuan Qi Powder. Remember! Regardless of which formula you choose, it is essential to add Ma Huang and Xing Ren for this pathocondition.

This patient will require long-term administration of TCM medicinals up until CT scan images reveal *no* pericardial or pleural effusion and the patient is able to exercise normally (consisting of walking at a slow pace for a mininum of 3–5 hours) without experiencing any discomfort or noticeable symptoms. That's when you know the patient's condition has been successfully treated, and at that time, you can gradually discontinue administration of TCM medicinals.

Case Study #6: Sweating from the Chest – Five Heart Sweating

Q: A 73 y/o male patient presented with mitral valve insufficiency (left atrial hypertrophy), arrhythmia, and occasional shortness of breath. He has been receiving treatment with Western medicine drugs for many years now.

Recently, he has experienced profuse sweating from the chest, and is concerned the condition could get worse, so he came to me for consultation. He hopes to wean away from Western medicine drugs and take TCM medicinals instead. What is your opinion? Would Fu Ling Bu Xin Tang variant be effective?

A: Sweating from the chest is one of the sweating of the five hearts (soles, palms, and center of the chest (heart region)), but it does *not* have any specific correlation with mitral valve insufficiency (left atrial hypertrophy), arrhythmia, and occasional shortness of breath.

If this condition derived from heart disease, the sweating would occur over the entire body and *not* just in the chest region. If the condition resulted from pleural effusion, sweating would flow profuse as rain and the patient would have difficulty breathing while lying in a recumbent position.

The key is that for any of these conditions you can prescribe Di Gu Pi Yin (nourishes blood and enriches yin) adding Zhi Mu, Qing Hao, and Sheng Mu Li; or Xiao Chai Hu Tang (harmonizes and resolves Shao Yang) adding Qing Hao, Zhi Mu, and Di Gu Pi. In the most severe cases, you can administer a liver-settling wind-extinguishing and yin-enriching yang-subduing such as Jian Ling Tang (including Gan Cao) adding Zhi Mu, Huang Bo, Qing Hao, Di Gu Pi, and Long Yan Gan. These formulas should be able to improve symptoms of profuse sweating.

Case Study #7: Coronary Artery Disease

Q: Coronary artery disease (CAD) can be life threatening if blood flow to the heart is severely blocked; thus, I am always particularly vigilant when treating these patients. I have treated a number of patients with this condition, from milder cases (e.g., arrhythmia, ischemia of coronary arterioles and capillaries) to severe cases (e.g., 80% coronary artery blockage), but unfortunately have never had very effective results.

In the past, for patients with severe myocardial ischemia, I have usually prescribed Bu Yang Huan Wu Tang adding Gan Jiang, Fu Zi, Rou Gui, and Ren Shen/Chuan Qi Powder for a duration of 2 weeks to 3 months. For arrhythmia and ischemia of the coronary arterioles and capillaries, I have prescribed the same main formula (including a large dose of Huang Qi (2.5 liang)) adding Gan Jiang, Fu Zi, and Rou Gui (large doses of 1 liang each), Huang Qin, and Ren Shen/Chuan Qi Powder for a duration of 1 1/2 months.

Do you have any suggestions about any changes that should be made to these treatment regimens? Please share your experience on treating this pathocondition.

A: Bu Yang Huan Wu Tang variant is the most effective formula for coronary artery disease (CAD)—aka coronary heart disease (CHD), coronary atherosclerosis, and ischemic heart disease (IHD).

If you have already prescribed large dosages of this formula over a period of time *without* effective results, then you can try having the patient soak this formula (decocting pieces) in rice wine for 30 minutes to 2 hours prior to decocting. This will increase the potency of the medicinals' active constituents, direct the medicinals into the upper burner, and enhance the overall blood-quickening and channel and network vessel-freeing capacity of this formula.

Remember! You do not need to add such a large dose (1 liang each) of The Three Great Yang-Supplementers for most cases. Sometimes if the dose is too large, paradoxically, it will act to inhibit heart function, resulting in PR interval lengthening, slow heart rate, irregular heartbeats, and sometimes even causing vasospasms. The best method is to start out at 5 qian each and maintain this dosage for 2–3 months, while continuing to assess the patient's condition. If there is *not* much improvement, then increase to 6 qian. Similarly, in another 2–3 months, if there still is *not* a lot of improvement, then increase to 7 qian.

Gradually increasing the dose is particularly relevant for Fu Zi due to its potential toxicity: long-term administration in large doses may induce adverse effects of slow heart rate, irregular heartbeats, dizziness, blurry vision and confusion, weakness of limbs, and cold sweats.

By starting out prescribing small doses, allowing the body to adapt, and then gradually increasing the dose, you can alleviate the potential of these adverse effects occurring. You can also consider adding Fu Ling, Ze Xie, Ting Li Zi, and Fang Ji to help neutralize the toxicity of Fu Zi. If the patient presents with pericardial effusion and/or cardiopulmonary disease, then you must add Ma Huang into your formula.

Case Study #8: Lower Limb Edema – Heart Disease, Deep Vein Thrombosis, or Peripheral Arterial Disease?

Q: A 60 y/o female patient developed left-sided lower limb edema. She went in for a thorough examination, but her doctors did *not* give her a diagnosis. She was administered diuretics *without* any efficacy.

That's when she came to me for consultation. This symptom has been present for over 1 year, and palpation on her shin revealed pitting edema that looked similar to lymphedema.

Do you think this could be deep vein thrombosis (DVT) or peripheral arterial disease (PAD)?

A: Lower limb edema could be a result of heart disease, with most cases arising from pericardial effusion, cardiopulmonary congestion (static blood), and pleural effusion.

This pathocondition can be identified as water accumulation with static blood pattern, requiring the prescription of a bland-percolating dampness- and water-disinhibiting formula such as Chai Ling Tang or Wu Ling San (Nephritis Formula) adding large doses of Fu Ling, Ze Xie, Ting Li Zi, Fang Ji, Ma Huang, and Ren Shen/Chuan Qi Powder. For longstanding chronic disease, you should also add The Three Great Yang-Supplementers and Huang Qin. Another approach would be to prescribe a blood-quickening qi-supplementing formula such as Bu Yang Huan Wu Tang adding Cang Zhu, Fu Ling, Ze Xie, Ting Li Zi, Fang Ji, and Ma Huang; and if vacuity heat presents, then add Huang Qin, Mu Dan Pi, Zhi Zi, Qing Hao, Zhi Mu, and Di Gu Pi.

Remember! Chronic conditions eventually evolve into cold pattern, and thus you must add The Three Great Yang-Supplementers and Huang Qin (as a counterbalance) into the main formula.

Your description of the patient's condition does *not* sound like DVT or PAD (aka peripheral vascular disease (PVD)) to me.

In patients with DVT, during the earlier stages, black and blue discoloration (or possibly redness) will appear and the skin is softer and looser, which in the later stages will later evolve into a feeling of tightness or heaviness, and the presentation of redness and tenderness with pain and swelling on exertion. DVT can be identified as blood stasis with water amassment pattern and qi and blood vacuity (or yang vacuity) with water amassment pattern. For DVT, the longer the patient stands or walks, the greater the swelling and pain; the swelling does not resolve easily; and the skin surrounding the thrombosed vessels tends to be itchy and tingly.

In patients with PAD, during the earlier stages (i.e., intermittent claudication), the skin may appear red, hard, swollen, and warm (or in some cases cool), which will later evolve into cool, dry, atrophic and shiny skin with a bluish tint. At the onset, PAD can be identified as blood stasis heat pattern, but over time, it will evolve into a true cold false heat pattern, and eventually in longstanding conditions it evolves into yang vacuity pattern. For PAD, when occlusion becomes severe enough the patient may feel a cramping pain in the distal aspect of the affected limb(s), which worsens at night and improves when the limb is lowered to promote circulation and upon standing. And in the critical stage, resting pain, ulceration, and tissue necrosis (gangrene) will be pronounced.

Case Study #9: Hyperglycemia Following Coronary Artery Stent Placement

Q: A 45 y/o male patient explained that 3 years ago he suffered from an acute myocardial infarction (MI) and received treatment that included placement of a coronary artery stent. Following surgery, the patient developed hyperglycemia (AC 200–300), prompting his doctors to prescribe Diaben (Glyburide), which was *not* effective. Subsequently, he has suffered from gout, facial palsy, glaucoma cataracta viridis (green cataract), and has distending pain in both eyes. How would you treat this patient?

A: I have already explained this to you previously on numerous occasions. Putting it simply, there are many precipitating factors for the presentation of hyperglycemia that you must consider—it can be caused by more than just islet cell inflammation, atrophy, and tumors!

Hyperglycemia can be caused by excessive release of glycogen and muscle glycogen or excessive absorption by the intestinal mucosa; dysfunction of hypothalamic endocrine regulation; vascular endothelial growth factor (VEGF), erythrocyte deformability, and lack of vascular permeability; and even vasculitis, myocarditis, and cardiac hypertrophy. Other causes of hypoglycemia include severe burns, contusions, and inflammation of the striated muscle, skeletal muscle, cranial nerves, and marrow; and cancer that induces hemolysis (e.g., leukemia).

Sometimes there is interference in the feedback system of the glycagon control centers in the brain, which essentially fools the brain into thinking that there is a deficiency, so it then works overtime to make up for the perceived loss by secreting large amounts of glycogen and muscle glycogen.

Therefore, you can see that it is necessary to clearly identify and understand the etiology and pathomechanisms involved in order to conduct accurate pattern identification as the basis for determining effective treatment.

If this patient's hyperglycemia really did result from coronary artery stent placement, then it can be identified as heart stasis heat and static blood with water amassment pattern. If pericardial effusion is inducing panting and palpitations or myocardial ischemia is inducing swelling and hypertrophy, then it can be identified as qi vacuity, blood stasis, and water amassment pattern. If the patient has been administered either TCM or Western medicine anti-inflammatory, antipyretic, anticoagulant, or diuretic medication for long durations *without* effectiveness, then this can be identified as cold damp with blood stasis heat pattern. All of these various patterns require the administration of different TCM medicinal therapeutic approaches.

Generally, for blood stasis heat pattern you can consider prescribing a blood-quickening stasis-transforming formula such as Ru Mo Si Wu Tang adding The Three Yellows; a blood-quickening blood-cooling and yin-nourishing formula such as Di Gu Pi Yin or Niu Jiao Di Huang Tang; or a diaphragm-cooling heat-eliminating formula such as Liang Ge San, Zhi Zi Bo Pi Tang, or Zhi Zi Chi Tang.

For water amassment pattern, it is essential to include Fu Ling, Zhu Ling, Ze Xie, Ting Li Zi, and Fang Ji in your main formula. For pericardial effusion, you can consider prescribing a bland-percolating dampness- and water-disinhibiting formula such as Chai Ling Tang, Wu Ling San, Ling Gui Zhu Gan Tang, Mu Fang Ji Tang, or Fang Ji Huang Qi Tang. Just make sure your formula includes the essential medicinals in Bu Yang Huan Wu Tang.

For cold damp with stasis heat pattern, you can consider prescribing a formula such as Wu Ling San (Nephritis Formula) combining Bu Yang Huan Wu Tang adding Ting Li Zi, Fang Ji, Ma Huang, Ren Shen/Chuan Qi Powder, Sang Bai Pi, and Sheng Shi Gao (or Mu Dan Pi, The Three Yellows, and Zhi Zi). If blood glucose levels *still* do *not* come down, then add Bai Jiang Can (or Wan Jiang Sha), Nu Zhen Zi, or Long Yan Gen.

These TCM formula variants are specifically for cardiac-related hyperglycemic conditions. Obviously, hyperglycemia resulting from other pathoconditions, pathomechanisms, and patterns may require different therapeutic approaches. The key is accurately identifying the pattern as the basis for determining treatment!

Case Study #10: Intermittent Claudication

Q: What is the etiology of intermittent claudication? Is it another kind of vascular occlusion? How should I treat this condition?

A: "Intermittent" means occurring occasionally or at intervals and "claudication" means to limp or walk with difficulty. This is a peripheral vascular disease (PVD) (aka peripheral arterial disease (PAD)) caused by arterial insufficiency (narrowing of an artery) and subsequent ischemia (arterial occlusion). For those with this condition, walking will induce pain, achiness, fatigue, cramping, and/or a burning sensation (paresthesia) in the leg(s) to the point the person must stop and rest for a while before they can continue.

The etiology of intermittent claudication is insufficient tissue perfusion resulting from atherosclerosis (e.g., coronary artery disease, renal disease, and hypertension). However, other types of conditions may present with similar symptoms such as the following:

1) CNS (brain, brainstem, spinal cord) damage resulting in the neural pain transmission of "pain signals" to the lower limb(s) remaining in the pain memory centers and thus manifesting as phantom pain (i.e., central memory theory). A classic example of this is the neurogenic claudication presenting in lumbar spinal stenosis.

2) A pain reflex resulting from administration of oral psychotropic drugs and thus manifesting as phantom pain (i.e., gate control theory).

3) Deep vein thrombosis (DVT), which is caused by the formation of a blood clot (thrombus) in a deep vein, typically the calves. Thrombus formation may be a result of endothelial damage, venous stasis, and/or hypercoagulability.

The swelling and pain arising from narrowing and spasm of an *artery* will typically be accompanied by heat and the skin will feel tauter upon palpation. In contrast, the swelling and pain arising from narrowing and spasm of a *vein* will feel suppler without pronounced heat (possibly even slightly cool). In the presence of fatigue, aching, cramping and/or pain after walking for moderate periods of time, you must first rule out the possibility of other pathoconditions before the diagnosis of intermittent claudication can be made.

Nearly all patients with intermittent claudication present with water amassment. Thus, when treating this condition, you must differentiate between blood stasis heat with water amassment pattern and qi vacuity with cold stasis and water amassment pattern. For blood stasis heat pattern, you can prescribe a formula variant such as Ru Mo Si Wu Tang adding Huang Qin, Huang Lian, Bai Zhu, Fu Ling, Ze Xie, and Chuan Qi; bleed the well points of the affected limb; and perform acupuncture on corresponding distal acupoints. For qi vacuity with cold stasis pattern, you can prescribe a formula variant such as Bu Yang Huan Wu Tang or Ru Mo Si Wu Tang adding Gan Jiang, Fu Zi, Huang Qin, Bai Zhu, Fu Ling, Ze Xie, and Chuan Qi; and administer acupuncture (warm needling) on corresponding distal acupoints.

Regarding the possiblity of intermittent claudication being caused by "pain signals" remaining in the pain memory centers and thus manifesting as phantom pain, you must sill differentiate between drug-induced phantom pain and CNS damage-induced phantom pain.

For drug-induced phantom pain, once the body develops tolerance, the phantom pain will gradually resolve; and if these symptoms do not resolve, then advise the patient to change medication.

For CNS damage-induced phantom pain, this condition will gradually resolve as the lesion heals. This type of phantom pain is unique in that every 3–4 weeks there will be recurring episodes of intensified pain for 1–2 days, and every 2.5–3 months there will be a period of about 2 weeks with symptoms of intensified, severe pain. After enduring a few of these intensified periods, the symptoms will rapidly improve, until there is no longer a pain signal of this memory stored in the brain. At this time, the symptoms of intermittent claudication will be remedied.

However, there are some cases of spinal stenosis that do *not* respond well to any type of treatment, including surgery, and these patients may experience recurring episodes of this phantom pain that will require long-term administration of TCM medicinals.

Case Study #11: Varicose Veins and Deep Vein Thrombosis

Q1: A 47 y/o female patient presented with swelling and bruising on both shins with localized pain, itch, and tingling. Symptoms are pronounced when her legs are draped in a sitting position or standing and improve when walking or with legs elevated.

I diagnosed this condition as varicose veins (VV) with concomitant deep vein thrombosis (DVT), and prescribed (Yu Sheng)

Wu Ling San (Nephritis Formula) (including large doses of Huang Qi, Fu Ling, and Ze Xie) adding Yin Xing Ye, Chuan Qi, Dang Gui, Chuan Xiong, Sheng Di Huang, and Chi Shao. Do you think this is the right approach?

A1: To put it simply, you can think of VV as veinous incompetency that may lead to tissue hypoperfusion, inflammation, swelling, atrophy and even ulceration; while DVT results from thrombus formation that causes swelling, progressive tenderness and pain, and can lead to pulmonary embolism. Patients with longstanding chronic venous insufficiency (i.e., VV) may also develop DVT over time.

This is an excellent approach for treating VV and DVT. However, this case clearly indicates secondary swelling (the tip) following the onset of venous insufficiency (the root) and thrombus formation (the root). The existing dose of Fu Ling and Ze Xie is enough for treating the tip, so you do *not* need to add larger doses. Just increase the dose of Huang Qi, which in combination with the Gan Jiang and Fu Zi already in this composition, will work towards promoting circulation (treating the root!).

Also, to accelerate the resolution of swelling, you can administer acupuncture (warm needling) on the distal extremity acupoints that correspond with the affected site.

Q2: After taking the TCM formula, the swelling in both lower legs improved, but there was still mild swelling in the right lower leg and the patient also felt fatigued. She explained that her husband told her he had heard people say, "If you don't have surgery for varicose veins you are susceptible to blood clots that could get stuck in your lungs and cause death." Thus, fearing the possibilty of pulmonary embolism, he encouraged his wife to go ahead with the surgical procedure (i.e., open surgery for partial removal of vein as opposed to vein ablation).

Unfortunately, her condition worsened following surgery to the point where simply sitting for 30 minutes would result in lower leg swelling and discomfort. So she came back to see me again, hoping that TCM treatment would help improve her condition. Is (Yu Sheng) Wu Ling San (Nephritis Formula) variant still the right formula to prescribe at this time?

A2: Increased swelling following surgery for VV is mainly due to compromised venous return and lymphatic circulation. DVT, as the name indicates, involves deeper veins and the risk of severe complications (i.e., pulmonary embolism) arising. Your treatment objective is to stimulate lower limb circulation, promoting venous return and preventing lymph and fluids from pooling.

Yes, you can still prescribe Wu Ling San (Nephritis Formula) variant; or possibly even Wu Ling San (Nephritis Formula) combining Bu Yang Huan Wu Tang adding large doses of The Three Great Yang-Supplementers; or Bu Yang Huan Wu Tang adding large doses of Gan Jiang, Fu Zi, The Four Lings, and Huang Bo.

Administer this formula up until the patient is able to walk continuously for long periods without resting, and sit continuously for up to 2–3 hours without swelling or stiffness. That's when you know the condition has been cured. Naturally, during the therapeutic regimen you should also urge the patient to walk for at least 1 hour every day to promote circulation and prevent blood, fluid, and lymph from pooling in the legs.

After any prolonged surgical procedure, venous return will likely be inhibited and swelling of the lower limbs may occur. For your patient, you must immediately stimulate lower limb circulation and promote venous return, preventing lymph and fluids from pooling. If left untreated, severe cases of DVT *can* lead to the formation of a blood clot, which *could* become dislodged and result in pulmonary embolism and fatality. You must be vigilant!

Case Study #12: Deep Vein Thrombosis

Q: A 50 y/o female developed symptoms of lower leg swelling, tightness and tenderness, prompting her to go in for examination. She was diagnosed with deep vein thrombosis (DVT), and not long after, underwent thrombectomy and was administered the anticoagulant drug Coumadin. Follow-up examination revealed no obstruction in the iliac vein, but the smaller venules located below Wei Zhong (UB40) are still blocked.

I happened to be reading a study about brain tumors sometimes causing this type of condition. Is this a viable scenario? What formula should I use to treat this condition?

A: DVT can be identified as stasis heat pattern and cold stasis pattern.

For stasis heat pattern, you can prescribe a blood-nourishing blood-quickening, stasis-dispelling pain-relieving, and network vessel-freeing channel-regulating formula such as Ru Mo Si Wu Tang adding Huang Lian, Mu Dan Pi, Niu Xi, and Chuan Qi. Also, bleed the well points on the affected limb(s) and needle the acupoints at the distal extremity that correspond with the affected site, such as Tai Chong (LV3), Zhong Feng (LV4), and Di Wu Hui (GB42).

For cold stasis pattern, you can prescribe the same main formula used for stasis heat pattern adding The Three Great Yang-Supplementers; or change the main formula to Bu Yang Huan Wu Tang (quickens the blood and supplements qi) adding The Three Great Yang-Supplementers, Huang Bo, Ni Xi, Chuan Qi, Cang Zhu, Fu Ling, and Ze Xie. Also, perform acupuncture (warm needling) on acupoints at the distal extremity that correspond with the affected site as mentioned above. Typically, cold stasis feels cool and supple on palpation and responds well to TCM treatment (medicinals and acupuncture (warm needling)) with swelling gradually resolving and the limb feeling light and uninhibited.

Most cases of DVT result from a history of immobilization, old age (e.g., due to poor circulation and sedentary lifestyle), malignancy (i.e., tumors produce proteins and cytokines with thrombophylic effects), and use of oral contraceptives. Blockage can occur in the arms (e.g., endothelial injury due to central venous catheters, pacemakers or injection drug use), but most often it occurs in the legs. The two factors that make countries such as Korea and Japan particularly susceptible to DVT are cold winters and the habit of sitting cross-legged.

In fact *The Yellow Emperor's Inner Canon* (黃帝內經 *Huang Di Nei Jing*) specifically mentions "a lack of walking (circulation)" as a factor involved in crippling wilt (痿躄 w□i bì) (i.e., limpness, weakness, and slackening of the limbs with loss of functional capacity). So you can see clearly here that exercising and maintaining good circulation (e.g., *not* sitting cross-legged) are essential for the prevention of DVT.

Case Study #13: Gangrene – Poor Circulation of the Lower Limbs

Q: A 48 y/o patient presented with darkened (black) skin on his left lower leg. The skin does *not* feel hot upon palpation and he has numerous large venous aneurysms bulging in this leg as well. The patient explained that he has been afflicted with this condition for 20 years. Despite evaluation and treatment by many specialists at major hospitals, *nothing* has proven effective.

Upon observation, his left lower leg is thinner than his right and the tissue feels noticeably tighter. I suspect the patient has gangrene, but I am not sure if it is cold type or heat type. Please offer your guidance and advice on this case. Thank you!

A: Based on the symptoms you have described, it sounds like cold type, but you must carefully differentiate between the skin discoloration of venous aneurysms (darkened skin with bruised appearance surrounding the site of the vessel) and gangrene (below a specific borderline, the entire lower extremity appears dark purple or black, almost like pig blood cake or charcoal).

If the leg is cool upon palpation and the skin tight, pale and lusterless, then this can be identified as congealing cold pattern. For this pattern, you can consider prescribing a blood-nourishing network vessel-freeing and cold-dissipating counterflow-downbearing formula such as Dang Gui Si Ni Jia Wu Zhu Yu Sheng Jiang Tang adding Fu Zi, Huang Qin, and Ren Shen/Chuan Qi Powder; or a qi- and blood-supplementing and kidney yang-supplementing formula such as Gui Qi Jian Zhong Tang adding Ren Shen/Chuan Qi Powder. If edema presents following administration, then also add Fu Ling and Ze Xie. This type of gangrene is commonly known as "dry gangrene" and is caused by inadequate arterial perfusion (e.g., peripheral artery disease, diabetes).

If the skin color is purplish brown or black-colored and putrid-smelling, and/or if purulent, bloody discharge oozes from the tissue smelling like a dead carcass, this can be identified as heat toxin with blood stasis pattern. For this pattern, you can consider prescribing a heat-clearing toxin-resolving, swelling-dispersing hardness-breaking, and blood-quickening pain-relieving formula such as Xian Fang Huo Ming Yin or Jie Du Ji Sheng Tang adding large doses of Pu Gong Ying and Huang Qin. This type of gangrene is commonly known as "wet gangrene" and is caused by bacterial infection or venous obstruction, which tends to spread rapidly and packs a greater risk of systemic infection.

Regardless of the specific pattern and type, you should always be vigilant and advise patients with gangrene to get a complete lab workup that includes BUN, Cr, WBC, PT, and APPT to rule out the possibility of systmetic toxicity (e.g., sepsis, kidney and liver failure, hemolytic anemia). Also, advise them to maintain a healthy lifestyle that includes adequate sleep, diet, and moderate exercise.

Case Study #14: Hyperlipidemia

Q: A 56 y/o female patient explained that she has many relatives who have become afflicted with chronic disease (e.g., liver, heart, diabetes) at around her age, and some have been fatal. With this family history, she has lived health consciously and goes for periodic medical checkups. Despite having only slightly elevated total cholesterol (T. Chol), triglyceride (TG), and blood sugar levels, she is still worried and wants to take TCM medicinals to regulate her constitution.

On the patient's initial consultation, her lab tests showed T. Chol/TG 264/232 and GLU AC 184. For 2 months now, I have been administering Sheng Yu Tang adding Shan Zha, Ji Nei Jin, Chuan Qi, Huang Qin, and Tu Si Zi. During her subsequent visits, lab test results were as follows: (second visit) Chol/TG 256/155 and GLU AC 175; (third visit) Chol/TG 238/203 and GLU AC 129; and (fourth visit) Chol/TG 275/274 and GLU AC 143. Do you think this is a good approach for treating hyperlipidemia? Please share your experiences in treating this condition?

A: This prescription looks good! However, you must be aware of a typical pattern that evolves when attempting to lower T. Chol, TG, GLU, BUA, BUN, and Cr levels. Initial treatment will usually result in successfully lowering these levels down to a threshold before rebounding (though not as high as before), leveling off for a period, and then progressively declining again.

This is the body's natural protection mechanism working here, ensuring that vital functions are maintained within viable homeostatic parameters and protecting the body against abrupt and dramatic changes that could be life threatening.

This is why it is safer and more logical to administer natural, multi-action, and reversible mediums of treatment, attuned to the body's physiological protection mechanisms. Once these physiological markers reach a threshold and level off, the only way to go beyond is change the formula or increase the dose.

Generally, for severe ascendant hyperactivity of liver yang, liver channel stasis obstruction, and deficiency of lipid metabolizing enzymes in the liver that results in increased T. Chol and TG levels, you can prescribe a formula such as Long Dan Xie Gan Tang (drains liver and gallbladder repletion fire and clears lower burner damp-heat), Huang Lian Jie Du Tang (clears heat and resolves toxin), or Da Chai Hu Tang (resolves exterior evil and frees interior repletion) adding medicinals with blood-quickening stasis transforming actions like Chi Shao, Dan Shen, Gu Sui Bu, Niu Xi, Shan Zha, and Sang Ji Sheng.

For patients with idiopathic hypercholesterolemia and hypertriglyceridemia, this condition can be identified as yang straying outward pattern. By "idiopathic" I mean that at some point in life the patient's lipid metabolism centers in the brain have been disrupted by toxin; the remnants (body or fragments) of the culled virus or bacteria (i.e., evil qi) disrupts the hosts metabolism; or the body produces too many antibodies, which interferes with the normal functioning of the endocrine system. The endocrine system then errantly perceives that it needs to produce large amounts of cholesterol and triglycerides in order to synthesize and produce cells, antibodies, antigens, and complements, resulting in their overabundance.

For patients with this type of yang straying outward pattern, you can prescribe liver-settling wind-extinguishing and yin-enriching yang-subduing formula variants such as Jian Ling Tang, Jian Ling Tang combining Huang Lian Jie Du Tang, Chai Hu Jia Long Gu Mu Li Tang, Zhi Bo Di Huang Tang, or Huang Lian Jie Du Tang. Just make sure to include Sheng Mu Li, Sheng Long Gu, Shan Zha, Dan Shen, and Chi Shao in your formula selection. All of these formulas have the potential to achieve effective results depending on further detailed pattern identification for each individual patient.

If the condition is caused by increased instestinal lipid absorption, in mild cases, this can be idenfitied as stomach heat food and oil accumulation pattern; and in severe cases, this can be identified as Yang Ming bowel repletion pattern. For these patients, you can consider prescribing formula variants such as Cheng Qi Tang, Ge Gen Qin Lian Tang, Huang Lian Jie Du Tang, Qing Wei San, or Bai Hu Tang adding food-dispersing stomach-fortifying medicinals such as Lai Fu Zi, Ji Nei Jin, Mai Ya, and Gu Ya.

In rare instances, a patient will develop hyperlipidemia as a result of an insufficient number of digestive enzymes produced in the pancreas, stomach, and bile (liver). This condition can be identified as binding depression of spleen qi pattern, requiring the administration of a depression-resolving, food-dispersing, and stomach-opening (digestion-promoting) formula such as Xiang Sha Liu Jun Zi Tang, Si Jun Zi Tang, Si Shen Tang, Yue Ju Wan, or Bao He Wan. Make sure to include Shen Qu in the mix!

In summary, regardless of the underlying cause, TCM can effectively treat hyperlipidemia (hypercholesterolemia and hypertriglyceridemia). Just remember! Do *not* discontinue TCM formula administration immediately after T. Chol and TG levels decrease. You must continue administering the formula for 1–2 more months to make sure levels do *not* rebound. Once you are certain that acceptable levels are being maintained, then, you can gradually reduce the dose until the formula is completely discontinued.

V. HEAD & NECK DISORDERS

Office workers and "smartphone" users are the demographic that most commonly experience stiffness, soreness, and aches in the head, shoulder, neck, and upper back region. However, there are many other potential causes of head and neck pain that the practitioner must be aware of!

Case Study #1: Foot Tai Yin Phlegm Reversal Headache – "I Don't Feel Right All Over"

Q: Today a 35 y/o female patient visited my clinic complaining of malaise saying, "I don't feel right all over." She explained her symptoms as follows: fatigue, distention and fullness in the lower abdomen (stool and urine normal), neck pain, lower back soreness, and increased perspiration when fatigued.

She has sought consultation and treatment from both Western medicine and TCM doctors, but *nothing* has been effective. Some TCM doctors said her condition was caused by postpartum wind, while Western medicine doctors diagnosed her with chronic pelvic inflammatory disease (PID).

Somewhat interestingly, I did note that during her visits to my clinic, these symptoms never seemed to be bothering her too much. What is your opinion about this case?

A: During the process of making a diagnosis, it is imperative to consider a full spectrum of potential pathologies based on both TCM pattern identification and results of Western medicine lab tests and imaging studies. It is possible that your patient my have chronic PID, but it sounds to me like she may also have concomitant foot Tai Yin phlegm reversal headache (**足太陰痰厥頭痛** zú tài y□n tán jué tou tong). Aspects of this pathocondition correlate with the constellation of commonly presenting symptoms of psychosomatic disorder defined in Western medicine.

I recommend prescribing a spleen- and stomach-supplementing, phlegm-damp-transforming, and wind-stabilizing formula such as Ban Xia Tian Ma Bai Zhu San adding Gan Cao, Long Yan Gan, Sheng Du

Zhong, Yuan Hu Suo, and Mu Xiang. If copious amounts of vaginal discharge (leukorrhea) presents, then add Sheng Mu Li, Bai Guo, and Yu Sheng Wan. If increased perspiration persists, then add Ma Huang Gen (or Qing Hao) and Zhi Mu.

Continue assessing the patient's condition on follow-up visits and adjust your formula accordingly. Naturally, you could also perform acupuncture, which may be effective for some patients.

Case Study #2: Psychosomatic Disorder, Fibromyalgia, or Foot Tai Yin Phlegm Reversal Headache?

Q: Three years ago, a 42 y/o male patient began having sudden attacks of neck stiffness and pain that radiated to the chest on both sides, the right eye socket, both shoulders, and the posterior aspect of the elbow (near Ching Leng Yuan (SJ11)). This pain was described as severe with episodes occurring 2–3 times per week and the pain worse at night. Occasionally, the patient felt hot flashes, dizziness, muzziness, headache, and blurred vision. Results of an MRI indicated no abnormalities in his cervical spine.

In an attempt to remedy these symptoms, the patient has received frequent injections of muscle relaxants and analgesics and has been taking oral sedatives for a long duration. Western medical doctors diagnosed him with psychosomatic disorder and fibromyalgia.

Do you think this patient could be suffering from cerebral atrophy or upper cervical spine problems? I carefully examined the MRI image myself and could *not* see any noticeable compression on the spinal cord or nerve roots. Please share your views on this case.

A: It sounds to me like this is another case of Foot Tai Yin phlegm reversal headache (**足太陰痰厥頭痛** zú tài y□n tán jué tou tong). Again, you can prescribe a spleen- and stomach-supplementing, phlegm-damp-transforming, and wind-stabilizing formula such as Ban Xia Tian Ma Bai Zhu San adding Gan Cao, Da Zao, Long Yan Gan, Tian Ma (a large dose, at least 1 liang), Gan Jiang, Fu Zi, and Wu Zhu Yu (5 qian each), Du Zhong (4 qian), and Yu Sheng Wan.

You can also administer acupuncture, selecting combinations of the following acupoints: Feng Chi (GB20), Tian Zhu (UB10), Feng Fu (DU16), Wan Gu (GB12), Guan Yuan Shu (UB26), He Gu (LI4),

Hou Xi (SI3), Zan Zhu (UB2), Si Zhu Kong (SJ23), and Ting Gong (SI19).

Case Study #3: Intractable Headache, Uterine Fibroids, and Endometrial Hyperplasia

Q: A 49 y/o female patient (a Western medical physician) has suffered from intractable headaches since she was a child. She explained that each time an episode occurs, the excrutiating distending pain in both eyes inhibits eye muscle rotation and the eyes remain fixed for 2–3 days. At that point, the pain goes away and normal movement is again possible.

A couple of years ago she incurred an abrubt elevation in blood pressure (190/110), but after being administered angiotensin II receptor blockers (ARBs) (i.e., decrease vasoconstriction) her systolic pressure dropped down to 140.

A few months ago, she experienced 2 weeks of continuous menstrual spotting, prompting her to go in for an examination. The exam revealed numerous uterine fibroids (the largest 6–7 cm in diameter), and lab tests results showed Hb 9 (12–16 g/dl) and insufficient Fe levels, which her gynecologist said was likely caused by excessive menstrual bleeding (menorrhagia or hypermenorrhea).

With so many different types of presenting symptoms, I am not sure where to focus my treatment. What would you do?

A: My impression is that the patient's gynecological symptoms are primarily induced by sleep deprivation combined with endometrial hyperplasia. The intractable headache, eye pain, and dizziness that have occurred since childhood most likely stem from cerebrovascular or brainstem circulatory irregularities inhibiting blood flow. This pathocondition can be identified as stasis obstructing the uterine vessels and the network vessels of the brain pattern.

I would prescribe a blood-nourishing blood-quickening, stasis-dispelling pain-relieving, and network vessel-freeing channel (menstruation)-regulating formula such as Ru Mo Si Wu Tang combining Wen Dan Tang adding Tian Ma (large dose), Ze Xie, Ce Bo Ye, Ou Jie, Chuan Qi (powder), Huang Qin (at least 8 qian), Huang Lian, and Huang Bo. If the patient still has continuous menstrual spotting, then mix Zhu Sha (powder) into the Chuan Qi (powder).

Additionally, you should perform acupuncture, selecting the acupoints Tai Chong (LV3), Zhong Feng (LV4), and San Yin Jiao (SP6). This approach should effectively stanch bleeding as well as promote good sleep and reduce the severity of her headaches. It is best for the patient to take this formula until the uterine fibroids completely disappear and the endometrial hyperplasia resolve, which generally takes about 6–10 months.

Remember! During the first 1–2 months of taking the formula, the uterine fibroids will appear "haloed" on CT scan images, enlarging at the onset and then gradually shrinking in size until they disappear. In the absence of the fibroids and hyperplasia, the patient will be primed for pregnancy so advise her to use contraception, unless of course, she wants to have a child.

Case Study #4: Swollen Lymph Node in Neck

Q: A 38 y/o male patient recently came down with a cold. Not long after, he discovered a slightly swollen nodule on the left side of his neck (near Tian Rong (SI17) and Tian Chuang (SI16)) with tenderness upon palpation. He does *not* have a fever. How would you treat this condition?

A: For a swollen nodule on the left side of the neck, I would prescribe a Shao Yang- harmonizing and -resolving formula such as Xiao Chai Hu Tang adding Huang Qin (large dose), Qing Hao, Zhi Mu, and Di Gu Pi. You can also bleed the three yang channel well points of the four limbs and needle acupoints on the Shao Yang channel. This approach should quickly resolve this condition.

Case Study #5: Elderly Patient Unable to Rotate Neck

Q: A 68 y/o male patient explained that starting 3 or 4 years ago he began having difficulty rotating his neck. He had a number of MRIs and CT scans performed *without* any irregularities found, and received treatment from both TCM and Western medicine doctors *without* success. Could this condition have derived from a transient ischemic attack (TIA) or a cerebrovascular accident (CVA)?

A: It is possible that this patient contracted tuberculosis (TB) at some point in his life, which resulted in a chronic cough that put wear-and-tear on his trachea, and neck and shoulder muscle tissues. After the TB infection resolved into a calcified granuloma, the tissues of the neck, shoulders, and trachea underwent fibrosis, leaving his neck too stiff and rigid to rotate. This is just one possibility that you can follow-up on.

If you do determine that this is the cause, then you can consider prescribing an yin-nourishing heat-clearing and lung-moistening phlegm-transforming formula such as Ba Xian Chang Shou Wan, Mai Men Dong Tang, or Bai He Gu Jin Tang. Just make sure to include Qing Hao, Yuan Shen, Zhi Mu, Di Gu Pi, and Chuan Qi.

You can also advise the patient to eat fresh South Korean homegrown Bei Sha Shen (Coastal Glehnia Root) and Hei Da Gen (aka Ge Gen)—the popular, inexpensive, and widely available "hangover" elixir in Korea—as well as lots of water chestnuts and Chinese turnips.

Case Study #6: Nuchal Rigidity

Q: A 39 y/o female patient explained that since about 1 year ago every time she lies flat on her back her legs spontaneously raise upwards, reaching a height of up to 50 cm. When this happens, the patient has tried laying both hands on her abdomen and pressing down on Tian Shu (ST25), but it has not been helpful. While lying down in other positions or during any other activity she does *not* experience any problems, only in a supine position.

She has already had an MRI performed on her neck and lumbar regions, which revealed no compression or other abnormalities. The only other significant complaint the patient mentioned was a stiff neck. Do you have any ideas or suggestions about this case?

A: These symptoms suggest increased intracranial pressure that compromises the foramen magnum, and thus induces nuchal rigidity (aka stretched stiffness of the nape and back (項背強几几 xiàng bèi qiáng sh□ sh□) in classical TCM pathologic terminology).

This condition can be identified as repletion or non-repletion pattern. For repletion pattern, you can prescribe Da Chai Hu Tang; Huang Lian Jie Du Tang combining Wu Ling San; or Jian Ling Tang combining Huang Lian Jie Du Tang adding Cang Zhu, Fu Ling, and Ze Xie. For non-repletion pattern, you can consider prescribing Ban Xia Tian Ma Bai Zhu San variant. For patients with hydrocephalus, you can prescribe a formula such as Wu Ling San (Nephritis Formula) adding Mang Xiao and Da Huang.

EPILOGUE

Our aim was to provide the reader with an insider's perspective on this subject matter through the compilation of these Q&A format case studies. We sincerely hope that TCM students, scholars, practitioners, physicians, and the interested layperson alike have gleaned valuable information on both the clinical application of TCM in primary and secondary care and as a first-line therapeutic option, as well as the integrative role TCM offers in neoadjuvant, adjuvant, complementary, and palliative therapy. This fluid introduction of a broad spectrum of pathologies is intended to inspire the reader to pursue further research and explore the vast potential for broader clinical applications. We recognize that the development and expansion of TCM clinical applications is in part influenced by prevailing cultural factors and institutional barriers existing within each respective society and nation. Amidst these dynamics, TCM's increasingly manifest scientific basis and overwhelming efficacy continues propelling this 3,000 year-old medical system to the forefront of inquiry and discovery into its promising possibilities. We hope that *Integrative Chinese Herbal Therapy Volume I Beyond the Being* has piqued your interests for learning more and encourage you to continue reading our upcoming volumes—*Volume II Surfaces in Motion* and *Volume III Roots of Life*—in the near future.

APPENDIX

DR. LEE'S MEDICINALS

This section introduces the medicinals Dr. Lee most commonly prescribes and includes details on processing, properties, actions, dosage and pharmacodynamics. All of the medicinals referred to in this text are either decocting pieces (majority) or pulverized medicinals (a few exceptions) that have been processed from raw plant or animal products and crude minerals or shells.

References from TCM classical texts are included, mostly from *The Essential Herbal Foundation* (**本草備要** *Ben Cao Bei Yao*), to provide insights into the foundations of Dr. Lee's medicinal applications. Contemporary sources that present commonly acknowledged medicinal attributes (e.g., flavor, nature, channel entry) and experimental findings are also included to provide examples of evidence-based biomedical support of clinical efficacy. The primary source texts for the contemporary medicinal attributes and experimental findings are *Chinese Materia Medica Grand Dictionary* (**新編中藥大辭典** *Xin Bian Zhong Yao Da Ci Dian*) and *Clinical Applications of Traditional Chinese Medicine* (**中藥臨牀應用** *Zhong Yao Lin Chuang Ying Yong*).

Frequently administered medicinal pairs and combinations are introduced both as single medicinals and together with their counterparts. It is important to reiterate that these profiles are intended to highlight and clarify some of the distinctive features and applications of Dr. Lee's commonly prescribed medicinals and does not attempt to present a complete listing of every medicinal Dr. Lee utilizes in clinical practice.

Bai Guo Ye (白果葉) – refer to **Yin Xing Ye**

Bai Jiang Can (白僵蠶/Bombyx Batryticatus/Silkworm/aka **Jiang Can)**

In classical literature on pharmacopoeia, it is described as follows: "[**Bai**] **Jiang** [**Can**] doesn't rot and obtains clearing and transforming qi, thus is able to treat wind and transform phlegm, and dissipate binds and move the channels…."

In contemporary texts, it is described as having a salty and acrid flavor and a balanced nature; entering the liver and lung channels; and having wind-extinguishing tetany-checking, wind-dispelling pain-relieving, and phlegm-transforming bind-dissipating actions. It is recognized as being particularly effective for treating pathoconditions involving fright-wind and epilepsy with phlegm-heat.

Traditionally, it is paired with **Quan Xie** for the treatment of infantile phlegm-heat acute fright. It can also be combined with **Quan Xie** and **Wu Gong** for the treatment of tetanus, spasm, and convulsion with arched-back rigidity, and intractable headache (e.g., migraine, cluster headache).

*For more details, refer to **The Three Insects** profile.

Bai Shao (白芍) – refer to **Chi Shao**

Bai Zhu (白术/Rhizoma Atractylodis Macrocephalae/White Atractylodes Rhizome)

In classical literature on pharmacopoeia, it is described as follows: "**Bai Zhu** is an essential medicinal for fortifying the spleen and stomach, expelling dampness, eliminating impediment, and dispersing food. [For] vacuous and unfortified spleen, [**Bai**] **Zhu** can supplement; and [for] stomach vacuity failing to absorb, [**Bai**] **Zhu** can assist."

In contemporary texts, it is described as having abitter and sweet flavor and a warm nature; entering the spleen and stomach channels; and having qi-supplementing spleen-fortifying, dampness-drying water-disinhibiting, sweat-checking, and fetus-quieting actions.

This medicinal contains the primary constituent atractylone as well as esters and carbohydrates (e.g., mannose, fructose) that strengthen the constitution (promote absorption of nutrients by the spleen), disinhibit urine, lower blood sugar levels, and provide anticoagulant, antimicrobial, and anti-inflammatory actions.

Cang Zhu (蒼朮/Rhizoma Atractylodis/Black Atractylodes Rhizome)

In classical literature on pharmacopoeia, it is described as follows: "Dries the stomach and strengthens the spleen, promotes sweating and eliminates dampness, and upbears and effuses yang qi in the stomach…an essential medicinal for dissipating wind-cold-damp in the treatment of wilting [pattern]. And [**Cang Zhu**] can also resolve the six depressions: phlegm, fire, qi, blood, dampness, and food."

In contemporary texts, it is described as having an acrid and bitter flavor and warm nature; entering the spleen and stomach channels; and having spleen-fortifying dampness-drying and wind-damp-dispelling sweat-promoting actions.

Cang Zhu has the spleen-fortifying action of **Bai Zhu**, along with the advantages of stomach dampness-drying and antimicrobial actions for the treatment of gastrointestinal disorders (e.g., sloppy stool, diarrhea, and dysentery) and other infectious diseases. Thus, this medicinal is ideal for Taiwan's humid subtropical climate.

Dr. Lee includes **Cang Zhu** in many Yu Sheng formulas, either added into the formula or substituted in place of **Bai Zhu** (unless the patient presents with qi vacuity). The spleen-fortifying dampness-drying action of **Cang Zhu** also counteracts the potential for digestion impairment and sloppy stools some patients experience when administered formulas containing large doses of certain medicinals (e.g., heat-clearing toxin-resolving, yin-nourishing blood-supplementing, blood-quickening stasis-transforming, and yin-enriching yang-subduing). Dr. Lee also prescribes this medicinal for the treatment of damp-heat pattern myasthenia gravis, which can be classified as wilting pattern.

The physiological mechanism of its dampness-drying action primarily involves its capacity to promote increased interstitial permeability of water between membranes throughout the body.

*For more details, refer to **The Four Lings** profile.

Chi Shao (赤芍/Radix Paeoniae Rubra/Red Peony Root)

In classical literature on pharmacopoeia, the attributes of **Chi Shao** and **Bai Shao (白芍)** are described as follows: "**Bai Shao** supplements and contracts and **Chi Shao** drains and dissipates. **Bai** [**Shao**] benefits the spleen and drains water from earth [spleen]; **Chi** [**Shao**] dissipates evil and moves stagnation in the blood."

In contemporary texts, **Chi Shao** is described as having a bitter flavor and slightly cold nature; entering the liver channel; and having heat-clearing blood-cooling and stasis-dissipating pain-relieving actions. **Bai Shao** is described as having a bitter, sour, and sweet flavor and slightly cold nature; entering the liver and spleen channel; and having yin-nourishing menstruation-regulating, liver-calming pain-relieving, and yin-consolidating sweat-checking actions.

A contemporary comparison of these two medicinals is as follows: "**Chi Shao** excels at quickening the blood and dissipating stasis and **Bai Shao** is better at tranquilizing and relieving pain; both have supplementing actions with **Bai Shao** superior at supplementing blood and nourishing yin, and **Chi Shao** superior at cooling the blood and expelling stasis."

Dr. Lee explains that most traditional formulas designed in times of antiquity originally included **Bai Shao** because the clinical presentation of dual qi and blood vacuity was far more prevalent back then, thus necessitating the emphasis of this medicinal's blood-nourishing actions. Our modern lifestyle, diet, and living environs have altered people's body constitutions with blood stasis and stagnation and a predilection towards blood heat more predominant nowadays. Thus, the blood-cooling stasis expelling actions of **Chi Shao** are more suitable for patients of today, and this is the reasoning behind **Chi Shao** replacing **Bai Shao** in Yu Sheng formula compsositions and variants. Dr. Lee also adds large doses of this medicinal into formulas during certain stages of cancer treatment to inhibit tumor angiogenesis (neovascularization).

Chuan Qi (川七/Radix Notoginseng/Notoginseng Root/aka **San Qi, Shan Qi)**

In classical literature on pharmacopoeia, it is described as follows: "Dissipates blood and settles pain. Treats blood ejection and spontaneous external bleeding, blood dysentery and flooding, red eyes and swollen welling-abscesses, and is an essential medicinal for knife, club, and incised wounds" and "**Chuan Qi**...excels at transforming static blood, [it] also excels at stanching the frenetic movement of blood, is an essential medicinal for blood ejection and spontaneous external bleeding, and following [treatment] and recovery no static blood is left behind in the channels and network vessels...and [it] transforms blood stasis without compromising the engendering of new blood, making it an exceptional blood-rectifying medicinal."

In contemporary texts, it is described as having a sweet and slightly bitter flavor and a warm nature; entering the liver and stomach channels; and having stasis-transforming blood-stanching and blood-quickening pain-settling actions.

Chuan Qi is clinically recognized as a blood-stanching and stasis-transforming essential medicinal and also has blood-quickening pain-relieving actions that can be prescribed for the treatment of pathoconditions involving a wide range of blood stasis pattern pathoconditions, such as compromised blood perfusion (e.g., cardiovascular disease (CVD), cerebrovascular disease (CVA)) and all types of bleeding and hemorrhage.

Chuan Qi is an expensive medicinal and the process of decoction diminishes potency, thus Dr. Lee typically administers it as a pulverized powder to minimize cost and maximize efficacy. This powder is either added directly into a formula after the decoction has cooled or taken separately. Since Dr. Lee prescribes **Chuan Qi** in pulverized powder form, it is omitted from Yu Sheng formula composition listings, which are decocting pieces only. This medicinal is often paired with **Ren Shen (powder)** to form **Ren Shen/Chuan Qi Powder**, one of the pillars of Dr. Lee's therapeutic approaches.

*For more details, refer to the **Ren Shen/Chuan Qi Powder** profile.

Cu Lu Rong (粗鹿茸) – refer to **Lu Rong**

Da Huang (大黃/Radix et Rhizoma Rhei/Rhubarb Root)

This medicinal is processed in Dr. Lee's in-house processing facility. Purchased raw, it is first steeped in rice wine over a period of 10 days (in warm weather) to 2 weeks (in cold weather), oven-dried, and then cut to be used as decocting pieces or pulverized into a powder for topical application.

In classical literature on pharmacopoeia, it is described as follows: "Great bitter [in flavor] and great cold [in nature]," "Enters the foot Tai Yin [channel] and hand and foot Yang Ming and Jue Yin [channels] blood aspect," and "Its nature is upbearing and thus does not sink, and its action is mobile and thus is not static. If steeped in wine [it] can also conduct upwards, [for] application in flushing the stomach and intestines and precipitating dryness-bind to eliminate static heat. It treats cold damage seasonal disease (**傷寒時疾** sh□ng hán shí jí), heat effusion (fever) with delirious speech, warm-heat miasmic malaria (瘴瘧 zhàng nüè), red and white dysentery, abdominal pain and urgency, jaundice and water-swelling (edema), concretions, conglomerations, accumulations and gatherings, lodged rheum and abiding food (留飲宿食 liú yǐn sù shí), distention and fullness in the heart [region] and abdomen, fecal and urinary stoppage, blood ejection and spontaneous external bleeding, blood block and blood desiccation, blood accumulation due to damage, and all [types of] repletion heat and latent heat in the blood (血分伏熱 xuè f□n fú rè). Moves water and eliminates phlegm, erodes pus and disperses swelling, and can remove the old and institute the new."

In contemporary texts, it is described as having a bitter flavor and cold nature; entering the spleen, stomach, large intestine, liver, and heart channels; and having draining and precipitating accumulation-attacking, heat-clearing toxin-resolving, fire-draining, blood-quickening stasis-transforming, and blood-stanching actions.

This medicinal is administered for patients with a wide range of pathoconditions from gastrointestinal disorders (e.g., constipation, gallstones) to elevated intracranial pressure. Its heat-clearing draining precipitation, fire-draining, accumulation-attacking, and blood-quickening stasis-transforming actions promote the removal of metabolic waste byproducts resulting from nerve cell damage and static blood; break down bile; reduce pressure of the portal vein and relax the diaphragm muscles; stimulate intestinal motility; and eliminate endothelial hyperplasia (e.g., inflammation from autoimmune disease, viral infection). For the treatment of increased intracranial pressure (ICP), initially small amounts are prescribed, increasing incrementally in 5 fen doses up to 7–8 qian until the desired draining precipitation action is achieved, which is typically 2–3 stools per day (sometimes as much as 5 stools per day depending on the pathocondition).

In addition to oral administration, **Da Huang** powder can be topically applied on open sores for its antimicrobial and blood-stanching actions. It dries and forms a protective barrier that prevents infectious agents from entering the wound and simultaneously fights infection within the lesion. For these reasons, Da Huang is often applied topically in Dr. Lee's clinic following bloodletting therapy. Da Huang can also be blended into either a petrolatum or an emulsifying hydrophilic ointment base for the treatment of inflammatory skin pathoconditions (e.g., streptococcal, staphylococcal).

Dan Shen (丹參/Radix Salviae Miltiorrhizae/Salvia Root)

In classical literature on pharmacopoeia, it is described as follows: "**Dan Shen** is bitter in flavor, engenders the new and dispels evil, breaks accumulations and regulates menstruation, and disperses welling- and flat-abscesses" and "...[its] actions are equivalent to Si Wu [Tang], and is an essential gynecological medicinal."

In contemporary texts, it is described as having a bitter flavor and slightly cold nature; entering the heart and liver channels; and having blood-quickening menstruation-regulating, blood-cooling welling abscess-dispersing, and spirit-quieting actions. Traditionally, it is one of the most commonly used medicinals for gynecological and obstetric pathoconditions.

Dr. Lee commonly includes **Dan Shen** decocting pieces in qi-supplementing, blood-supplementing, and stasis-dispeling formulas instead of **Ren Shen** to improve cerebrovascular, cardiovascular, and peripheral vascular circulation and diffuse depressed heat. This substitution is founded in the TCM classical theory of enduring illness results in stasis, which applies to many of Dr. Lee's patients who seek treatment for their chronic pathoconditions. Depending on the presenting signs, symptoms, and pattern, Dr. Lee may prescribe **Ren Shen** (powder) (or **Ren Shen/Chuan Qi Powder**) and **Dan Shen** together with their respective qi- and blood-supplementing actions forming a complementary medicinal combination that adheres to the TCM classical theory of qi is the commander of blood and blood is the mother of qi.

Dang Gui (當歸/Radix Angelicae Sinensis/Chinese Angelica Root)

This medicinal is processed in-house in Dr. Lee's own medicinal processing and decoction facility. Raw **Dang Gui** (head, body, and tail) is first washed and cleaned and then placed in barrels where it is steeped in cooking rice wine until the roots are fully saturated (anywhere from 10 days (hot weather) up to 2 weeks (cold weather)). The saturated roots are then oven-dried at low temperatures to preserve freshness and ensure longer storage life.

In classical literature on pharmacopoeia, it is described as follows: "Supplements the blood, moistens dryness, and lubricates the intestines," "**Dang Gui** is sweet [in flavor] and warm [in nature], engenders blood and supplements the heart, supports vacuity and boosts detriment, and expels stasis and engenders the new," and

"**Dang Gui** is sweet in flavor and heavy, thus specializes in supplementing blood; it is acrid [in flavor] and its qi is light, thus it also moves blood. Movement in supplementation and supplementation in movement, indeed, it is a qi-in-blood medicinal (血中氣藥 xuè zhòng qì yào) and an in-blood sage medicinal."

In contemporary texts, it is described as having a sweet and acrid flavor and a warm nature; entering the liver, heart, and spleen channels; and having blood-supplementing blood-harmonizing, menstruation-regulating pain-checking, and dryness-moistening intestine-lubricating actions. Prescribed in small doses (≤ 2 qian), it nourishes blood; in large doses (3–4 qian), it has blood-quickening stasis-transforming actions.

Dang Shen (黨參/Radix Codonopsis/Codonopsis Root)

In classical literature on pharmacopoeia, it is described as follows: "Enters the hand and foot Tai Yin channel qi aspect" and "Supplements the center and boosts qi, harmonizes the spleen and stomach, and eliminates vexation-heat. [For] slight vacuity of center qi, use [**Dang Shen**] to regulate and supplement, it's the most appropriate."

In contemporary texts, this medicinal is described as having a sweet flavor and a slightly warm nature; entering the spleen and lung channels; and having center-suplementing qi-boosting, spleen-fortifying lung-boosting, and liquid-engedering actions.

Considering the comparatively high cost of **Ren Shen**, many TCM physicians will substitute **Dang Shen** for mild cases of center qi vacuity. However, for the types of severe acute diseases and chronic disorders that Dr. Lee commonly treats presenting with pronounced blood stasis and qi vacuity, **Dang Shen** is generally *not* a viable substitute. Instead, Dr. Lee will prescribe **Dan Shen** (blood-quickening stasis-transforming and blood-cooling actions) decocting pieces in place of **Dang Shen**, and either add **Ren Shen** (powder) separately for its potent qi-supplementing and nourishing actions or **Ren Shen/Chuan Qi Powder** for its qi-supplementing, nourishing, and stasis-dispelling actions. Dr. Lee *does* include **Dang Shen** in formulas such as Gui Zhi Jia Long Gu Mu Li Tang, Pu Xiao Dang Bao Tang, and Sheng Hua Tang to improve the flavor of the formula, supplement qi, fortify the stomach, and promote digestion.

Di Huang (地黃) – refer to **Sheng Di Huang**

Di Long (地龍/Lumbricus/Earthworm/aka **Qiu Yin**)

In classical literature on pharmacopoeia, it is described as follows: "Cold in nature but descending, cold in nature thus resolves all types of heat diseases, descending thus disinhibits urine, and treats lower extremity diseases and frees the channels and network vessels. Indicated for cold damage malaria, great heat mania and vexation, urinary stoppage in adults and children, acute and chronic fright wind (**急慢驚風** jí màn jǐng f□ng), and joint-running wind pain (**歷節風痛** lì jié f□ng tòng)."

In contemporary texts, it is described as having a salty flavor and cold nature; entering the liver, spleen, and urinary bladder channel; and having heat-clearing wind-extinguishing, channel-freeing network vessel-quickening, panting-calming, and urine-disinhibiting actions.

Dr. Lee commonly pairs this medicinal with **Ma Huang** for pathoconditions affecting the respiratory and vasomotor centers in the brainstem (e.g., cerebral vasuclar accident (CVA), trauma, microbial infection, and enduring illness) and for the treatment of wind-cold-damp impediment.

Ding Shu Xiu (丁豎杇/Scaber Elephantopus/Elephant's Foot)

In contemporary texts, it is described as having an acrid flavor and cool nature; entering the liver, kidney, stomach, and small intestine; and having urine-disinhibiting swelling-dispersing, blood-cooling toxin-resolving, phlegm-dispelling, and pain-relieving actions.

In Dr. Lee's pharmacopeia it is an essential medicinal for inhibiting the synthesis of blood urea nitrogen (BUN) and serum creatinine (Cr) in the treatment of pathological conditions that result from hypoperfusion of blood through functionally normal kidneys (prerenal), structural damage to the renal parenchyma (intrinsic renal), and urinary tract obstruction (postrenal).

Dr. Lee commonly prescribes **Ding Shu Xiu** paired with **Ren Dong Teng**, adding them into Wu Ling San (Nephritis Formula), Chai Ling Tang, or other formula variants based on presenting signs, symptoms, and pattern identification.

Fu Ling (茯苓/Sclerotium Poriae Cocos/Poria)

In classical literature on pharmacopoeia, it is described as follows: "**Fu Ling** is sweet [in flavor] and warm [in nature], engenders liquid and checks thirst, abates heat and quiets the fetus, and boosts the spleen and aides yang" and "…percolates dampness and disinhibits the orifices and eliminates dampness…."

In contemporary texts, it is described as having a sweet and bland flavor and balanced nature; entering the heart, spleen, and kidney channels; and having water-disinhibiting dampness-percolating, and spleen-fortifying spirit-quieting actions. It is experimentally proven to increase the urinary excretion of electrolytes (e.g., potassium, sodium, and chloride), lower blood sugar levels, and provide sedative actions.

As a general rule, if large doses of this medicinal are prescribed (≥ 8 qian), Dr. Lee will include a comparable dose of **Ze Xie** to enhance water-disinhibiting actions.

*For more details, refer to **The Four Lings** profile.

Fu Zi (附子/Radix Aconiti Lateralis Carmichaeli Praeparata/ Aconite)

In this book, the medicinal referred to as **Fu Zi** is actually **Tian Xiong (天雄)**, which is the root tuber of this plant without the daughter (accessory) roots. The processing of this medicinal entails steeping in a solution of magnesium chloride ($MgCl_2$), sodium chloride ($NaCl$), and water, and then it is dried and sliced into small pieces.

In classical literature on pharmacopoeia, it is described as follows: "The mother [root] is **Wu Tou (烏頭)**, the [peripheral] accessory roots are **Fu Zi**, the [peripheral] extensions [of the accessory roots] are **Ce Zi (側子)**, and the long slender part [extending from the mother root] is **Tian Xiong**," "…great drying and yang returning, kidney- and life fire-supplementing, and wind-cold-damp-expelling [actions]," and "…frees the twelve channels [with] no limits beyond its reach."

In contemporary texts, it is described as having an acrid and sweet flavor, hot nature, and toxicity; entering the heart, kidney, and spleen channels; and having yang-returning counterflow-stemming, yang-reinforcing fire-supplementing, and cold-dissipating pain-relieving actions.

*For more details, refer to **The Three Great Yang-Supplementers** profile.

Gan Di Huang (乾地黃) – refer to **Sheng Di Huang**

Gan Jiang (乾薑/Rhizoma Zingiberis Officianalis/Dried Ginger)

This medicinal is processed by steaming **Sheng Jiang** with sulfur. In classical literature on pharmacopoeia, it is described as having "drying, yang-returning, diffusing, and vessel-freeing [actions]" and the complementary relationship between **Gan Jiang** and **Fu Zi** is expressed as follows: "**Fu Zi** is mobile [extends throughout body] and **Gan Jiang** is both mobile and static [long-lasting effect]."

In contemporary texts, it is described as having a bitter and astringent flavor and a warm nature, entering the spleen and liver channels, and having center-warming cold-expelling and yang-returning vessel-freeing actions.

*For more details, refer to **The Three Great Yang-Supplementers** profile.

Gui Zhi (桂枝) – refer to **Rou Gui**

Huang Bai (黃柏) – refer to **Huang Bo**

Huang Bo (黃柏/Cortex Phellodendri/Phellodendron Bark/aka **Huang Bai)**

In classical literature on pharmacopoeia, it is described as follows: "Drains ministerial fire and supplements kidney water," "**Huang Bo** is bitter [in flavor] and cold [in nature], drains fire and nourishes yin, and can be used [to treat] steaming bone with damp-heat and precipitation of blood," "Foot Tai Yang channel conductor medicinal," and "Combined with **Cang Zhu** [this pair] is called Er Miao Wan (二妙丸) (aka Mysterious Two Powder), [with its] heat-clearing dampness-disinhibiting actions forming an essential medicinal [pair] for treating wilting [pattern]."

In contemporary texts, this medicinal is described as having a bitter flavor and cold nature; entering the kidney, urinary bladder, and large intestine channels; and having heat-clearing dampness-drying, fire-draining toxin-resolving, and heat-abating steam-eliminating actions.

*For more details, refer to **The Three Yellows** profile.

Huang Lian (黃連/Rhizoma Coptidis/Coptis Rhizome)

In classical literature on pharmacopoeia, it is described as follows: "**Huang Lian** is bitter in flavor, drains the heart and eliminates impediment, drains heat and resolves toxin, and thickens the intestines and checks diarrhea" and "It has six actions: one, drains heart fire; two, eliminates middle burner heat; three, indispensable for [treating] all sores; four, eliminates wind-damp; five, treats fulminant fire eye (**暴發火眼** bao f□ huǒ yǎn); and six, checks blood in the stool."

In contemporary texts, it is described as having a cold nature and bitter flavor; entering the heart, liver, stomach, and large intestine channels; and having heat-clearing dampness-drying and fire-draining toxin-resolving actions.

The market price of this medicinal frequently fluctuates and is considerably more expensive than **Huang Qin** and **Huang Bo**, thus Dr. Lee tends to either prescribe smaller doses of this medicinal, or substitutes **Huang Qin** and/or **Huang Bo** instead, or prescribe a combination of all three (aka **The Three Yellows**) depending on the pattern and pathocondition being treated. Typically, larger doses of **Huang Lian** are reserved for severe heat patterns or specific pathoconditions such as vasculitis, gastrointestinal ulcers, and inflammatory autoimmune disorders.

*For more details, refer to **The Three Yellows** profile.

Huang Qi (黃耆/Radix Astragali/Astragalus Root)

Dr. Lee only administers premium quality raw northern **Huang Qi**, which is distinguishable by its reddish phloem that encircles the xylem of the vascular tissue of the plant.

In classical literature on pharmacopoeia, it is described as follows: "**Raw** [**Huang Qi**] secures the exterior, effuses in the absence of sweating, checks in the presence of sweating, warms the seam of the flesh (肉分 ròu f□n), fortifies the interstices of the flesh, drains yin fire, and resolves flesh heat. **Mix-fried** [**Huang Qi**] supplements the center and boosts original qi, warms the triple burner, strengthens the spleen and stomach, engenders blood and flesh, expels pus and internally draws, and is a sore and welling-abscess sage medicinal."

In contemporary texts, it is described as having a sweet flavor and a slightly warm nature; entering the spleen and lung channels; and having qi-supplementing yang-upbearing, water-disinhibiting swelling-dispersing, and sore-expressing flesh-engendering actions.

For the treatment of qi vacuity pattern pathoconditions, Dr. Lee typically starts out with a dose of 1 liang and increases incrementally by 5 qian every 1–2 weeks depending on the patient's presenting signs and symptoms, eventually peaking at a maximum dose of 2.5 liang. Excessive doses of beyond 3–5 liang may cause compromised blood vessels to rupture or paroxysmal increases in intracranial pressure in the presence of arteriosclerosis, atheroclerosis, hematoma, or adhesions in the subarachnoid space of the meninges

Dr. Lee explains that **Huang Qi** promotes accelerated exchanges across membranes throughout the body and regulates the permeability of the glomerular membrane thus inhibiting protein loss. This medicinal has been experimentally and clincally proven to eliminate nephritic proteinuria, increase myocardial contractility, contain estrogen-like effects, and provide broad-spectrum antimicrobial efficacy.

Among its bioactive constituents, astragalus saponins lower blood pressure, promote erythrocyte membrane stability, increase c-AMP concentration of blood plasma and tissues, boost immune function, and promote the regeneration of liver DNA synthesis; and astragalus polysaccharides enhance immune function, regulate blood sugar levels, protect the cardiovascular system, and accelerate regeneration of tissue growth in patients suffering from radiotherapy complications.

Huang Qin (黃芩/Radix Scutellariae/Scutellaria Root)

In classical literature on pharmacopoeia, it is described as follows: "**Huang Qin** is bitter [in flavor] and cold [in nature], bitter drains liver fire, engenders and clears the large intestine, and [treats] both damp and heat," "Bitter [flavor] enters the heart, cold [nature] overcomes heat, drains the middle burner fire [and] eliminates spleen domain damp-heat…," "[Zhu (朱)] Dan Xi (丹溪) uses **Huang Qin** to downbear phlegm as a means of downbearing fire," and "**Huang Qin** is an upper and middle burner medicinal."

In contemporary texts, it is described as having a cold nature and bitter flavor; entering the lung, stomach, gallbladder, and large intestine channels; and having heat-clearing dampness-drying, fire-draining toxin-resolving, blood-cooling blood-stanching, and heat elminating fetus-quieting actions.

*For more details, refer to **The Three Yellows** profile.

Ji Nei Jin (雞內金/Endothelium Corneum Gigeriae Galli/Chicken Gizzard/aka Ji Zhun Pi)

In classical literature on pharmacopoeia, it is described as follows: "Sweet and balanced [in flavor] and astringent in nature" and "Disperses grain and water, eliminates heat and relieves vexation, and frees the small intestine and urinary bladder. Treats diarrhea and dysentery and frequent defecation, enuresis and bloody urine, flooding and vaginal discharge and intestinal wind, diaphragm dispersion and stomach reflux, and food malaria in children."

In contemporary texts, it is described as having a sweet flavor and neutral nature; entering the spleen, stomach, small intestine, and urinary bladder channels; and having food-dispersing stomach-fortifying and essence-astringing (seminal) emission- and enuresis-checking actions.

Dr. Lee commonly adds the medicinal pair **Ji Nei Jin** and **Shan Zha** into formulas (e.g., heat-clearing toxin-resolving, yin-nourishing blood-supplementing, blood-quickening stasis-transforming, and yin-enriching yang-subduing) that may impair digestion and cause sloppy stools in some patients. This medicinal pair is also added into formula variants for the treatment of hyperlipidemia and hypertrigliceridemia.

Jiang Can (僵蠶) – refer to **Bai Jiang Can**

Lu Jiao (鹿角) – refer to **Lu Rong**

Lu Jiao Shuang (鹿角霜) – refer to **Lu Rong**

Lu Rong (鹿茸/Cornu Cervi Pantotrichum/Deer Antler)

In classical literature on pharmacopoeia, it is described as follows: "Sweet [in flavor], warm [in nature], and pure yang" and "Engenders essence and supplements marrow, nourishes blood and assists yang, and strengthens the sinews and fortifies bone. Treats lumbar and kidney vacuity cold, aching and pain in the extremities, dizzy head and black eyes, flooding and vaginal discharge and seminal emission, and all [types of] vacuity-detriment taxation damage. Suitable for patients with a fine sunken pulse and debilitation of the ministerial fire."

In contemporary texts, it is described as having a sweet and salty flavor and warm nature; entering the kidney and liver channels; and having yang-invigorating, blood essence-supplementing, sinew- and bone-strengthening, thoroughfare and controlling vessel-harmonizing, and toxin- and sore-expressing actions.

Lu Rong is the whole cartilaginous antler in a pre-calcified stage, with hair that looks and feels like velvet. It contains many growth factors (e.g., NT-3, NGF, IGF) and has been experimentally and clinically proven to increase hormone levels (e.g., testosterone and luteinizing hormone), stimulate adrenal cortical function, and promote hematopoiesis.

In his clinical practice, Dr. Lee prescribes either **Cu Lu Rong** or **Xi Lu Rong** depending on the pathocondition and presenting signs, symptoms, and pattern.

Cu Lu Rong (粗鹿茸/Coarse-Haired Deer Antler)

This is a type of **Lu Rong** that is fully developed, but *not* yet completely calcified (hormone level production low), for which Dr. Lee identifies as **Cu Lu Rong** with the "coarse" (粗 c□) antler hairs describing its texture and appearance. This medicinal is less expensive than **Xi Lu Rong** and requires larger doses (typically, 8 qian/3x/day) to achieve efficacy, thus Dr. Lee administers this medicinal in decocting piece form rather than powder.

Cu Lu Rong is *inferior* to **Xi Lu Rong** at increasing hormone levels and promoting hematopoiesis, but *superior* to **Lu Jiao** at quickening the blood and transforming stasis. This medicinal has been experimentally and clinically proven to inhibit tumor vasculature from generating hormones and thus functioning to inhibit tumor angionesis and tumerogenesis.

Dr. Lee typically prescribes **Cu Lu Rong** for cancer patients at high risk of bone metastasis or with existing metastasis, and for bone cancers, spinal cord tumors, and fractures that fail to heal properly (i.e., delayed union, nonunion).

Xi Lu Rong (細鹿茸/Fine-Haired Deer Antler)

This is a premium quality **Lu Rong** (reaching 60% to 70% growth at peak hormone production levels) offering superior medicinal efficacy, for which Dr. Lee identifies as **Xi Lu Rong** with the "fine" (細 xi) velvet sheen of the antler describing its texture and appearance. **Lu Rong** is a precious natural resource, very expensive, and typically only requires small doses (typically, 5 fen/3x/day) to achieve efficacy, thus Dr. Lee administers this

medicinal only in pulverized powder form rather than decocting pieces.

Xi Lu Rong offers superior efficacy for severe cases of thrombocytopenia (low platelet count), whether it is caused by *impaired platelet production* resulting from bone marrow failure (e.g., aplastic anemia), bone marrow suppression (e.g., chemotherapy, radiotherapy, immunotherapy), infection (e.g., cytomegalovirus (CMV), Epstein-Barr virus (EBV), hepatitis C virus (HCV), HIV), and malignancy (e.g., leukemia, lymphoma, myelodysplastic syndrome); *increased platelet turnover* resulting from immune thrombocytopenia (ITP) and other autoimmune diseases (e.g., systemic lupus erythematosus (SLE), rheumatoid arthritis (RA)), drug-induced drug side effects (e.g., heparin, quinine, sulfa drugs, NSAIDS, anticonvulsants), pregnancy, and infection; or *redistribution and dilution* (e.g., liver disease, splenomegaly, gestational, post-transfusion).

Lu Jiao (鹿角/Cervi Cornu/Mature Deer Antler)

Lu Jiao is the completely calcified antler whose coarse hairs have shed and it contains high calcium phosphate content.

In classical literature on pharmacopoeia, it is described as follows: "Salty [in flavor] and warm [in nature]. …dissipates heat and moves blood, disperses swelling and repels evil…."

In contemporary texts, it is described as having a salty flavor and a warm nature; entering the liver and kidney channels; and having blood-quickening stasis transforming actions. Traditionally, it is prescribed for the treatment of all types of vacuity taxation and offers exceptional efficacy for flat-abscesses and cold-type pus sores.

Lu Jiao can be processed into **Lu Jiao Shuang (Cervi Cornu Degelatinatum/degelatinated deer antler)**, which Dr. Lee uses in powder form combined with **Fu Zi** and **Gan Jiang** for the treatment of chronic (dry) skin ulcerations (e.g., diabetic ulcers). **Lu Jiao** can also be processed into **Lu Jiao Jiao (Cervi Cornus Gelatinum/deer antler glue)** combined with **Gui Ban Jiao (tortoise plastron glue)** to make Gui Lu Er Xian Jiao (Tortoise Shell and Deerhorn Two Immortals Glue), which Dr. Lee typically includes in formulas treating pathoconditions such as true origin vacuity detriment, extreme exhaustion of essence, extreme exhaustion of bone (e.g., osteoporosis), emaciation and shortage of qi, and dim vision (e.g., presbyopia). **Lu Jiao Jiao** can also be administered in small doses and eaten like candy (soft and chewy) as a method of regulating the constitution for the elderly.

Ma Huang (麻黃/Herba Ephedrae/Ephedra Stem)

In classical literature on pharmacopoeia, it is described as follows: "Enters Tai Yang [channel] along with hand Shao Yin [and] Yang Ming [channels], and is a lung domain (家 ji□) chief medicinal" and "Promotes sweating and resolves flesh, and dispels cold evil at the construction [level] and wind-heat at the defense [level]. It regulates blood vessels, frees the nine orifices, and opens the pores; treats wind strike and cold damage, headache and warm malaria, cough and counterflow qi ascent, phlegm wheezing and panting, red and black macule toxin, toxic wind papules (measles) impediment (毒風疹痹 dú f□ng zh□n bì), skin insensitivity, sore red swollen eyes, and water swelling and wind swelling."

In contemporary texts, it is described as having an acrid and slightly bitter flavor and a warm nature; entering the lung and urinary bladder channels; and having sweating-promoting exterior-resolving, lung-diffusing panting-calming, water-disinhibiting swelling-dispersing, nasal orifice-freeing, papule-outthrusting, and itch-relieving actions. However, this medicinal takes on an even broader role in Dr. Lee's pharmacopoeia.

Dr. Lee interprets **Ma Huang**'s action of opening the pores (開竅 k□i qiào) broadly to mean it can "open up" and transport other medicinals across all membranes of the body at the cellular level, which makes it an effective systemic channel conductor for all types of diseases (e.g., dermatology, rheumatology, cardiology, neurology). And he also interprets **Ma Huang**'s action of "opening the nine orifices" as innervating the nervous system (i.e., CNS, PNS, ANS), prompting its application for neurological disorders of the brain and nervous system.

Of course, Dr. Lee utilizes the revered bronchodilation action of **Ma Huang** for the treatment of respiratory tract pathoconditions (e.g., sinusitis, bronchitis, COPD, pneumonia). He also commonly pairs this medicinal with **Di Long** for pathoconditions affecting the respiratory and vasomotor centers in the brainstem (e.g., cerebrovasuclar accident (CVA), trauma, microbial infection, enduring illness) and for the treatment of wind-cold-damp impediment.

As for dosage, it depends on the individual's constitution and the particular season. Typically, I would start out with a small dose of anywhere from 5 fen to 1.5 qian, incrementally increasing in 5 fen doses up until the patient notices difficulty sleeping, and then, adjusting the dose back down a bit to where sleep is unaffected. A typical dose would be 1.5 qian to 3 qian.

Mang Xiao (芒硝/Mirabilitum/Glauber's Salt)

The primary constituent of this medicinal is sodium sulfate decahydrate ($Na_2SO_4 \cdot 10H_2O$). However, depending on availability and physician preference, **Mang Xiao** may be substituted with **Epsom salt** (aka **Magnesium Sulfate**). In the past, a distinction was made establishing different grades of processed crude mirabilite based on the level of purity, with **Po Xiao (朴消)** classified as having the most *impurities*, **Mang Xiao** as a *purer* form, and **Xuan Ming Fen (玄明粉)** as the *purest* form. Nowadays, there is no such distinction made, and if *less refined* medicinals are used, it is standard practice to denote these medicinals as **Po Xiao** in the prescription.

In classical literature on pharmacopoeia, it is described as follows: "**Po Xiao** settles at the bottom, the crystals are coarse, and turbid and heavy in substance. **Mang Xiao** and **Ya Xiao (牙消)** form [float] on the top, the crystals are refined, and clear and light in substance…, "**Mang Xiao** is salty [in flavor] and cold [in nature], can eliminate abiding grime, transform accumulations and disperse phlegm, and abate all [types of] heat," and "Acridity can moisten dryness, saltiness can soften hardness, bitterness can precipitate diarrhea, and great cold can eliminate heat…. [It] can flush away triple burner and gastrointestinal repletion heat, and remove the old and institute the new…."

In contemporary texts, it is described as having a salty, bitter flavor and a cold nature; entering the stomach and large intestine channels; and having heat-draining stool-freeing, dryness-moistening hardness-softening, and fire-clearing swelling-dispersing actions.

This medicinal has the action of inhibiting the large intestine's capacity to absorb water and thus promotes the excretion of large amounts of water. It must be prescribed prudently in small doses to prevent excessive watery diarrhea that may lead to malabsorption. Dr. Lee only prescribes this medicinal in cases where large doses (5–7 qian) of **Da Huang** have already been administered for a period of time without efficacy to promote defecation and maintain 2–3 stools per day.

Po Xiao (朴消) – refer to **Mang Xiao**

Qiu Yin (蚯蚓) – refer to **Di Long**

Quan Xie (全蝎/Buthus Martensi/Scorpion/aka **Xie)**

In classical literature on pharmacopoeia, it is described as follows: "Green-blue is associated with wood, thus [**Quan Xie**] treats all [types of] wind with shaking and dizzy vision, fright epilepsy and pulling, deviated eyes and mouth, malarial wind sores, deafness, vaginal discharge, and hernia, and Jue Yin wind and wood diseases."

In contemporary texts, it is described as having an acrid flavor, balanced nature, and toxicity; entering the liver channel; and having wind-extinguishing tetany-checking, toxin-attacking bind-dispersing, and network vessel-freeing pain-relieving actions.

Traditionally, it is commonly paired with **Wu Gong** for the treatment of pathoconditions involving spasm and convulsion (e.g., acute and chronic fright wind, tetanus, wind striking the channels and network vessels with deviated eyes and mouth). It is also combined with **Wu Gong** and **Bai Jiang Can** for the treatment of neuropathic pain (e.g., trigeminal neuralgia) and intractable headache (e.g., migraine, cluster headache).

*For more details, refer to **The Three Insects** profile.

Ren Dong Teng (忍冬藤/Caulis Lonicerae/Honeysuckle Stem)

In classical literature on pharmacopeia, it is described as follows: "Sweet and bitter flavor and slightly cold nature," "Enters the heart and lung channels," and "Governs heat-toxin, blood dysentery, and water dysentery."

Traditionally this medicinal is prescribed for its heat-clearing toxin-resolving and network vessel-freeing actions. In Dr. Lee's pharmacopeia it is an essential medicinal for inhibiting the synthesis of blood urea nitrogen (BUN) and serum creatinine (Cr) for the treatment of pathological conditions that result from hypoperfusion of blood through functionally normal kidneys (prerenal), structural damage to the renal parenchyma (intrinsic renal), and urinary tract obstruction (postrenal).

Dr. Lee commonly prescribes **Ren Dong Teng** paired with **Ding Shu Xiu**, adding them into Wu Ling San (Nephritis Formula), Chai Ling Tang, or other formula variants based on presenting signs, symptoms, and pattern identification.

Ren Shen (人參/Radix Ginseng/Ginseng Root)

In classical literature on pharmacopoeia, it is described as follows: "**Ren Shen** is sweet [in flavor] and balanced [in nature], greatly supplements original qi, checks thirst and engenders fluid, and regulates construction and nourishes defense."

In contemporary texts, it is described as having a sweet and slightly bitter flavor and mildly warm nature; entering the heart, lung, and spleen channels; and having great original qi-supplementing vacuity desertion-stemming, spleen-supplementing lung-boosting, liquid-engendering, and spirit-quieting actions.

Ren Shen is an expensive medicinal and the process of decoction diminishes potency, thus Dr. Lee typically administers it as a pulverized powder to minimize cost and maximize efficacy. This powder is either added directly into a formula after the decoction has cooled or taken separately. Since Dr. Lee prescribes **Ren Shen** in pulverized powder form, it is omitted from Yu Sheng formula composition listings, which are decocting pieces only. This medicinal is often paired with **Chuan Qi (powder)** to form **Ren Shen/Chuan Qi Powder**, one of the pillars of Dr. Lee's therapeutic approaches.

Dr. Lee explains in a more modern biomedical perspective: "As an adaptogenic medicinal, **Ren Shen** has the capacity to regulate cell metabolism throughout the entire body, down-regulating and up-regulating whenever it is necessary, and offers exceptional efficacy in repairing and maintaining physiological function of spinal nerves."

*For more details, refer to the **Ren Shen/Chuan Qi Powder** profile.

Ren Shen/Chuan Qi Powder (人參/川七粉)

This medicinal pair forms one of the pillars of Dr. Lee's therapeutic approaches. These two medicinals have qi-boosting fluid-engendering, origin-supporting desertion-stemming, blood-quickening stasis-transforming, and blood-stanching actions that exemplify the TCM classical theory of qi is the commander of blood and blood is the mother of qi.

Together, they can be prescribed for the treatment of a wide spectrum of pathoconditions that involve compromised vasculature leading to insufficient blood perfusion, excessive blood loss or hemorrhage, and chronic diseases in which taxation and desertion present. Specific pathoconditions include cardiovascular disease (e.g., coronary heart disease (CHD), aortic aneurysm, peripheral artery disease (PAD), deep vein thrombosis (DVT)), cerebrovascular disease (e.g., stroke, transient ischemic attack (TIA), vascular dementia), autoimmune disorders (e.g., systemic lupus erythematosus (SLE), dermatomyositis), gynecological disorders (e.g., menorrhagia, hypermenorrhagia, spotting), and end-stage cancer patients among others.

For severe blood stasis, **Dan Shen** decocting pieces are commonly prescribed along with this medicinal pair to further enhance the blood-quickening stasis-transforming actions and complement the pair with blood-cooling actions. The administration of medicinals with blood-quickening stasis-transforming actions in chronic pathoconditions is based on the TCM classical theory of enduring illness results in stasis.

The raw, pulverized powder of these medicinals are mixed together and placed in ziplock packets with a typical dosage of 7g/3x/day (a total of 21 g/day).

Rou Gui (肉桂/Cortex Cinnamoni Cassiae/Cinnamon Bark/aka Yu Gui)

In classical literature on pharmacopoeia, it is described as follows: "Acrid and sweet [in flavor] and great heat [in nature] and thick qi pure yang," "Enters the blood aspect of the liver and kidney [channels]," and "Supplements insufficiency of the life gate ministerial fire and boosts yang to disperse yin. Treats intractable cold and deep cold, can promote sweating, free the blood vessels, and perfuses and conducts the hundred medicinals. Eliminates construction and defense wind-cold, exterior vacuity spontaneous sweating, cold pain in the abdomen, and cough and counterflow qi bind…."

In contemporary texts, it is described as having an acrid and sweet flavor and hot nature; entering the spleen, kidney, heart, and liver channels; and having fire-supplementing yang-assisting, cold-dissipating pain-relieving, and channel-warming vessel-freeing actions.

The majority of formulas Dr. Lee prescribes are variants of classical formulas derived from *On Cold Damage and Miscellaneous Diseases* (傷寒雜病論 *Shang Han Za Bing Lun*) (which was subsequently divided into two books called *On Cold Damage* (傷寒論

Shang Han Lun) and *Essential Prescriptions of the Golden Coffer* (**金匱要略方論** *Jin Gui Yao Lue Fang Lun*)). In this text, the instructions to "remove the skin" (i.e., scrape away the thin layers of fungal growth on the surface of the bark) from **Gui Zhi** suggests that the bark (**Rou Gui**) with its higher volatile oil content was in fact used instead of the twig (**Gui Zhi**). Also, due to logistical considerations during the Eastern Han Dynasty (25-220 CE), it would have been much more viable to transport the relatively lighter bark (**Rou Gui**) up to northern China, where Zhang Zhong-Jing wrote his TCM classic, from southern China (or Vietnam), where the cinnamon tree (*Cinnamomum cassia* Presl.) grows.

And from a practical perspective, it is also much simpler to decoct the entire formula composition together, instead of adding the medicinals containing volatile oils towards the end of decoction to mitigate the extent of evaporation. Since **Rou Gui** contains a much higher volatile oil content than **Gui Zhi**, a higher potency of the bioactive constituents in these volatile oils will be retained during decoction. Thus, Dr. Lee predominantly prescribes **Rou Gui** in place of **Gui Zhi** even in exterior-resolving formulas such as Gui Zhi Tang, and with the exception of **Chai Ling Tang**, the only other time he prescribes **Gui Zhi** is for its function as an upper extremity channel-conducting medicinal. Amidst this dynamic, **Rou Gui**'s actions can be interpreted as encompassing those of **Gui Zhi** (e.g., exterior-resolving, spleen-fortifying, pain-relieving, antimicrobial), while also containing vasodilation actions that more effectively promote blood circulation.

*For more details, refer to **The Three Great Yang-Supplementers** profile.

San Qi (三七) – refer to **Chuan Qi**

Sang Bai Pi (桑白皮/Cortex Mori Albae Radicis/Mulberry Root Bark)

In classical literature on pharmacopoeia, it is described as follows: "Sweet and acrid [in flavor] and cold [in nature]," "Drains lung fire, disinhibits urine and stool, dissipates static blood, precipitates qi and moves water, and suppresses cough and clears phlegm. It treats lung heat panting and fullness, spitting of blood and heat thirst, and water swelling and cranium distention. Made into string it can [be used for] sewing incised wounds," and "Drains fire evil in the lung, but not lung qi. Fire and original qi are incompatible, and once fire is eliminated then qi will be calm."

In contemporary texts, it is described as having a sweet flavor and cold nature; entering the lung channel; and having lung-draining panting-calming and water-disinhibiting swelling-dispersing actions.

Dr. Lee describes this medicinal as having the capacity to "clean up the metabolic waste that clogs cell membranes throughout the entire body." Metabolic waste build-up may derive from normal metabolic processes or from inflammatory responses to disease, which may inhibit (or further exacerbate) the normal function of cellular mechanisms, disrupt homeostasis, and lead to heat pattern pathoconditions such as diabetes. For this reason, **Sang Bai Pi** is an essential medicinal for the treatment of diabetes and it is also prescribed for other heat pattern pathoconditions of the respiratory tract (e.g., acute bronchitis, emphysema) and skin (e.g., atopic dermatitis).

Shan Qi (山七) – refer to **Chuan Qi**

Shan Zha (山楂/Fructus Crataegi/Hawthorn Fruit/aka **Xian Zha)**

In classical literature on pharmacopoeia, it is described as follows: "Sour, sweet, and salty [in flavor] and warm [in nature]," "Shan Zha is sour and sweet [in flavor], grinds and disperses meat-type food, treats mounting (疝 shàn) and moves stasis, and disperses bloating and fortifies the stomach," and "Fortifies the spleen and moves qi, dissipates stasis and transforms phlegm, disperses food and grinds accumulations, effuses infantile pox, and relieves infant's-pillow [postpartum abdominal] pain."

In contemporary texts, it is described as having a sour and sweet flavor and a slightly warm nature; entering the spleen, stomach, and liver channels; and having food-dispersing accumulation-transforming actions and qi-moving stasis-dispersing actions.

Shan Zha is an essential medicinal for promoting digestion of greasy, rich and meat-type food accumulation and stagnation; and its **seed (pit)** (核 hé) is also prescribed in combination with **Li Zhi He** and **Ju He** for the treatment of stomach pain and mounting qi (hernia) pain.

Dr. Lee commonly adds the medicinal pair **Shan Zha** and **Ji Nei Jin** into formulas (e.g., heat-clearing toxin-resolving, yin-nourishing blood-supplementing, blood-quickening stasis-transforming, yin-enriching yang-subduing) that may impair digestion and cause sloppy stools in some patients. This medicinal pair is also added into formula variants for the treatment of hyperlipidemia and hypertrigliceridemia. Additionally, Dr. Lee adds **Shan Zha** into formula variants for the treatment of static blood pattern pathoconditions, such as postpartum infant's-pillow pain (postpartum abdominal pain) and coronary artery spasm.

*For more details, refer to **The Seeds** profile.

Sheng Di Huang (生地黃/Radix Rehmanniae/Rehmannia Root/aka Gan Di Huang)

Clarification is warranted for the confusing parallel nomenclature used to describe the **Rehmannia Root (Di Huang)** throughout history. To clarify this ambiguity, contemporary texts make the clear distinction of **Xian Di Huang** (鮮 xi□n = fresh) as opposed to **Sheng Di Huang** (生 sh□ng = raw), a term that is now used synonymously in reference to **Gan Di Huang** (乾 g□n = dried). **Gan Di Huang** is the term used at Dr. Lee's clinic for this medicinal; however, since most readers may be more familiar with the term **Sheng Di Huang**, it is referred to as such for the purpose of this text.

In classical literature on pharmacopoeia, it is described as follows: "Sweet and bitter [in flavor] and cold [in nature] and sinks yin and downbears," "Enters the hand and foot Shao Yin and Jue Yin and hand Tai Yang channels," and "Enriches yin, abates yang, and engenders and cools blood. It treats blood vacuity heat effusion, taxation damage cough, wilting and impediment fright palpitations, blood ejection and bloody urine, blood dizziness and flooding, heat and pain on the underside of the foot, and sinew expiration from fractures and falls. It replenishes the bone marrow, generates flesh, disinhibits stool and urine, regulates menstruation, and quiets the fetus. It can also kill worms and treats acute pain in the heart [region] and abdomen."

In contemporary texts, it is described as having a sweet and bitter flavor and cold nature; entering the heart, liver, and lung channels; and having heat-clearing blood-cooling and yin-nourishing liquid-engendering actions.

Xian Di Huang (鮮地黃/Fresh Rehmannia Root)

It has a sweet and bitter flavor and a cold nature; enters the heart, liver and lung channels; and has heat-clearing blood-cooling and yin-nourising liquid-engendering actions. Due to the cost concerns of shipping and storage, Dr. Lee does *not* keep **Xian Di Huang** in his dispensary and uses **Sheng Di Huang** instead. In cases where the heat-abating action of **Xian Di Huang** is preferred, Dr. Lee will typically pair **Sheng Di Huang** with **Huang Bo**.

Shu Di Huang (熟地黃/Cooked Rehmannia Root)

It has a sweet flavor and a slightly warm nature; enters the liver and kidney channels; and has blood-supplementing yin-enriching and essence-boosting marrow-replenishing actions. The traditional processing method (involving steeping **Sheng Di Huang** in yellow wine mixed with **Sha Ren (砂仁)** and steaming and sun-drying repeatedly a total of nine times) is extremely time-consuming, labor-intensive and expensive, and thus seldom implemented anymore. The modern method of processing **Shu Di Huang** results in inferior quality that differs in nature and property compared to its predecessor.

Taking these factors into consideration, in cases where the blood-supplementing yin-enriching and essence-boosting marrow-replenishing actions of **Shu Di Huang** are preferred, Dr. Lee typically pairs **Sheng Di Huang** with medicinals such as **Fu Zi** (frees the twelve channels), **Rou Gui** (enters the liver and kidney blood aspect and supplements life gate ministerial fire), **Ma Huang** (frees the nine orifices), and **Shi Chang Pu (石菖蒲)** (opens heart hole [passage] and disinhibits the nine orifices).

However, Dr. Lee *does* keep traditionally processed **Shu Di Huang** in his dispensary for inclusion in Du Huo Ji Sheng Tang, which is typically prescribed for impediment pattern (痹症 bì zhèng) pathoconditions such as postpartum blood vacuity engendering wind, pulling of the extremities, hypertonicity of the sinews and vessels, intermittent convulsions, and hemiparesis.

Shu Di Huang (熟地黃) – refer to **Sheng Di Huang**

The Four Lings (四苓)

This medicinal combination derives from Si Ling Tang (四苓湯)—**Fu Ling**, **Ze Xie**, **Zhu Ling**, and **Bai Zhu**—recorded in the *Teachings of Dan Xi* (丹溪心法 *Dan Xi Xin Fa*). However, Dr. Lee usually substitutes **Cang Zhu** in place of **Bai Zhu** for its spleen-fortifying, stomach dampness-drying, and antimicrobial actions, which are ideal for Taiwan's humid subtropical climate.

Fu Ling, **Ze Xie**, and **Zhu Ling** all have similar flavor and nature (sweet, bland, and balanced); enter the kidney and urinary bladder channels; and share the complementary actions of disinhibiting water, percolating dampness, fortifying the spleen, and discharging heat. **Cang Zhu** has an acrid and bitter flavor and warm nature; enters the spleen and stomach channels; and has spleen-fortifying dampness-drying and wind-damp-dispelling sweat-promoting actions. The combination of these medicinals fortifies the spleen, disinhibits water, and percolates dampness for the treatment of water-damp collecting internally, inhibited urination, diarrhea, swelling (edema), and bloody urine.

These medicinals form one of the pillars of Dr. Lee's therapeutic approaches administered for a broad scope of pathoconditions involving water amassment or water-rheum collecting internally, which causes obstruction or stagnation and leads to the disruption of physiological mechanisms and pathological disorders. The resulting homeostatic imbalance may manifest in pathoconditions such as generalized edema, ascites, pericardial effusion, pleural effusion, and increased intracranial pressure (ICP) (e.g., traumatic injury, hemorrhage, tumor, herniation, heart failure, obstruction of cerebrospinal fluid).

Dr. Lee typically includes these medicinals in Wu Ling San (Calculi Formula), Wu Ling San (Nephritis Formula), and Chai Ling Tang or adds them into a formula variant based on presenting signs, symptoms, and pattern identification. For pathoconditions such as diarrhea, ascites, and ICP, Dr. Lee commonly includes **Da Huang** to enhance the draining precipitation action and adds **Ren Shen** as a counterbalance that aides the reabsoprtion of nutrients and electrolytes.

Depending on the specific pathocondition, Dr. Lee may prescribe large doses (up to 8 qian–1 liang each) of **The Four Lings** (especially **Fu Ling** and **Ze Xie**) to ensure an adequate level of water disinhibition is achieved.

The Three Great Yang-Supplementers (三大補陽)

The medicinal combination of **Gan Jiang**, **Fu Zi**, and **Rou Gui** comprise one of the pillars of Dr. Lee's therapeutic approaches. These great spleen and kidney yang-supplementing medicinals are prescribed for the post-acute and chronic stages that present with yang vacuity and cold stasis pattern. They are also prescribed following surgery, radiotherapy, and the administration of chemotherapeutic agents—*suppress* bone marrow function, thus *inhibiting* hematopoiesis—and corticosteroids—*suppress* the hypothalamic-pituitary-adrenal (HPA) axis, thus *decreasing* corticotropin-releasing hormone (CRH), adrenocorticotropic hormone (ACTH), and endogenous cortisol)—which result in yang vacuity and cold stasis pattern.

Additionally, Dr. Lee may prescribe this medicinal combination when the therapeutic regimen has reached a point where marginal or no significant improvement is being made. In this instance, the treatment method of returning and reinforcing yang is applied to "boost" the metabolism and immune system, giving the body the strength and capacity to bolster right qi and win the struggle between right and evil.

These great yang-supplementing medicinals boost the metabolism and immune system by innervating the central nervous system (CNS), peripheral nervous system (PNS), and autonomic nervous system (ANS) and by engaging a cascade of endocrine and hormonal factors. And when **Ren Shen**, **Huang Qi**, and **Lu Rong** are prescribed together with **The Three Great Yang-Supplementers** in a formula, this combination stimulates the body's capacity for self-repair, regeneration (e.g., nerves, skin, tissue, bone), and hematopoiesis.

An initial dose of 2–3 qian for each medicinal will be prescribed, increasing incrementally up to 5–8 qian each. Once the combined dose reaches 10–12 qian, then 3–5 qian of either one or a combination of **The Three Yellows** (**Huang Qin**, **Huang Bo**, and **Huang Lian**) are added to counteract excessive heat and mitigate the potential adverse effects.

The Three Insects (三蟲)

This term refers to the combination of **Quan Xie**, **Wu Gong**, and **Bai Jiang Can**. These arthropods have evolutionary ancestry dating back nearly 500 million years and are composed of relatively smaller, more basic fundamental amino acid and protein archetypes, offering exceptional efficacy at regulating the transmission of neurotransmitters across chemical synapses.

These three medicinals all enter the liver channel and share common actions of extinguishing wind and checking tetany, with **Quan Xie** and **Wu Gong** attacking toxins, dissipating binds, and freeing the network vessels and relieving pain, and **Bai Jiang Can** dispeling wind and relieving pain and transforming phelgm and dissipitating binds.

Dr. Lee typically adds **The Three Insects** into formula variants for the treatment of neuropathic pain (e.g., trigeminal neuralgia) and intractable headache (e.g., migraine, cluster headache).

The Three Yellows (三黃)

This term refers to the combination of **Huang Qin**, **Huang Bo**, and **Huang Lian**. The heat-clearing toxin-resolving (antimicrobial and anti-inflammatory) actions of these medicinals make them among the most important and commonly used medicinals in Dr. Lee's pharmacopoeia, comprising one of the pillars of Dr. Lee's therapeutic approaches. They provide exceptional efficacy for the treatment of all kinds of infections and inflammation (e.g., nasal, upper respiratory tract, gastrointestinal, hepatic, renal, autoimmune), and are also added into Yu Sheng formula variants to counteract the great heat of **The Three Great Yang-Supplementers** (**Gan Jiang**, **Fu Zi**, and **Rou Gui**).

Classical literature on pharmacopoeia differentiates the specific actions of these three medicinals as follows: "…**Huang Lian** drains heart fire and middle burner fire, **Huang Qin** drains upper burner fire, **Huang Bo** drains lower burner fire…." Dr. Lee also acknowledges these differentiations, using **Huang Lian** for the gastrointestinal tract, **Huang Qin** for the upper respiratory tract, and **Huang Bo** for the kidneys and genitourinary tract. However, from his clinical experience, these specific distinctions are *not* vital to achieve efficacy, and when evil qi (i.e., microbial infection) is being treated, the combination of **The Three Yellows** provides effective broad-spectrum antimicrobial action.

Tian Ma (天麻/Rhizoma Gastrodiae Elatae/Gastrodia Rhizome)

In classical literature on pharmacopoeia, it is described as follows: "Acrid [in flavor] and warm [in nature]," "Enters the liver channel qi aspect," and "Boosts qi and strengthens yin, frees the blood vessels, strengthens the sinews, and courses phlegm qi. Treats all types of wind dizziness and shaking, dizzy head and eye blackening [spots in visual field], speech not complying (語言不逐 yǔ yán bù zhú), wind-damp insensitive impediment (**頑痹** wán bì) [paralysis of the extremities], and infantile fright epilepsy."

In contemporary texts, it is described as having a sweet flavor and balanced nature; entering the liver channel; and having wind-extinguishing tetany-checking, liver yang uprising-repressing, wind-dispelling, and network vessel-freeing actions.

Tian Ma shares many common properties with **The Three Insects**, thus Dr. Lee typically administers this medicinal either along with them or in combination with **Chuan Xiong**, **Chai Hu**, **Ban Xia**, and **Ge Gen** for the treatment of dizziness, vertigo (e.g., Meniere's disease, benign paroxysmal positional vertigo (BPPV), idiopathic), and intractable headache (e.g., migraine, cluster headache). Dr. Lee also prescribes this medicinal for the treatment of neurogenic hypertension caused by brainstem dysfunction.

Depending on the severity of the patient's signs and symptoms, Dr. Lee may prescribe a dose of 3 qian up to 1 liang.

Tian Xiong (天雄) – refer to **Fu Zi**

Tu Si Zi (菟絲子/Semen Cuscutae Chinensis/Cuscuta)

This medicinal is processed in-house in Dr. Lee's own medicinal processing and decoction facility. **Sheng Tu Si Zi** (**生** sh□ng = raw) is mix-fried over a low flame until faint crackling sounds can be heard and an aromatic scent arises. At this time, these seeds will be dark yellow to light brown in color. The purpose for processing in this way is to crack open the seed coat, thus allowing the constituents to be easily extracted upon decoction.

In classical literature on pharmacopoeia, it is described as follows: "Sweet and acrid [in flavor] and harmonious and balanced [in nature] and condenses qi of right yang (**凝正陽之氣** níng zhèng yáng zh□ qì)," "Enters the three yin [channels] of the foot," and "Strengthens yin and boosts essence, warms without drying, and does not reinforce ministerial fire. Treats the five taxations and seven damages, seminal cold and dribbling, and bitterness of mouth with dryness and thirst. Dispels wind and brightens the eyes, supplements defense qi, aides the sinews and vessels, boosts qi and bodily strength, and fattens and fortifies the body."

In contemporary texts, it is described as having a sweet flavor and a warm nature; entering the liver, kidney and spleen channels; and having kidney-supplementing essence-securing, liver-nourishing eye-brightening, diarrhea-checking, and fetus-quieting actions.

Dr. Lee includes the medicinal pair **Tu Si Zi** and **Sha Yuan Ji Li** (supplements the kidney and secures essence and nourishes the liver and brightens the eyes) in Atopic Dermatitis Formula and Blood Desiccation Formula; and commonly adds the pair into formula variants for their balanced and moderate liver and kidney yin-nourishing actions. Together, these medicinals offer superior capacity for retaining moisture (cellular hydration) and maintaining cell metabolic activity.

Wu Gong (蜈蚣/Scolopendra Subspinipes/Centipede)

In classical literature on pharmacopoeia, it is described as follows: "Mobile and able to dissipate, [it] treats umbilical wind clenched jaw, fright epilepsy and scrofula, snake concretions and nail sores, and kills worms and aborts the fetus."

In contemporary texts, it is described as having an acrid flavor, a warm, mobile and penetrating nature able to reach the interior and exterior, and toxicity; entering the liver channel; and having wind-extinguishing tetany-checking, toxin-attacking bind-dissipating, and network vessel-freeing pain-relieving actions. Traditionally, it is commonly paired with **Quan Xie** for the treatment of pathoconditions presenting with spasm and convulsion, such as acute and chronic fright wind, tetanus, and wind striking the channels and network vessels with devitated eyes and mouth.

Dr. Lee combines this medicinal with **Quan Xie** and **Bai Jiang Can** for the treatment of neuropathic pain (e.g., trigeminal neuralgia) and intractable headache (e.g., migraine, cluster headache). Due to its high market price, Dr. Lee typically only prescribes it in cases where the pain is "unbearable."

*For more details, refer to **The Three Insects** profile.

Xi Lu Rong (細鹿茸) – refer to **Lu Rong**

Xian Di Huang (鮮地黃) – refer to **Sheng Di Huang**

Xian Zha (仙楂) – refer to **Shan Zha**

Xie (蠍) – refer to **Quan Xie**

Xiong Huang (雄黃/Realgar)

In classical literature on pharmacopoeia, it is described as follows: "Acrid [in flavor] and warm [in nature] with toxicity and obtains qi of right yang," "Enters the liver channel qi aspect," and "Tracks (down) the liver (搜肝 s□u g□n) and strengthens the spleen, dissipates great wind of the hundred joints (百節大風 bǎi jié dà f□ng), kills hundred toxin, and repels ghosts and goblins. Treats fright epilepsy and phlegm-drool, headache and dizziness, summerheat malaria and afflux dysentery (澼痢 pì lì), and diarrhea and accumulations and gatherings. [It] can also transform blood into water, dry dampness and kill worms, and treat taxation gan (勞疳 láo g□n), sores and boils, and snake bite."

In contemporary texts, it is described as having an acrid flavor, warm nature, and toxicity; entering the heart, liver and stomach channels; and having toxin-resolving worm-killing, dampness-drying, and wind-dispelling actions.

This medicinal contains the toxic constituent arsenic sulfide (As2S2). To mitigate the potential for harmful side effects and ensure safety, a time-consuming and rigorous traditional water grind (water-refining) processing method must be performed (calcination is strictly prohibited!). This processed pulverized powder form of **Xiong Huang** is then used for clinical application. It is experimentally and clinically proven to contain potent and effective toxin-resolving, worm-killing (i.e., antimicrobial), and anticancer actions (i.e., suppresses cell differentiation, induces apoptosis, inhibits tumor growth and angiogenesis).

Administered orally, this medicinal can only be prescribed in minuscule doses and added within a well-balanced formula composition due to the potential risk of adverse effects if taken in excessive dosages (e.g., suppression of hematopoiesis). **Xiong Huang** powder is included in the Yu Sheng formula compositions of Bao An Wan Ling Dan, Sai Ji (Vaginal Suppository), Xi Ji (Vaginal Wash/Douche), Shuang Shen Fen, and Medicated Thread (Yao Xian).

Dr. Lee also uses this medicinal as an external application for the treatment of herpes zoster skin rash.

Yin Xing Ye (銀杏葉/Folium Ginkgo/Ginkgo Leaf/aka **Bai Guo Ye)**

This medicinal is the leaf of *Ginkgo biloba* L. and its seed is **Bai Guo**.

In classical literature on pharmacopoeia, it is described as follows: "Grind into powder, knead into dough, make into cake, roast and eat cooked, [it] checks diarrhea and dysentery."

In contemporary texts, it is described as having a bitter, sweet and astringent flavor, balanced nature, and mild toxicity; entering the heart, lung, and spleen channels; and having blood-quickening heart-nourishing and lung-constraining intestine-astringing actions.

Traditionally, it is prescribed for the treatment of chest impediment heart pain, panting with phlegm cough, diarrhea and dysentery, and white vaginal discharge. Experimental animal studies have shown that the flavonols (i.e., quercetin, kaempferol, and isorhamnetin) and biflavonols in **Yin Xing Ye** have the capacity to dilate coronary blood vessels, increase coronary blood flow, lower serum cholesterol, and inhibit platelet aggregation. Dr. Lee explains that one of its main physiological mechanisms involves increasing exchanges across blood vessel membranes.

This is a commonly prescribed medicinal in Dr. Lee's pharmacopoeia and is prescribed for the treatment of such conditions as coronary artery disease (CAD), angina pectoris, hyperlipidemia, atherosclerosis, hypertension, cerebral vasospasm, and aneurysms. It is also an essential medicinal in (Yu Sheng) Bu Yang Huan Wu Tang, which is typically prescribed for sequelae of cerebrovascular accident (CVA), Parkinson's disease (PD), Alzheimer's disease (AD), and other cerebrovascular, cardiovascular and neurodegenerative pathoconditions.

Yu Gui (玉桂) – refer to **Rou Gui**

Ze Xie (澤瀉/Rhizoma Alismatis Orientalitis/Alisma)

In classical literature on pharmacopoeia, it is described as follows: "Enters the urinary bladder [channel], disinhibits urine, drains fire evil in the kidney channel, and specializes in disinhibiting dampness and moving water."

In contemporary texts, it is described as having a sweet and bland flavor and cold nature; entering the kidney and urinary bladder channels; and having water-disinhibiting dampness-percolating and heat-discharging actions. It is experimentally proven to increase urine output along with the excretion of urea and chloride, lower blood pressure, and lower blood sugar levels.

As a general rule, if large doses of this medicinal are prescribed ($\geq$ 8 qian), Dr. Lee will include a comparable dose of **Fu Ling** to enhance water-disinhibiting actions.

*For more details, refer to **The Four Lings** profile.

Zhu Ling (豬苓/Sclerotium Polyporus Umbellati/Polyporus)

In classical literature on pharmacopoeia, it is described as follows: "Bitter [in flavor] drains stagnation, bland [in flavor] disinhibits the orifices, and sweet [in flavor] assists yang. Enters the urinary bladder kidney channel, upbears thus can downbear, opens the interstices and promotes sweating, disinhibits urine and moves water, and has similar actions as **Fu Ling** except that it doesn't supplement...."

In contemporary texts, it is described as having a sweet and bland flavor and a balanced nature; entering the kidney and urinary bladder channels; and having water-disinhibiting dampness-percolating actions. **Zhu Ling** has a stronger water-disinhibiting action compared to **Fu Ling**, but not as strong of a supplementing action. The physiological mechanism of its urine-disinhibiting (diuretic) action primarily involves inhibiting the absorption of water and electrolytes (specifically potassium (K+), sodium (Na+), and chlorine (Cl-)) in the renal tubules of the nephron.

*For more details, refer to **The Four Lings** profile.

DR. LEE'S FORMULAS

This section introduces the formulas Dr. Lee commonly prescribes and includes details about the dose and action of each medicinal, the composite action of each formula, and the types of pathoconditions for which each formula is typically administered. Many of these formulas are variants on Han dynasty classical formulas from the *On Cold Damage and Miscellaneous Diseases* (傷寒雜病論 *Shang Han Za Bing Lun*), some are variants on more contemporary classic formulas from the Tang, Song, Ming, and Qing dynasties, and others are original formulas designed by Dr. Lee. Additionally, other formulas that Dr. Lee mentions as alternatively effective therapeutic options within the text are also listed for reference with only the compositions provided.

Throughout the text, the name "(Yu Sheng)" may be included in front of a formula's name to distinguish that it is a Dr. Lee variant on an existing formula or his own unique composition. Even when not included, it is still implied that all of the formulas Dr. Lee prescribes are indeed (Yu Sheng) formulas. The term Yu Sheng simply refers to Yu Sheng Chinese Medicine Clinic of which Dr. Lee is the founder, director, and chief physician.

The following formulas are set compositions designed to treat the extensive scope of pathoconditions that Dr. Lee commonly incurs in his clinical practice. The medicinals comprising the formulas are either purchased already processed or processed in-house, and then pre-weighed and pre-packaged into semiporous decocting packets (not yet sealed) for convenient storage and administration. Dr. Lee makes modifications to these formulas by adding medicinals based on each individual patient's symptoms, signs, and pattern identification. The packets are then sealed and ready for administration and decoction. This is not an exhaustive listing: when special cases present, Dr. Lee will compose formulas specifically designed for a particular case.

As time evolves, social and environmental factors affect the manifestation of maladies in the human body and mind. Dr. Lee continues to search for the best approaches to provide the most effective treatment in our modern world.

*__Disclaimer__: The formula compositions and medicinal doses provided in Dr. Lee's commonly prescribed formulas listed below and throughout this entire book are *for reference purposes only* and are *not* intended for indiscriminate administration by other individuals or parties. Prescription of these formulas should only be administered by a licensed traditional Chinese medicine (TCM) physician or practitioner who has carefully evaluated the patient's history, signs, and symptoms, and conducted pattern identification as the basis for determining treatment. Licensed TCM practitioners must be aware that these formula compositions and medicinal doses are for reference purposes only and are solely intended for administration by Dr. Lee in his own clinical practice.

Asthma Formula (氣喘方 / Qi Chuan Fang)

Ma Huang	1.5 qian
Dan Shen, Cang Zhu, Fu Ling, Gan Cao	3 qian each
Mu Xiang, Sha Ren, Wu Wei Zi	3 qian each
Chen Pi, Ban Xia, Xing Ren, Bai Guo	4 qian each
Shan Yao, Rou Gui	5 qian each

This original Yu Sheng formula contains the qi-boosting spleen-fortifying and qi-moving phlegm-transforming actions of **Xiang Sha Liu Jun Zi Tang** adding Ma Huang, Wu Wei Zi, Xing Ren, Bai Guo, Shan Yao, and Rou Gui. Ma Huang promotes sweating and resolves the exterior; Wu Wei Zi constrains the lung and stabilizes panting; Xing Ren suppresses cough and calms panting; Bai Guo constrains the lung and dispels phlegm; Shan Yao supplements the spleen, lung, and kidneys and nourishes yin; and Rou Gui supplements fire and assists yang for the treatment of vacuity asthma debilitation of the life gate fire. Dr. Lee will also add Ren Shen (powder), which enters the lung and spleen channels, greatly supplements original qi, and supplements the spleen and boosts the lung. As its name indicates, this formula is designed for the treatment of asthma, and specifically for the spleen yang vacuity pattern type that presents with panting (asthma) and shortness of breath (dyspnea).

Spleen yang vacuity pattern presents in the early stages of this pathocondition, when it can be more readily managed and often even cured. If this pathocondition progresses to the more severe, chronic stage of kidney yang vacuity pattern, Dr. Lee typically prescribes **You Gui Yin** variant. For acute flare-ups, heat-clearing toxin-resolving, lung-depurating phlegm-transforming, and cough-suppressing panting-calming medicinals will be added to the formula; or the original formula will be substituted with a heat-clearing, cough-suppressing, and panting-calming formula variant (e.g., **Ma Xing Gan Shi Tang**, **Da Qing Long Tang**) until the flare-up subsides.

Atopic Dermatitis Formula (異位性皮膚炎方/Yi Wei Xing Pi Fu Yan Fang)

Ma Huang	1.5 qian
Dan Shen, Cang Zhu, Fu Ling, Gan Cao	3 qian each
Chen Pi, Ban Xia, Mu Xiang, Sha Ren	3 qian each
Xing Ren, Bai Guo, Wu Wei Zi, Shan Yao	3 qian each
Dang Gui, He Shou Wu, Tu Si Zi, Sha Yuan Zi	5 qian each

This is an Yu Sheng original compound formula derived from **Asthma Formula (Qi Chuan Fang)** (subtracting Rou Gui) and **Blood Desiccation Formula (Xue Ku Fang)** (subtracting Ci Ji Li). **Asthma Formula** supplements the spleen, lung, and kidneys, nourishes yin, resolves the exterior, opens the pores, and dispels phlegm; and **Blood Desiccation Formula** nourishes blood, enriches yin, and dispels wind. As its name indicates, Dr. Lee administers this formula for the treatment of atopic dermatitis and specifically spleen yang vacuity patttern type.

Depending on the patient's presenting signs, symptoms and pattern, the following medicinals are commonly added: for severe pruritus—Shi Gao, Lu Lu Tong, and Hua Shi; for flare-ups with excessive suppuration—Bai Xian Pi, Huang Qin, Yi Yi Ren; and for chronic persistent cases with erythematous lesions (in body creases or generalized), cracking, suppuration, pruritus, and agitation—the medicinal doses in **Blood Desiccation Formula** will be increased with small amounts of The Three Great Yang-Supplementers (Gan Jiang, Fu Zi, and Rou Gui) added to supplement kidney and spleen vacuity and return and reinforce yang.

Ba Xian Chang Shou Wan (八仙長壽丸)

Sheng Di Huang, Shan Zhu Yu, Huai Shan, Fu Ling, Mu Dan Pi, Ze Xie, Mai Men Dong, Wu Wei Zi

Bai He Gu Jin Tang (百合固金湯)

Bai He, Sheng Di Huang, Shu Di Huang, Yuan Shen	3 qian each
Jie Geng, Gan Cao, Mai Men Dong	3 qian each
Dang Gui, Chi Shao, Cang Zhu	3 qian each

Bai Hu Tang (白虎湯)

Zhi Mu, Shi Gao, Gan Cao, Jing Mi

Bai Tou Weng Tang (白頭翁湯)

Bai Tou Weng, Qin Pi, Huang Lian, Huang Bo

Ban Xia Hou Po Tang (半夏厚朴湯)

Ban Xia, Hou Po, Fu Ling, Sheng Jiang, Gan Su Ye

Ban Xia Tian Ma Bai Zhu San (半夏天麻白朮散)

Dang Gui	2 qian
Ban Xia, Bai Zhu, Fu Ling, Cang Zhu	3 qian each
Ze Xie, Chen Pi, Shen Qu	3 qian each
Mai Ya, Gan Jiang, Huang Bo	3 qian each
Fu Zi, Tian Ma	5 qian each
Huang Qi	1 liang

The Yu Sheng version is virtually the same as the original formula except for the addition of Dang Gui and Fu Zi, and the fact that Ren Shen (powder) is either taken separately or added into the formula after decoction. Dang Gui supplements and quickens the blood and Fu Zi returns yang and stems counterflow, supplements fire and reinforces yang, and dissipates cold and relieves pain. These additions complement this foot Tai Yin spleen channel formula's overall spleen and stomach-supplementing, phlegm-damp transforming, and wind-stabilizing actions. The classical TCM pathomechanisms of this formula are explained as follows: "Phlegm reversal [refers to] phlegm-damp reverse flow ascending. Phlegm counterflow leads to upper body repletion, causing headache, dizzy head, and black [spots] in front of the eyes [visual field]."

This is among Dr. Lee's most commonly prescribed formulas, administered for a wide range of pathoconditions including Meniere's disease, benign paroxysmal positional vertigo (BPPV), psychosomatic symptoms (e.g., abdominal distention, malaise, and fatigue), migraine and cluster headaches, traumatic brain injury resulting in increased intracranial pressure, and benign brain tumors. It is also one of the commonly prescribed formulas in Dr. Lee's cancer treatment protocol, specifically administered for malignant brain tumors.

Bao An Wan Ling Dan (保安萬靈丹/Safeguard Unlimited Efficacy Elixir)

Tian Ma, Chuan Xiong, Chuan Wu, Wu Cao	1 liang each
Fang Feng, Jing Jie, Ma Huang, Xi Xin	1 liang each
Qiang Huo, He Shou Wu, Dang Gui	1 liang each
Shi Hu, Quan Xie, Gan Cao	1 liang each
Cang Zhu	8 liang
Xiong Huang	6 qian

Dr. Lee uses the *Orthodox Manual of External Medicine* (外科正宗 *Wai Ke Zheng Zong*) version of this formula and commonly abbreviates the name, calling it simply **Wan Ling Dan**. This is a pill specially prepared for Dr. Lee by an outsourced medicinal processing facility. It is composed of medicinals that dispel wind, eliminate dampness, dissipate cold, extinguish wind, quicken the blood, supplement the blood, check tetany, free the network vessels, open the orifices, resolve toxin, dissipate binds, and relieve pain. Xiong Huang is among the principal medicinals in this composition with its antimicrobial and anticancer actions (e.g., suppresses cell differentiation, induces apoptosis, and inhibits tumor growth and angiogenesis).

As its name implies, this formula has been traditionally administered for the treatment of a broad spectrum of pathoconditions including welling- and flat-abscesses, deep pus sores, clove toxin, mouth-level nape flat abscess, jowl effusion, damp phlegm streaming sore, bone flat-abscesses, crane's-knee wind, wind-cold-damp impediment, paralysis, tetanus, and migraine headaches.

Dr. Lee prescribes this formula for various types of acute, chronic, and intractable pathoconditions including innominate toxin-swelling, benign tumors, and paralysis resulting from parasitic infection. It also constitutes one of the pillars of Dr. Lee's cancer treatment protocol, prescribed as a part of the regimen for all types of solid tumors (e.g., carcinoma, sarcoma) and hematological cancers (i.e., leukemia, lymphoma, myeloma). Combined with other formulas, **Wan Ling Dan** has the capacity to induce partial or complete remission and lower the chances of recurrence and metastasis.

Bao He Wan (保和丸)

Shen Qu, Shan Zha, Fu Ling, Ban Xia, Chen Pi, Lian Qiao, Lai Fu Zi

Bie Jia Jian Wan (鱉甲煎丸)

Bie Jia, She Gan, Huang Qin, Chai Hu, Di Shi, Gan Jiang, Da Huang, Chi Shao, Gui Zhi, Ting Li Zi, Shi Wei, Hou Po, Mu Dan Pi, Qu Mai, Zi Wei, Ban Xia, Ren Shen, Zhe Chong, E Jiao, Feng Wo, Mang Xiao, Tang Lang, Tao Ren

Blood Desiccation Formula (血枯方 /Xue Ku Fang)

Cang Zhu, Ci Ji Li	4 qian each
Dang Gui, He Shou Wu, Tu Si Zi, Sha Yuan Zi	8 qian each

The term blood desiccation first appears in the *The Yellow Emperor's Inner Canon* (黃帝內經 *Huang Di Nei Jing*) and refers to this pathocondition as blood vacuity following hemorrhage. Indeed, Dr. Lee's adaptation of this term covers a much broader scope of applications. This Yu Sheng original formula has similar actions and clinical applications as **Dang Gui Yin Zi** containing the essential medicinals Dang Gui, He Shou Wu, and Ci Ji Li. However, it replaces Shao Yao, Chuan Xiong, and Sheng Di Huang with large doses of Dang Gui and He Shou Wu; subtracts Fang Feng, Jing Jie, and Huang Qi; and adds Sha Yuan Zi, Tu Si Zi, and Cang Zhu.

Sha Yuan Zi and Tu Si Zi both supplement the kidney, secure essence, and nourish the liver; and Cang Zhu dispels wind-damp and dries dampness and fortifies the spleen to counteract the potential for digestion impairment and loose stools resulting from the blood-nourishing yin-enriching medicinals. These additions complement this formula's overall actions of nourishing the blood, moistening dryness, dispeling wind, and relieving itch for the treatment of yin vacuity, blood vacuity, and blood desiccation patterns. For the treatment of skin pathoconditions, the relatively hardier Ma Huang is added to resolve the exterior instead of Fang Feng and Jing Jie (their volatile oils readily vaporize upon decoction and thus require large doses to achieve efficacy); and if itch presents, add Ci Ji Li, Zao Jiao Ci, and Lu Lu Tong.

Dr. Lee typically prescribes this formula for wind-dryness presenting as dry, itchy skin, and possibly mild redness (e.g., pruritus, erythema, urticaria, eczema, atopic dermatitis), liver blood vacuity (e.g., late stage hepatic cirrhosis with darkened skin and compromised hematopoiesis), and endometrial hypoperfusion (e.g., causing infertility and miscarriage).

Bu Yang Huan Wu Tang (補陽還五湯)

Dang Gui, Chuan Xiong, Chi Shao	4 qian each
Dan Shen, Yin Xing Ye	4 qian each
Huang Qi	2 liang

The Yu Sheng version is based on the original formula, but only contains 2 liang of Huang Qi as opposed to 4 liang; excludes Di Long, Tao Ren, and Hong Hua; and adds Yin Xing Ye and Dan Shen. Though not listed above, Ren Shen *is* included in this composition just as in the original formula, except in pulverized powder form, and is often paired with Chuan Qi (aka Ren Shen/Chuan Qi Powder). This medicinal pair serves to complement the qi-supplementing action of Huang Qi and the blood-quickening action of Dan Shen. Dr. Lee has chosen a relatively smaller dose of Huang Qi for this composition, because starting out with an excessive dose may result in the rupture of compromised blood vessels or a sudden increase in intracranial pressure in patients with arteriosclerosis, atherosclerosis, hematoma, or adhesions in the subarachnoid space of the meninges.

Yin Xing Ye is an essential medicinal in this formula and Dr. Lee utilizes its capacity of increasing exchanges across blood vessel membranes (e.g., promotes lymphatic circulation) and phlegm-transforming actions to reduce blood viscosity and eliminate plaque for patients with cerebrovascular accident (CVA) (stroke) sequelae, transient ischemic attack (TIA) sequelae, Parkinson's disease (PD), Alzheimer's disease (AD), and other cerebrovascular and neurodegenerative pathoconditions. Tao Ren, Hong Hua, and Di Long are excluded, because unlike stroke patients in the 18th and 19th centuries when this formula was designed, modern biomedicine has already intervened during the acute stage to accelerate reperfusion with drugs and surgical decompression. This intervention obviates the need for these potent blood-quickening stasis-dispeling and network vessel-freeing medicinals.

Nowadays, the primary role of TCM is to treat the neurological sequelae and prevent subsequent attacks. This requires the administration of dual supplementation of blood and qi, blood-quickening, and phlegm-transforming medicinals to reduce blood viscosity, maintain plaque-free vasculature, and prevent the development of emboli or thrombi. Prescribed for the treatment of neurodegenerative diseases (e.g., AD, PD, Huntington's disease), this formula slows down the rate of degeneration, enhances quality of life, and extends life expectancy.

Bu Zhong Yi Qi Tang (補中益氣湯)

Huang Qi	1 liang
Dang Gui	2 qian
Dan Shen, Cang Zhu, Chen Pi	3 qian each
Gan Cao, Sheng Ma, Chai Hu	3 qian each

The Yu Sheng version is similar to the original formula except that Dan Shen replaces Ren Shen for its blood-quickening stasis-dispelling action, and Cang Zhu replaces Bai Zhu for its spleen-fortifying dampness-drying action, which aids digestion and is more suitable for Taiwan's humid subtropical climate. However, depending on the presenting signs, symptoms, and pattern, Dr. Lee may also add Ren Shen (powder) (or Ren Shen/Chuan Qi Powder).

Dr. Lee prescribes this qi-boosting, yang-upbearing fall-raising, and spleen-supplementing stomach-regulating formula for pathoconditions such as anal prolapse, uterine prolapse, gastroptosis, nephroptosis, inguinal hernia, anal fissures, hemorrhoids, myasthenia gravis (qi-vacuity type), leukorrhea (qi-vacuity type), and proteinuria (intrinsic renal disease) in pediatric patients. Additionally, this formula's exceptional efficacy at promoting tissue repair and mucous membrane healing makes it an essential formula for patients with post-surgical wounds and cancer patients who have undergone (or are currently receiving) radiotherapy or chemotherapy.

Chai Hu Gui Zhi Tang (柴胡桂枝湯)

Chai Hu, Gui Zhi, Ren Shen, Gan Cao, Ban Xia, Huang Qin, Shao Yao, Da Zao, Sheng Jiang

Chai Hu Jia Long Gu Mu Li Tang (柴胡加龍骨牡蠣湯)

Chai Hu, Long Gu, Huang Qin, Sheng Jiang, Qian Dan, Ren Shen, Gui Zhi, Fu Ling, Ba Xia, Da Huang, Mu Li, Da Zao

Chai Ling Tang (柴苓湯)

Huang Qin, Fu Ling, Zhu Ling, Ze Xie	3 qian each
Cang Zhu, Yuan Hu Suo, Mu Xiang, Gui Zhi	3 qian each
Dan Shen, Ban Xia, Gan Cao, Sheng Jiang	5 qian each
Da Zao	3 pieces
Chai Hu	6 qian

The Yu Sheng version is similar to the original formula with the addition of Yuan Hu Suo, Mu Xiang, and Dan Shen, and the replacement of Bai Zhu with Cang Zhu; Ren Shen pulverized powder is used instead of decocting pieces; and unlike other Yu Sheng formulas, Gui Zhi *is* included (instead of Rou Gui) for its yang-assisting qi-transforming actions. Yan Hu Suo and Mu Xiang relax smooth muscle and thus relieve pain.

This is a compound formula that includes elements of **Xiao Chai Hu Tang (小柴胡湯)** and **Wu Ling San (Calculi Formula) (五苓散) (結石方)** and functions to eliminate heat, disinhibit water, and transform phlegm for the treatment of symptoms and patterns involving water amassment collecting above and below the diaphragm, amassed phlegm and collecting rheum, cold damage with residual Shao Yang heat, chest and rib-side distention and impediment, difficult urination, and vomiting and diarrhea upon drinking water.

Dr. Lee typically prescribes this formula for pathoconditions that manifest as ascites, portal hypertension, pleural effusion, pleuritis, pericardial effusion, cerebral edema, and increased intracranial pressure, such as in chronic liver disease (e.g., hepatitis, cirrhosis, fulminant hepatitis, hepatorenal syndrome (HRS), hepatocellular carcinoma), encephalitis, trauma, and radiotherapy. It is also one of the commonly prescribed formulas in Dr. Lee's cancer treatment protocol, specifically administered for Shao Yang cancers, which are identified as membranous tissue cancers manifesting in organs such as the liver, kidney, and lung.

Chang Shan Wan (常山丸)

Chang Shan, Cao Guo, Bing Lang, Zhi Mu, Bei Mu, Wu Mei, Sheng Jiang, Da Zao

Cheng Qi Tang (承氣湯) – refer to **Xiao Cheng Qi Tang**, **Da Cheng Qi Tang**, and **Tiao Wei Cheng Qi Tang**

Chi Shi Zhi Yu Yu Liang Tang (赤石脂禹餘糧湯)

Chi Shi Zhi, Yu Yu Liang

Chun Ze Tang (春澤湯)

Zhu Ling, Ze Xie, Bai Zhu, Fu Ling, Gui Zhi, Ren Shen

Da Chai Hu Tang (大柴胡湯)

Chai Hu, Huang Qin, Ban Xia, Zhi Shi, Da Huang, Shao Yao, Sheng Jiang, Da Zao

Da Cheng Qi Tang (大承氣湯)

Da Huang, Hou Po, Zhi Shi, Mang Xiao

Da Qing Long Tang (大青龍湯/Major Green-Blue Dragon)

Ma Huang	2 qian
Xing Ren, Cang Zhu	4 qian each
Rou Gui, Sheng Jiang, Gan Cao	3 qian each
Sheng Shi Gao	1 liang
Da Zao	5 pieces

The Yu Sheng version is virtually identical to the original formula, which is a derivative of **Ma Huang Tang** that includes large doses of Ma Huang and Gan Cao and adds Sheng Shi Gao, Sheng Jiang, and Da Zao. However, as is the case in many of Dr. Lee's formulas, Rou Gui replaces Gui Zhi, and Cang Zhu is added due to considerations for Taiwan's humid subtropical climate. Its name, **Major Green-Blue Dragon**, refers to the fact that after taking this formula, sweat flows and evil abates as if a dragon rose up to the skies and brought rain pouring down, thus resulting in the immediate elimination of depressed heat.

This formula is traditionally prescribed for the treatment of external contraction wind-cold exterior repletion with interior heat pattern, presenting in pathoconditions such as the common cold, influenza, bronchitis, measles papules, wind papules, urticaria, and itchy skin. Similarly, Dr. Lee prescribes this formula for the treatment of Tai Yang cold damage with vexation and agitation from interior heat; however, for external medicine (i.e., dermatology) manifestations he may also consider prescribing formula variants such as **Yue Bi Tang**, **Gui Zhi Ma Huang Ge Ban Tang**, or **Ma Xing Gan Shi Tang** instead.

Da Xian Xiong Tang (大陷胸湯)

Da Huang, Mang Xiao, Gan Sui

Dan Dong Shen You Wan (舟東神佑丸)

Da Huang, Gan Sui, Da Ji, Yuan Hua, Qing Pi, Bing Lang, Chen Pi, Mu Xiang, Qian Niu, Qing Fen

Dang Gui Liu Huang Tang (當歸六黃湯)

Dang Gui, Sheng Di Huang, Shu Di Huang, Huang Qin, Huang Lian, Huang Bo, Huang Qi

Dang Gui San (當歸散)

Dang Gui, Chuan Xiong, Sheng Bai Shao	3 qian each
Sheng Di Huang, Chao Bai Zhu, Xu Duan	3 qian each
Du Zhong, Gan Cao	3 qian each
Shan Yao, Ai Cao	5 qian each
Huang Qin	2 qian

The Yu Sheng version is composed of the same essential medicinals as the original formula—Dang Gui, Chuan Xiong, Sheng Bai Shao, Chao Bai Zhu, and Huang Qin—along with the addition of Shan Yao, Ai Ye, Sheng Di Huang, Xu Duan, Du Zhong, and Gan Cao.

Sheng Di Huang clears heat and cools the blood and nourishes yin and engenders liquid; Xu Duan quickens the blood and stanches bleeding and supplements the liver and kidney and quiets the fetus; Du Zhong serves as a channel conductor directing medicinals downwards to the lumbus and lower limbs and supplements the liver and kidney and quiets the fetus; Ai Ye warms the channels and stanches bleeding, dissipates cold and regulates menstruation, and quiets the fetus; Shan Yao boosts qi and nourishes yin, supplements the spleen, lung, and kidney, and secures essence and checks vaginal discharge; and Gan Cao supplements the center and harmonizes the nature of medicinals. These additions enhance and complement the blood-nourishing blood-harmonizing, blood quickening stasis-moving, liver-emolliating construction aspect harmonizing, heat-clearing blood-cooling, and spleen-fortifying dampness-drying actions of this formula's essential medicinals.

This blood-nourishing fetus-quieting formula promotes a healthy pregnancy and treats all types of prenatal and postpartum pathoconditions. It is traditionally prescribed for women with a history of habitual abortion and/or premature labor, stirring fetus, scant blood with heat, heat vexation and thirst, hysteria, and aching lumbus and abdominal pain. This is Dr. Lee's first-line formula for a broad spectrum of obstetric pathoconditions such as the prevention of spontaneous abortions due to poor implantation of the blastocyst embryo during the first two weeks of pregnancy, absence of cervical mucous, ovulation disorders (e.g., anovulation, oligoovulation), thin endometrial lining, absence of cervical mucous, morning sickness, preeclampsia, and gestational diabetes; and also postpartum pathoconditions (e.g., "baby blues" (depression), perineal pain, uterine infection, mastitis).

Dang Gui Shao Yao San (當歸芍藥散)

Dang Gui, Shao Yao, Chuan Xiong, Fu Ling, Ze Xie, Bai Zhu

Dang Gui Si Ni Jia Wu Zhu Yu Gan Jiang Tang (當歸四逆吳茱萸湯)

Dang Gui, Gui Zhi, Bai Shao, Xi Xin, Gan Cao, Tong Cao, Da Zao, Wu Zhu Yu, Sheng Jiang

Dang Gui Si Ni Tang (當歸四逆湯)

Dang Gui, Gui Zhi, Bai Shao, Xi Xin, Gan Cao, Tong Cao, Da Zao

Dao Tan Tang (導痰湯)

Ban Xia, Ju Hong, Fu Ling, Gan Cao, Tian Nan Xing, Zhi Shi, Sheng Jiang

Di Dang Tang (抵擋湯)

Tao Ren	1 g
Meng Chong	2 g
Shui Zhi	2 g
Da Huang	3 g

Note: This formula is administered as a pulverized medicinal powder.

Di Gu Pi Yin (地骨皮飲)

Dang Gui, Chuan Xiong, Chi Shao	3 qian each
Sheng Di Huang, Gan Cao, Huang Qin	3 qian each
Cang Zhu	4 qian
Di Gu Pi, Mu Dan Pi	5 qian each

The Yu Sheng version is based on the *On Blood Pathoconditions* (血症論 *Xue Zheng Lun*) formula. It is composed of a **Si Wu Tang** variant (Dang Gui, Chuan Xiong, Chi Shao, Sheng Di Huang) adding Di Gu Pi, Mu Dan Pi, Huang Qin, and Cang Zhu. **Si Wu Tang** supplements and quickens the blood; Di Gu Pi nourishes yin, cools the blood, downbears latent heat in the lung, and supplements right qi; Mu Dan Pi drains latent heat in the blood and harmonizes, cools, and engenders blood; Huang Qin clears heat and dries dampness and drains fire and resolves toxin; and Cang Zhu fortifies the spleen and dries dampness to counteract the digestion impairment and loose stools some patients experience when administered blood-nourishing yin-enriching medicinals.

The blood-nourishing yin-enriching and heat-clearing blood-cooling actions of this formula are traditionally prescribed for the treatment of fire effulgence due to yin-vacuity, steaming bone taxation heat, heat entering the blood chamber, antepartum heat, and alternating tidal heat. Similarly, Dr. Lee typically prescribes this formula for yin-vacuity blood heat with stasis heat (or Shao Yang heat) pattern and steaming bone taxation heat (fever) pattern that manifests in pathoconditions such as autoimmune diseases, leukemia, lymphoma, idiopathic thrombocytopenic purpura (ITP), menopausal transition symptoms, sweating of the five hearts, dengue fever, tuberculosis, and vasculitis.

Di Long San (地龍散)

Rou Gui, Di Long, Huang Bo, Gan Cao, Qiang Huo, Su Mu, Ma Huang, Tao Ren, Dang Gui, Du Huo

Di Tan Tang (滌痰湯)

Ban Xia, Tian Nan Xing, Ju Hong, Zhi Shi, Fu Ling, Ren Shen, Shi Chang Pu, Zhu Ru, Gan Cao, Sheng Jiang, Da Zao

Diao Fen Gao (吊粉膏/Suspension Powder Paste)

Da Huang, Huang Bo	1 part
Ru Xiang, Mo Yao	1 part
Xu Duan, Gu Sui Bu	1 part
Chuan Wu, Cao Wu	1 part
Rice Wine	

These medicinals are pulverized into medicinal powder and then mixed with rice wine (27% alcohol) to form a medicinal paste (藥膏 yào g□o) that is applied topically in the acute stage of inflammation. This is the stage presenting with heat, pain, redness (or purplish), and swelling in traumatic injuries (e.g., sprains, subluxation, fractures). It comprises equal parts of heat-dispersing inflammation-resolving; blood-quickening stasis-transforming and swelling-dispersing flesh-engendering; sinew- and bone-strengthening and injury-treating breakage-mending; and anesthetic and pain-relieving medicinals.

This medicinal paste is spread on fine burlap cloth, covered with gauze, and then sufficiently wrapped with bandage and secured with tubular elastic net dressing (wrapped just tight enough to secure the cloth in place without adversely affecting circulation). For best efficacy, it is recommended that the medicinal paste be left on for 6 to 8 hours; however, in the rare case of mild allergic reaction (e.g., patient feels itchiness, tingling, and discomfort), it should be removed ahead of the recommended time.

Du Huo Ji Sheng Tang (獨活寄生湯)

Shu Di Huang	8 qian
Ren Shen, Gan Jiang, Fu Zi, Qin Jiao, Xu Duan	5 qian each

Gu Sui Bu, Gui Ban, Bie Jia, Du Zhong	5 qian each
Niu Xi, Chen Pi, Du Huo, Wu Jia Pi	5 qian each
Fu Ling, Chao Shao Yao, Chao Bai Zhu	4 qian each
Dang Gui, Chuan Xiong, Rou Gui, Huang Qin	3 qian each
Fang Feng, Xi Xin, Gan Cao	3 qian each
Dang Shen, Huang Qi, Sang Ji Sheng	1 liang each

Er Chen Tang (二陳湯)

Huang Qin	3 qian
Chen Pi, Ban Xia, Fu Ling, Gan Cao	4 qian each

The Yu Sheng version is similar to the original except for the subtraction of Sheng Jiang and Wu Mei and the addition of Huang Qin, whose heat-clearing dampness-drying actions are acclimated for Taiwan's humid subtropical climate, complementing this formula's overall dampness-drying phlegm-harmonizing and qi-normalizing center-harmonizing actions. The derivatives of **Er Chen Tang**—**Wen Dan Tang** and **Ban Xia Tian Ma Bai Zhu San**—are frequently prescribed for a broad scope of pathoconditions ranging from external contraction (common cold), psychosomatic symptoms (e.g., abdominal distention, malaise, and fatigue) to infertility, glaucoma and brain tumors.

Er Miao San (二妙散)

Huang Bo, Cang Zhu, Sheng Jiang Zhi (Raw Ginger Juice)

Fang Ji Huang Qi Tang (方己黃耆湯)

Fang Ji, Huang Qi, Bai Zhu, Gan Cao, Sheng Jiang, Da Zao

Feng Shi Fang (風濕方)

Ma Huang	1.5 qian
Rou Gui, Chi Shao, Gan Cao, Gan Jiang	3 qian each
Fu Zi, Huang Qin, Huang Bo, Fu Ling	3 qian each
Zhu Ling, Ze Xie, Cang Zhu, Sheng Shi Gao	3 qian each
Jin Yin Hua, Wu Wei Zi, Yin Yang Huo	3 qian each
Da Zao	5 pieces

This Yu Sheng original formula was designed by Dr. Lee early on in his clinical practice and was specifically administered for patients with rheumatic disorders (e.g., osteoarthritis (OA), rheumatoid arthritis (RA)) either currently receiving or having recently received administration of immunosuppressants (e.g., corticosteroids).

In years past, Western medical doctors in Taiwan indiscriminately prescribed systemic corticosteroids for the treatment of all types of inflammatory pain, including rheumatic disorders, without any consideration given to the deleterious side effects. This practice has been largely superseded by a more responsible approach that has in part been driven by the advent of new drugs and drug combinations.

Attuned to the pulse of our ever-evolving modern environment, nowadays, Dr. Lee typically prescribes **(Yu Sheng) Hyperactive Immune Formula** for these types of pathoconditions instead.

Fu Ling Bu Xin Tang (茯苓補心湯)

Fu Ling, Rou Gui, Da Zao, Zi Shi Ying, Gan Cao, Ren Shen, Chi Xiao Dou, Mai Men Dong

Gan Jiang Ren Shen Ban Xia Wan (乾薑人參半下丸)

Gan Jiang, Ren Shen, Ban Xia, Sheng Jiang

Gan Mai Da Zao Tang (甘麥大棗湯)

Gan Cao, Xiao Mai, Da Zao

Gan Mai Da Zao Tang Combining Ban Xia Hou Po Tang (甘麥大棗湯合併半夏厚朴湯)

Ban Xia, Hou Po, Zi Su Zi, Fu Ling	4 qian
Gan Cao	5 qian
Da Zao	10 pieces
Fu Xiao Mai	1 liang

This is a compound formula with a composition almost identical to the original formulas except for the subtraction of Sheng Jiang. **Gan Mai Da Zao Tang** has the actions of harmonizing the center and quieting the spirit and relaxing tension and calming agitation, and is traditionally prescribed for the treatment of visceral agitation. **Ban Xia Hou Po Tang** has the actions of moving qi and downbearing counterflow and dissipating stagnation and transforming phlegm, and is traditionally prescribed for the treatment of seven-affect binding depression (七情鬱結 q□ qíng yù jié) (e.g., mood disorders such as anxiety, depression, hypomania), insomnia, palpitations, gastrointestinal neurosis, vocal cord nodules and polyps, plum-pit qi, and menopausal transition symptoms.

Since the actions and indications of these two formulas are complementary, Dr. Lee has combined them for the treatment of a broad spectrum of mood, psychosomatic, and neuropsychiatric disorders (e.g., mild cases of Tourette syndrome) including those mentioned above. For some presenting with phlegm reversal and ascending counterflow symptoms (e.g., abdominal distention, headache, malaise, fatigue), Dr. Lee will prescribe this compound formula in combination with another formula, such as **Ban Xia Tian Ma Bai Zhu San**. And for relatively mild pathoconditions, he may prescribe one of these simple formulas on its own.

Ge Gen Qin Lian Tang (葛根芩連湯)/aka **Ge Gen Huang Qin Huang Lian Tang (葛根黃芩黃連湯)**

Ge Gen, Huang Qin, Huang Lian, Gan Cao

Ge Gen Tang (葛根湯)

Ma Huang	1.5 liang
Huang Qin, Cang Zhu	3 qian each
Ge Gen, Chi Shao, Gan Cao, Rou Gui, Sheng Jiang	5 qian each
Da Zao	5 pieces

The Yu Sheng version is very similar to the original formula, which is a derivative of **Gui Zhi Tang**. But as in Dr. Lee's other formulas, Rou Gui replaces Gui Zhi and Chi Shao replaces Bai Shao, and Cang Zhu and Huang Qin are added due to considerations for Taiwan's humid subtropical climate. This formula promotes sweating and resolves the exterior and upbears liquid and courses the channels.

Dr. Lee commonly prescribes variants of this formula for external contraction with Yang Ming headache and body ache, heat effusion (fever) without sweating, aversion to cold, stretched stiffness of the nape and back (項背強几几 xiàng bèi qiáng sh□ sh□), crick in the neck, and sinusitis. This formula is also prescribed for patients with acute stage facial palsy (caused by trauma or tumor), Bell's palsy (caused by a virus such as herpes simplex), or trigeminal neuralgia, who have *not* been prescribed corticosteroids.

The inclusion of Huang Qin and Cang Zhu in the Yu Sheng version of this formula also makes it easily modified into **Ge Gen Huang Qin Huang Lian Tang** (by adding Huang Lian) for the treatment of heat evil entering the interior causing diarrhea or dysentery (gastroenteritis) and exterior evil that has not yet resolved.

Gong Zhen Dan (拱振丹)

Lu Rong, Shan Zhu Yu, Dang Gui, She Xiang

Gui Ma Ge Ban Tang (桂麻各半湯) – refer to **Gui Zhi Ma Huang Ge Ban Tang (桂枝麻黃各半湯)**

Gui Pi Tang (歸脾湯)

Ren Shen, Huang Qi, Bai Zhu, Fu Ling, Dang Gui, Suan Zao Ren, Gui Yuan Rou, Yuan Zhi, Mu Xiang, Gan Cao, Sheng Jiang, Da Zao

Gui Qi Jian Zhong Tang (歸耆建中湯)

Dang Gui	2 qian
Gan Jiang, Huang Qin, Cang Zhu	3 qian each
Rou Gui, Chi Shao, Gan Cao, Fu Zi	5 qian each
Da Zao	5 pieces
Huang Qi	1 liang

This formula is derived from **Xiao Jian Zhong Tang** adding Dang Gui and Huang Qi. The Yu Sheng version of this formula is similar to the original version, but includes large doses of Huang Qi; replaces Bai Shao with Chi Shao, Sheng Jiang with Gan Jiang, and Gui Pi with large doses of Rou Gui (superior quality and efficacy); and adds Cang Zhu, Da Zao, and a large dose of Fu Zi. Huang Qin is also added for its heat-clearing dampness-drying and fire-draining toxin-resolving actions that counteract the great heat medicinals of Gan Jiang, Rou Gui, and Fu Zi. Huang Qi functions as a channel conductor for the upper limbs and Rou Gui as a channel conductor for the four extremities (the limbs).

The additions to the Yu Sheng version of this formula enhance its qi-supplementing center-fortifying, tension-relaxing interior-harmonizing, and blood supplementing actions, while also equipping it with the capacity to treat vacuity cold pathoconditions of the upper body.

Dr. Lee commonly prescribes this formula for cold impediment of the Tai Yang small intestine channel, neuropathy, frozen shoulder, and Raynaud's disease (and phenomenon); and for skin pathoconditions (e.g., non-erupting papules (acne), menopausal pruritus).

Gui Zhi Jia Ling Zhu Fu Tang (桂枝加苓朮附湯)

Gui Zhi, Fu Ling, Bai Zhu, Fu Zi, Sheng Jiang, Gan Cao, Da Zao

Gui Zhi Jia Long Gu Mu Li Tang (桂枝加龍骨牡蠣湯)

Cang Zhu	4 qian
Rou Gui, Chi Shao, Gan Cao, Sheng Jiang	5 qian each
Sheng Long Gu, Sheng Mu Li, Shan Yao, Dang Shen	5 qian each
Da Zao	5 pieces

The Yu Sheng version contains all of the essential medicinals of the original formula with the exception of Rou Gui replacing Gui Zhi and the addition of Dang Shen, Shan Yao, and Cang Zhu. The qi-boosting spleen-fortifying and essence-securing dampness-drying actions of these additional medicinals complement this formula's overall action of neutrally supplementing yin and yang, subduing and settling, and securing essence and containing urine.

This formula is traditionally prescribed for pathoconditions such as vacuity taxation with dual yin and yang vacuity, dreaming with seminal emission, hypertonicity of the lesser abdomen, lower burner vacuity cold, stirring palpitations below the umbilicus resulting from urinary incontinence, and hysteria.

In addition to these pathoconditions, Dr. Lee also prescribes this formula for the treatment of juvenile acne, stress-related hair loss (e.g., alopecia areata, hair shedding (telogen effluvium), hair pulling disorder (trichotillomania)), and children with hyperactivity or impulsivity (e.g., attention deficit hyperactivity disorder (ADHD)). Early on in Dr. Lee's clinical practice, he would prescribe this formula for obstetrics pathoconditions, but in recent years he typically prescribes **Dang Gui San** variants instead.

Gui Zhi Ma Huang Ge Ban Tang (桂枝麻黃各半湯)

Gui Zhi, Ma Huang, Shao Yao, Sheng Jiang, Xing Ren, Gan Cao, Da Zao

Gui Zhi Tang (桂枝湯) – refer to **Yang Dan Tang (陽但湯)**

Huang Lian Jie Du Tang (黃連解毒湯)

Huang Lian, Huang Qin, Huang Bo, Zhi Zi	3 qian each
Cang Zhu	4 qian
Gan Cao	5 qian

The Yu Sheng version is virtually the same as the original formula except for the addition of Cang Zhu and Gan Cao. Cang Zhu fortifies the spleen and dries dampness and Gan Cao supplements the center and harmonizes the nature of medicinals—a pair that combines to promote digestion and protect the stomach from the bitter flavor and cold nature of the essential medicinals. The essential medicinals of this formula are The Three Yellows (Huang Qin, Huang Bo, and Huang Lian), which Dr. Lee commonly utilizes for their heat-clearing toxin-resolving (antimicrobial and anti-inflammatory) actions.

This is a commonly administered formula for triple burner heat toxin congestion. Huang Lian drains heart fire and middle burner fire; Huang Qin drains upper burner fire; Huang Bo drains lower burner fire; and Zhi Zi frees and drains heat in all three burners, abducting heat downward where the heat evil is excreted in the urine. These medicinals contain powerful heat-clearing toxin-resolving (antimicrobial and anti-inflammatory) actions, and when combined together into one formula provide exceptional efficacy for the treatment of all types of infections and inflammation throughout the body (e.g., upper respiratory, gastrointestinal, hepatic, renal, genitourinary, autoimmune disorders).

It is important to note here that long-term administration (≥ 3 months) of Zhi Zi may cause transient grayish yellow skin pigmentation in some patients. In cases where long-term administration is necessary, Dr. Lee will either subtract Zhi Zi or prescribe another formula, such as the heat-clearing toxin-resolving and yin vacuity-heat clearing yin-enriching **Hyperactive Immune Formula**, instead.

Huo Luo Dan (活絡丹/Network-Quickening Elixir)

Dang Gui, Ru Xiang, Mo Yao	5 jin each
Dan Shen, Di Long, Chuan Wu	5 jin each
Wu Cao, Tian Nan Xing, Ma Huang	5 jin each

The Yu Sheng version is identical to the original formula, which is also known as **Xiao Huo Luo Dan (小活絡丹/Minor Network-Quickening Elixir)**, except for the addition of Dang Gui, Dan Shen, and Ma Huang. Dang Gui supplements and quickens the blood; Dan Shen quickens the blood and dispels stasis; and Ma Huang "opens up" and transports medicinals across all membranes. These additions complement and further enhance this formula's overall wind-dispeling dampness-dispersing, blood-quickening stasis-dispeling, and network vessel-freeing pain-relieving actions.

This formula is traditionally prescribed for the treatment of wind-cold-damp evil invading the channels and network vessels, contraction and pain of the sinews and vessels, inhibited bending and stretching of the joints, and wandering aches and pain; insensitivity of the limbs following stroke and phlegm-damp dead blood in the channels and network vessels; and knocks and falls (traumatic injury) and stasis obstruction in the channels and network vessels causing pain.

Dr. Lee utilizes this pill's blood-quickening stasis-dispelling and channel- and network vessel-freeing actions for its exceptional efficacy in relieving pain, particularly for wind-damp impediment and traumatic injuries involving the lumbus and lower limbs. This pill is produced and processed in-house, using a strictly controlled fermentation method and oven-roast process that safely ensures elimination of the potential for toxicity.

Hyperactive Immune Formula (免疫過抗方/Mian Yi Guo Kang Fang)

Huang Lian, Huang Qin, Huang Bo, Cang Zhu	5 qian each
Qing Hao, Zhi Mu, Di Gu Pi	5 qian each

This formula was designed relatively later in Dr. Lee's clinical practice primarily for the treatment of connective tissue diseases, degenerative disorders, and systemic inflammation in patients who are *not* being administered immunosuppressants (e.g., systemic corticosteroids, high dose methotrexate (MTX)) or those who *have* been administered immunosuppressants for ≤ 1 week.

It is composed of the essential medicinals from **(Yu Sheng) Huang Lian Jie Du Tang** (Huang Lian, Huang Qin, Huang Bo, and Cang Zhu) along with the additions of Qing Hao, Zhi Mu, and Di Gu Pi. These medicinals combine to form a potent combination of heat-clearing toxin-resolving (anti-inflammatory), vacuity heat-clearing steaming bone-eliminating, yin-enriching dryness-moistening, and blood-cooling fire-draining actions.

As mentioned in the **Feng Shi Fang** profile, the changing practice of Western medicine in Taiwan has seen a trend away from indiscriminate administration of systemic corticosteroids. In response, Dr. Lee now commonly prescribes this formula for treating patients with a broad scope of pathoconditions presenting with acute stage inflammation and chronic autoimmune and degenerative diseases (e.g., including osteoarthritis (OA), rheumatoid arthritis (RA), ankylosing spondylitis (AS), systemic lupus erythematosis (SLE), polymyositis, dermatomyositis, scleroderma, multiple sclerosis (MS), Behcet's disease (BD), Sjogren's syndrome (SS), immune thrombocytopenic purpura (ITP), inflammatory bowel disease (IBS), vasculitis).

In addition to applying eight-principle and six-channel pattern identification methods, inflammatory indices (e.g., erythrocyte sedimentation rate (ESR), antinuclear antibody (ANA), rheumatoid factor (RF)) are invaluable diagnostic tools for determining the severity of inflammation and gauging clinical efficacy. This formula provides reliable and lasting effectiveness in resolving inflammation and relieving symptoms (i.e., treat the tip). Once the inflammation is under control, the patient can proceed on to other supplementing and nourishing TCM formulas in the process of bringing the pathocondition into complete remission (i.e., treat the root).

Jia Wei Er Miao San (加味二妙散)

Cang Zhu, Huang Bo, Gui Ban, Bi Xie, Zhi Mu

Jia Wei Gui Pi Tang (加味歸脾湯)

Ren Shen, Huang Qi, Fu Shen, Gan Cao, Bai Zhu, Mu Xiang, Yuan Zhi, Suan Zao Ren, Long Yan Rou, Dang Gui, Mu Dan Pi, Shan Zhi

Jian Ling Tang (健瓴湯)

Ci Shi	3 qian
Bo Zi Ren	4 qian
Niu Xi, Chi Shao, Sheng Long Gu	5 qian each
Sheng Mu Li, Sheng Di Huang, Shan Yao	5 qian each
Dai Zhe Shi	8 qian

The Yu Sheng version is virtually the same as the original formula with the exception of Chi Shao replacing Bai Shao and the addition of Ci Shi. As in many Yu Sheng formulas, Chi Shao is selected for its superior blood-quickening stasis-dispeling actions. The primary constituents of this spirit-quieting by heavy settling formula are Dai Zhe Shi—enters the blood aspect of the liver and heart channels, eliminates heat, calms the liver and subdues yang, and downbears counterflow by heavy settling; Ci Shi—enters the liver and kidney channels, governs the lung and kidney, settles fright and quiets the spirit, and calms the liver and subdues yang; Sheng Long Gu—enters the heart, liver, and kidney channels, subdues yang, and quiets the spirit; and Sheng Mu Li—calms the liver and subdues yang, softens hardness and dissipates binds, and astringes and secures.

Dr. Lee typically reserves this formula for only the most severe cases of ascendent hyperactivity of yang, manifesting in pathoconditions such as hyperglycemia (diabetes), hypertension, hyperthyroidism, insomnia, schizophrenia, and Tourette syndrome. This includes cases in which Western medicine drug therapy has been administered without efficacy, or with initial efficacy, but is no longer able to effectively control the pathocondition.

Jie Du Ji Sheng Tang (解毒劑生湯)

Chuan Xiong, Dang Gui, Huang Bo, Zhi Mu, Tian Hua Fen, Jin Yin Hua, Mai Men Dong, Yuan Zhi, Chai Hu, Huang Qin, Xi Jiao (or Shui Niu Jiao), Fu Shen, Gan Cao, Hong Hua

Jin Suo Gu Jing Wan (金鎖固精丸)

Sha Yuan Zi, Qian Shi, Lian Xu, Long Gu, Mu Li, Lian Zi Fen

Liang Ge San (凉膈散)

Lian Qiao, Huang Qin, Bo He Ye	3 qian each
Zhu Ye, Shan Zhi Zi, Gan Cao	3 qian each
Da Huang, Mang Xiao	1 qian each
Cang Zhu	4 qian

Ling Gui Zhu Gan Tang (苓桂朮甘湯)

Fu Ling, Gui Zhi, Bai Zhu, Gan Cao

Liu Wei Di Huang Wan (六味地黃丸)

Shu Di Huang, Shan Zhu Yu, Shan Yao, Ze Xie, Fu Ling, Mu Dan Pi

Long Dan Xie Gan Tang (龍膽瀉肝湯)

Long Dan Cao, Huang Qin, Zhi Zi, Dang Gui	3 qian each
Sheng Di Huang, Mu Tong, Chai Hu, Che Qian Zi	3 qian each
Cang Zhu, Ze Xie	4 qian
Sheng Gan Cao	5 qian

The Yu Sheng version is identical to the original except for the addition of Cang Zhu, with its wind-damp dispelling actions further enchancing this formula's potent overall liver-clearing dampness-disinhibiting actions, as it drains liver and gallbladder repletion fire and clears lower burner damp-heat.

Traditionally, this formula is prescribed for liver and gallbladder repletion fire flaming upward pattern pathoconditions presenting with rib-side pain (e.g., herpes zoster) and headache (e.g., acute hepatitis, acute cholecystitis), red eyes (e.g., acute conjunctivitis, keratitis) and bitter taste in mouth, and deafness and swelling of the ear (e.g., otitis media, sinusitis); and liver channel damp-heat pouring downward pattern presenting with urinary dribbling and stranguary-turbidity (e.g., urinary tract infection, enlarged prostate), pudendal itch, genital swelling (e.g., acute epididymitis), and vaginal discharge (e.g., vaginitis). In addition to these pathoconditions, Dr. Lee also administers this formula for pain wind (gout and pseudogout).

Ma Gui Wen Dan Tang (麻桂溫膽湯)

Ma Huang, Gui Zhi, Ban Xia, Ju Hong, Fu Ling, Gan Cao, Zhu Ru, Zhi Shi, Sheng Jiang, Da Zao

Ma Xing Gan Shi Tang (麻杏甘石湯)

Ma Huang	1.5 qian
Cang Zhu	3 qian
Xing Ren	4 qian
Gan Cao	5 qian
Shi Gao	1 liang

The Yu Sheng version is identical to the original formula except for the addition of Cang Zhu, which is included for its wind-damp dispelling dampness-drying actions. This formula's heat-draining, lung-diffusing panting-calming, and cough-suppressing actions are traditionally administered for the treatment of externally contracted wind-cold and exuberant lung heat, failure to resolve generalized heat (fever), and panting counterflow and rapid breathing.

Dr. Lee typically prescribes this formula for the treatment of the common cold (exterior wind-heat external contraction), acute bronchitis, and pneumonia. Additionally, Dr. Lee may also add Yi Yi Ren to form a variant of **Ma Xing Yi Gan Tang** used for the treatment of wind-damp exterior pattern external medicine (dermatological) pathoconditions (e.g., eczema, urticaria, seborrheic dermatitis).

Ma Xing Yi Gan Tang (麻杏薏甘湯)/aka **Ma Huang Xing Ren Yi Yi Ren Gan Cao Tang (麻黃杏仁薏苡甘草湯)**

Ma Huang, Gan Cao, Yi Yi Ren, Xing Ren

Mai Men Dong Tang (麥門冬湯)

Ma Huang	1.5 qian
Xing Ren, Cang Zhu	4 qian each
Mai Men Dong, Xuan Shen, Ban Xia	5 qian each
Gan Cao, Shan Yao, Sheng Jiang	5 qian each
Da Zao	5 pieces

The Yu Sheng version is the same as the original formula except for the subtraction of Jing Mi; Ren Shen pulverized powder is used instead of decocting pieces; and the addition of Ma Huang, Xing Ren, Cang Zhu, Xuan Shen, Shan Yao, and Sheng Jiang. As in **Jia Wei Mai Men Dong Tang**, the qi-boosting yin-enriching, spleen- and lung-supplementing, and kidney-supplementing essence-securing actions of Shan Yao replaces Jing Mi. Xuan Shen's heat-clearing blood-cooling and yin-enriching toxin-resolving actions complement Mai Men Dong (nourishes yin, engenders liquid, and moistens the lung) and Ren Shen (supplements the spleen, boosts the lung, and engenders liquid). Ma Huang suppresses cough and counterflow qi and opens the nine orifices; Xing Ren downbears and drains lung qi and suppresses cough and calms panting; and Cang Zhu has the action of drying dampness and fortifying the spleen.

Mai Men Dong Tang is traditionally prescribed to clear heat, nourish the lung and stomach, downbear counterflow, and precipitate qi for the treatment of lung yin vacuity, lung wilting, upflaming vacuity fire, and qi counterflow panting and coughing. These types of pathoconditions result from microbial infections (i.e., bacteria, virus, fungus) damaging the mucous membranes of the respiratory tract (e.g., larynx, trachea, bronchi) and inhibiting the secretion of epithelial lining fluid (ELF). In health, this fluid maintains epithelial moisture, traps particulate material and pathogens moving through the airway, and transports mucous (e.g., metabolic waste, pus, phlegm-rheum) upwards through the trachea towards the mouth, where it is either coughed out or swallowed.

This formula functions to promote healing of these mucous membranes and serves to restore normal regulation of fluid secretion in the respiratory tract. Dr. Lee classifies these types of pathoconditions as yin vacuity cough (**陰虛發咳** y□ n x□ f□ ké) (aka dryness cough) in the lung and kidney channels, and he will also prescribe this formula for side effects resulting from radiotherapy (e.g., head and neck cancers) such as dry mouth and throat and skin redness, blistering and peeling.

Meng Shi Gun Tan Wan (礞石滾痰丸)

Meng Shi, Chen Xiang, Da Huang, Huang Qin, Pu Xiao

Mu Fang Ji Tang (木防己湯)

Fang Ji, Shi Gao, Gui Zhi, Ren Shen

Niu Jiao Di Huang Tang (犀角地黃湯)

Xi Jiao (or Shui Niu Jiao), Sheng Di Huang, Shao Yao, Mu Dan Pi

Paralysis Formula Series (截癱方系)

These three formulas were specially designed early on in Dr. Lee's clinical practice for the treatment of paresis and paralysis, which correlates with wilting pattern (痿證 w□ i zhèng) in TCM classical pathologic terminology, resulting from traumatic injury (including iatrogenic), microbial infection, and degenerative diseases of automimmune and hereditary etiology.

Each formula in this series has a specific function throughout the various stages of the pathocondition. Since the determination of treatment is based on signs, symptoms, and pattern identification, in addition to the selections in this **Paralysis Formula** series, Dr. Lee may also prescribe other formulas for the treatment of paresis, paralysis, and neuropathies. For instance, in cases involving paralysis induced by viral infection, if the patient has not yet been administered corticosteroids and it is still in the acute stage (approximately < 3 to 4 days), Dr. Lee will approach this as an external contraction wind-heat pattern, prescribing a formula such as **Ge Gen Tang** variant with its cool acrid exterior resolution actions combined with other medicinals such as Di Long that free the orifices.

The typical protocol is as follows: **Paralysis Formula #1 (Di Long San Variant) (截癱一號方) (地龍散加方)**—acute stage (approximately ≤ 1 week following the onset of symptoms, unless corticosteroids have already been administered) with static blood and metabolic waste (e.g., hyaline degeneration, inflammatory factors) congesting the vasculature, channels, and network vessels that can be identified as collection of static blood pattern; **Paralysis Formula #2 (Shi Quan Da Bu Tang Variant) (截癱二號方) (十全大補湯加方)**—post-acute and chronic stage (approximately ≥ 1 week) with enduring symptoms that can be identified as dual qi and blood vacuity pattern, and specifically for cases involving cervical and thoracic spine injuries; and **Paralysis Formula #3 (You Gui Yin Variant) (截癱三號方) (右歸飲加方)**—post-acute and chronic stages (approximately ≥ 1 week) with enduring symptoms that can be identified as kidney yang vacuity pattern, and specifically for cases involving lumbar spine injuries.

Formula Paralysis #1 (Di Long San Variant) (截癱一號方) (地龍散加方)

Ma Huang, Hong Hua	1.5 qian each
Tao Ren, Gan Cao, Gan Jiang, Rou Gui	3 qian each
Di Long, Dang Gui, Huang Bo	3 qian each
Du Zhong	4 qian
Wei Ling Xian, Niu Xi, Fu Zi	5 qian each

The Yu Sheng version is composed of the original formula's essential medicinals—Di Long, Tao Ren, Rou Gui, Huang Bo, Gan Cao, Ma Huang, and Dang Gui—along with the addition of Hong Hua, Niu Xi, Wei Ling Xian, Gan Jiang, Fu Zi, and Du Zhong. Hong Hua, Niu Xi, and Wei Ling Xian enhance the formula's blood-quickening stasis-dispeling, blood-supplementing blood-breaking, and channel-freeing actions. Wei Ling Xian is a Tai Yang urinary bladder channel medicinal that perfuses the twelve channels and network vessels; and Du Zhong and Niu Xi are channel conductors directing medicinals into the lumbar spine and lower limbs. Fu Zi and Gan Jiang combine with Rou Gui to form one of the pillars of Dr. Lee's treatment approaches—The Three Great Yang-Supplementers—that boost the metabolism by innervating the central nervous system (CNS) and peripheral nervous system (PNS), repairing damaged cells, rejuvenating weakened cells, and promoting tissue regeneration. Ma Huang "opens up" and transports other medicinals across all membranes of the body down to the cellular level, thus making it an effective channel-conductor, while its action of opening the nine orifices innervates the nervous system (i.e., CNS, PNS, ANS). Di Long is a Tai Yang urinary bladder channel medicinal that extinguishes wind, clears heat and disinhibits urine, and frees the channels and quickens the network vessels; Huang Bo clears heat and resolves toxin, abates heat and dries dampness, drains fire and elminates steam in the lower burner, and counteracts the heat of The Three Great Yang-Supplementers; and Gan Cao supplements the center and harmonizes the nature of medicinals.

The original formula is traditionally prescribed for the treatment of knocks and falls, pain in the cervical, thoracic, and lumbar spine, pain in the arms, accumulations and gatherings in the abdomen, and blood stasis and static blood pain.

As mentioned in the **Paralysis Formula Series** introduction, Dr. Lee typically administers this formula during the acute stage (approximately ≤ 1 week following the onset of symptoms, unless corticosteroids have already been administered) with static blood and metabolic waste (e.g., hyaline degeneration, inflammatory factors) congesting the vasculature, channels, and network vessels that can be identified as collection of static blood pattern.

Paralysis Formula #2 (Shi Quan Da Bu Tang Variant) (截癱二號方) (十全大補湯加方)

Da Huang	5 fen
Ma Huang	1.5 qian
Dan Shen, Chao Bai Zhu, Fu Ling, Gan Cao	3 qian each
Dang Gui, Chuan Xiong, Chi Shao	3 qian each
Sheng Di Huang, Huang Qi, Rou Gui	3 qian each
Di Long, Niu Xi, Huang Qin, Gan Jiang	3 qian each
Fu Zi	5 qian

This formula is composed of **(Yu Sheng) Shi Quan Da Bu Tang** with Chao Bai Zhu replacing Cang Zhu for its emphasis on supplementing qi and fortifying the spleen, along with the addition of Da Huang, Ma Huang, Di Long, and Niu Xi. Da Huang drains precipitation and damp heat, quickens the blood and transforms stasis, and disperses accumulation to effectively lower intracranial pressure, relieve tension in the diaphragm, and promote lysis of hyaline degeneration and the removal of metabolic waste that obstructs neurotransmitters. Ma Huang "opens up" and transports other medicinals across all membranes of the body down to the cellular level, thus making it an effective channel-conductor, and its action of opening the nine orifices innervates the nervous system (i.e., CNS, PNS, ANS). Di Long is a Tai Yang urinary bladder channel medicinal that extinguishes wind, clears heat and disinhibits urine, and frees the channels and quickens the network vessels. Niu Xi quickens the blood and frees the channels, supplements the liver and kidney, strengthens the sinews and bones, conducts fire (blood) downward, and serves as a channel conductor directing medicinals into the lumbar spine and lower limbs.

The addition of the precipitation-draining, water-disinhibiting, accumulation-dispersing, blood-quickening stasis-transforming, and wind-extinguishing channel-freeing network vessel-quickening medicinals complements and enhances the blood-quickening blood-supplementing, qi-boosting spleen-fortifying, and kidney yang-supplementing actions of **Shi Quan Da Bu Tang**.

As mentioned in the **Paralysis Formula Series** introduction, Dr. Lee typically administers this formula during the post-acute and chronic stage (approximately ≥ 1 week) with enduring symptoms that can be identified as dual qi and blood vacuity pattern, and specifically for cases involving cervical and thoracic spine injuries.

Paralysis Formula #3 (You Gui Yin Variant)
(截癱三號方) (右歸飲加方)

Da Huang	5 fen
Ma Huang	1.5 qian
Fu Ling, Dang Gui	2 qian each
Gou Qi Zi, Niu Xi, Du Zhong, Huang Bo	3 qian each
Di Long, Gan Jiang, Rou Gui	3 qian each
Sheng Di Huang, Shan Zhu Yu, Shan Yao, Tu Si Zi	4 qian each
Fu Zi	5 qian

This formula is derived from **(Yu Sheng) You Gui Yin** subtracting Cang Zhu and adding Di Long, Da Huang, and Ma Huang, just as in the **Paralysis #2 Formula (Shi Quan Da Bu Tang Variant)** above. Ma Huang "opens up" and transports other medicinals across all membranes of the body down to the cellular level, thus making it an effective channel-conductor, and its action of opening the nine orifices innervates the nervous system (i.e., CNS, PNS, ANS). Di Long is a Tai Yang urinary bladder channel medicinal that extinguishes wind, clears heat and disinhibits urine, and frees the channels and quickens the network vessels. Da Huang drains precipitation and damp heat, quickens the blood and transforms stasis, and disperses accumulation to effectively lower intracranial pressure, relieve tension in the diaphragm, and promote lysis of hyaline degeneration and the removal of metabolic waste that obstructs neurotransmitters.

The addition of the precipitation-draining, water-disinhibiting, accumulation-dispersing, blood-quickening stasis-transforming, and wind-extinguishing channel-freeing network vessel-quickening medicinals complements and enhances the overall kidney yang-warming and -supplementing, blood-quickening stasis-dissipating, sinew- and bone-strengthening, and dampness-eliminating pain-relieving actions of this formula.

As mentioned in the **Paralysis Formula Series** introduction, Dr. Lee typically administers this formula during the post-acute and chronic stage (approximately ≥ 1 week) with enduring symptoms that can be identified as kidney yang vacuity pattern, and specifically for cases involving lumbar spine injuries.

Ping Wei San (平胃散)

Chen Pi, Hou Po, Cang Zhu, Gan Cao, Sheng Jiang, Da Zao

Po Xiao Dang Bao Tang (朴硝盪胞湯)

Da Huang, Mang Xiao	1 qian each
Rou Gui, Fu Ling, Mu Dan Pi, Chi Shao	3 qian each
Tao Ren, Dang Shen, Gan Cao	3 qian each
Niu Xi, Dang Gui, Hou Po, Xi Xin	3 qian each
Jie Geng, Huang Qin, Qing Pi, Shui Zhi	3 qian each
Cang Zhu	4 qian
Gan Jiang, Fu Zi	5 qian each
Meng Chong	20 pieces

The Yu Sheng version is virtually identical to the original formula with the exception of Dang Shen replacing Ren Shen and the addition of Huang Qin, Cang Zhu, and Gan Jiang. Meng Chong, Shui Zhi, Hou Po, Da Huang, and Mang Xiao are among the essential medicinals combining to provide an effective formula for treating female infertility with its draining-precipitation, stasis-dispeling accumulation-breaking, phlegm-transforming accumulation-dispersing, qi-moving downwards, and channel-freeing actions. Po Xiao is a less refined low grade of mirabilite and generally *not* used for medicinal purposes anymore; instead, it has been replaced by the refined high-grade form called Mang Xiao.

As its name indicates—**Dang Bao (盪胞)** means to "flush the uterus." This formula functions to "flush away" the residual metabolic waste (e.g., pus, cellular matter, blood clots) that may stagnate on the uterine lining and fallopian tube junctions (i.e, uterotubal junction) as a result of inflammation, adhesions, polyps, endometrial hyperplasia, endometriosis, and leiomyomas. This formula also elicits uterine contractions, which sends a definitive feedback signal to the hypothalamus and pituitary gland so that the body clearly recognizes it should recalibrate normal hormone regulation and continue the regeneration process once again (e.g., a pathophysiological phenomenon occurring in some women whom have already given birth or have had a spontaneous abortion, either knowingly or unknowingly).

Dr. Lee administers this formula specifically as a first-line treatment for female infertility—defined as *absence* of a live birth despite ≥ 1 years of efforts with a male partner (primary infertility), during which they have *not* used contraceptives; or in women who *have* consummated a live birth previously, but are subsequently *unable* to despite ≥ 1 years of efforts (secondary infertility), during which they have *not* used contraceptives.

The treatment regimen involves administration of this formula for 1 week starting a few days before menstruation, with the couple subsequently proceeding in an attempt at natural insemination over a 6-month period. In approximately 70% of these cases, this approach will lead to pregnancy within that 6-month period. If this treatment does *not* result in pregancy, then Dr. Lee will advise the couple to undergo further evaluation (e.g., ultrasound to determine the thickness of the endometrial lining, scrotal ultrasound) and testing (e.g., postcoital test (PCT), semen analysis to determine the presence of anti-sperm antibodies) prior to conducting further pattern identification and proceeding with other therapeutic approaches.

Qi Bao Mei Ran Dan (七寶美髯丸)

He Shou Wu, Fu Ling, Niu Xi, Dang Gui, Gou Qi Zi, Tu Si Zi, Po Gu Zhi

Qi Chuan Fang (氣喘方) – refer to **Asthma Formula**

Qing Wei San (清胃散)

Huang Lian, Sheng Ma, Dang Gui	3 qian each
Sheng Di Huang, Mu Dan Pi	3 qian each

Qing Xin Niu Huang Wan (清心牛黃丸)

Huang Lian, Huang Qin, Shan Zha Ren, Yu Jin, Chen Sha, Niu Huang

Qing Zao Jiu Fei Tang (清燥救肺湯)

Sang Ye, Shi Gao, Gan Cao, Ren Shen, Hua Ma Ren, E Jiao, Mai Men Dong, Xing Ren, Pi Pa Ye

Ren Shen Yang Rong Tang (人參養榮湯)

Ren Shen, Bai Zhu, Huang Qi, Gan Cao, Chen Pi, Rou Gui, Dang Gui, Shu Di Huang, Wu Wei Zi, Fu Ling, Yuan Zhi, Bai Shao, Da Zao, Sheng Jiang

Ru Mo Si Wu Tang (乳沒四物湯)

Dang Gui, Chuan Xiong, Chi Shao	3 qian each
Sheng Di Huang, Ru Xiang, Mo Yao	3 qian each
Cang Zhu, Gan Cao, Tao Ren	3 qian each
Hong Hua	1.5 qian

This Yu Sheng formula is a variant of **Tao Hong Si Wu Tang** with Sheng Di Huang replacing Shu Di Huang, Chi Shao replacing Bai Shao, and adding Cang Zhu and Gan Cao. Sheng Di Huang supplements yin and cools the blood; Chi Shao cools the blood and expels stasis; Tao Ren quickens the blood and dispels stasis; and Hong Hua quickens the blood, dispels stasis, and frees the channels (menstruation). The addition of the medicinal pair Ru Xiang (quickens the blood and moves qi, disperses swelling and engenders flesh, and relieves pain) and Mo Yao (dissipates the blood and transforms stasis, disperses swelling and engenders flesh, and relieves pain) complements **Tao Hong Si Wu Tang**'s blood-nourishing blood-quickening, network vessel-freeing channel (menstruation)-regulating, and stasis-dispeling pain-relieving actions

This is a commonly prescribed formula for gynecological pathoconditions presenting with blood stasis and concretions, conglomerations, accumulations, and gatherings (e.g., uterine fibroids (leiomyomas), endometrial hyperplasia, ovarian cysts, menstrual irregularities). Dr. Lee prescribes this formula for treating a broad spectrum of pathoconditions involving blockage of the flow of blood both inside the vessels (e.g., thrombus, embolus) and outside in the interstitium (e.g., hemorrhage) where it is capable of promoting absorption of blood and stanching bleeding. And it is also one of the main formulas prescribed in Dr. Lee's cancer treatment protocol, specifically administered for malignant (or benign) tumors of the smooth muscle (soft tissue) (e.g., carcinomas, fibromas, leiomyosarcomas, hamartomas) involving the breast, urinary bladder, uterus, gastrointestinal tract, and respiratory tract.

Sai Ji (塞劑 /Vaginal Suppository)

She Chuang Zi	1 g
Xiong Huang, Liu Huang, Da Huang	0.3 g each

Sai Ji is a vaginal suppository prescribed for various types of vaginal infections including bacterial vaginosis (i.e., *Gardnerella vaginalis*), yeast (candidiasis), parasites (trichomoniasis), and sexually transmitted diseases (STDs) (e.g., genital herpes, gonorrhea, Chlamydia) that present with itching, irritation, and watery or viscous vaginal discharge.

This formula is typically prescribed as part of a therapeutic regimen that includes decocted formulas taken orally such as **Long Dan Xie Gan Tang**, **Jin Suo Gu Jing Wan**, or **Bu Zhong Yi Qi Tang**.

San Bi Tang (三痹湯)

Ren Shen, Huang Qi, Fu Ling, Gan Cao, Dang Gui, Chuan Xiong, Bai Shao, Sheng Di Huang, Du Zhong, Niu Xi, Xu Duan, Gui Xin, Xi Xin, Qin Jiao, Du Huo, Fang Feng

San Miao Wan (三妙丸)

Huang Bo, Cang Zhu, Niu Xi

Seborrheic Dermatitis Formula (脂漏方 /Zhi Lou Fang)

Ma Huang	1.5 qian
Huang Qin	3 qian

Cang Zhu	4 qian
Gan Cao, Jin Yin Hua	5 qian each
Lu Lu Tong	10 pieces
Shi Gao, Yi Yi Ren	1 liang each

This Yu Sheng original formula is composed of **(Yu Sheng) Ma Xing Yi Gan Tang** adding Huang Qin, Jin Yin Hua, and Lu Lu Tong. Huang Qin clears heat and resolves toxin, dries dampness, and drains fire; Jin Yin Hua clears heat and resolves toxin, courses wind and dissipates heat, disperses welling-abscesses and swelling, and is an essential medicinal for the treatment of all types of yang pattern swollen welling-abscess and clove sores (carbuncles, furuncles, boils); and Lu Lu Tong dispels wind, eliminates dampness, and resolves toxin for the treatment of wind-damp streaming sores, welling-abscesses, scab, and lichen.

As the name indicates, this Yu Sheng formula is designed for the treatment of seborrheic dermatitis, and specifically for the acute and post-acute stages that can be identified as exterior wind-heat or exterior wind-heat-damp pattern. Seborrheic dermatitits correlates with the classical TCM pathologic terms wandering wind of the face (**面游風** miàn yóu feng) and white scaling wind (**白屑風** bái xiè feng).

Sha Shen Mai Dong Tang (沙參麥冬湯)

Sha Shen, Yu Zhu, Gan Cao, Sang Ye, Mai Men Dong, Bian Dou, Hua Fen

Shen Ling Bai Zhu San (參苓白朮散)

Bian Dou, Ren Shen, Bai Zhu, Fu Ling, Gan Cao, Shan Yao, Lian Zi, Yi Yi Ren, Jie Geng, Sha Ren, Da Zao

Shen Qi Wan (腎氣丸)

Sheng Di Huang, Shan Zhu Yu	4 qian each
Shan Yao, Cang Zhu, Du Zhong	4 qian each
Fu Ling, Ze Xie, Mu Dan Pi, Huang Bo	2 qian each
Niu Xi, Fu Zi, Rou Gui	5 qian each
Gan Cao, Gan Jiang	3 qian each

Sheng Yang Yi Wei Tang (升陽益胃湯)

Huang Qi, Ban Xia, Ren Shen, Gan Cao, Du Huo, Fang Feng, Bai Shao, Qiang Huo, Ju Pi, Fu Ling, Chai Hu, Ze Xie, Bai Zhu, Huang Lian, Sheng Jiang, Da Zao

Sheng Yu Tang (聖愈湯)

Dang Gui, Chuan Xiong, Chi Shao	3 qian each
Sheng Di Huang, Cang Zhu	3 qian each
Dan Shen	5 qian
Huang Qi	1.5 liang

The Yu Sheng version is similar to the original formula except that Sheng Di Huang replaces Shu Di Huang and Dan Shen replaces Ren Shen, and Chi Shao and Cang Zhu are added. Due to the time-consuming and costly method of traditional processing, the Shu Di Huang on the market today is either very expensive or uses modern processing methods resulting in inferior quality; thus, Dr. Lee typically substitutes it with Sheng Di Huang, which has yin-enriching, blood-nourishing, and blood-cooling actions.

Chi Shao cools the blood and expels stasis; Dan Shen quickens the blood and dispels stasis and regulates menses and relieves pain; and Cang Zhu fortifies the spleen and dries dampness, thus counteracting the potential for digestion impairment and loose stools induced by the blood-nourishing yin-enriching medicinals. These additions complement and enhance this formula's overall blood-nourishing menstruation (blood)-regulating, blood-cooling stasis-dispelling, and yin-enriching qi-supplementing actions. Depending on the presenting signs, symptoms, and pattern, Dr. Lee may also add Ren Shen (powder) or Ren Shen/Chuan Qi Powder.

Dr. Lee utilizes this formula's stasis-dispelling blood-cooling actions for the treatment of vascular wall pathologies such as chemotherapy-induced nephrototoxicity (e.g., interstitial nephritis), chemotherapy-induced hepatotoxicity (e.g., hepatitis), aneurysm, and retinopathy (e.g., diabetic). For the treatment of chemotherapy side effects manifesting as vascular wall pathoconditions, Dr. Lee will typically prescribe **Xiao Chai Hu Tang** combined with **Sheng Yu Tang**. **Sheng Yu Tang** is an excellent formula for providing *stable* and *lasting* effects in the promotion of blood perfusion, but it neither *controls* blood as effectively as **Blood Desiccation Formula**, nor does it *promote* blood perfusion as rapidly as **Bu Yang Huan Wu Tang**.

Shi Quan Da Bu Tang Tang (十全大補湯)

Huang Qin	2 qian
Dan Shen, Cang Zhu, Fu Ling, Gan Cao	3 qian each
Dang Gui, Chuan Xiong, Chi Shao	3 qian each
Sheng Di Huang, Gan Jiang, Fu Zi	3 qian each
Rou Gui	5 qian
Huang Qi	1 liang

This formula combines the blood-quickening blood-supplementing actions of **(Yu Sheng) Si Wu Tang** (Dang Gui, Chuan Xiong, Chi Shao, and Sheng Di Huang) and the qi-boosting spleen-fortifying actions of **(Yu Sheng) Si Jun Zi Tang** (Dan Shen, Cang Zhu, Fu Ling, and Gan Cao) adding Gan Jiang, Fu Zi, Huang Qin, and a large dose of Huang Qi. Huang Qin is added to counteract the heat of The Three Great Yang-Supplementers.

The Yu Sheng version of this formula provides enhanced blood-quickening blood-supplementing, qi-boosting spleen-fortifying, and kidney yang-supplementing actions applicable for the treatment of a broad range of dual qi and blood vacuity with yang vacuity pattern pathoconditions. In addition to other applications, Dr. Lee commonly prescribes this formula for pediatric patients with delayed growth (i.e., height and weight), cerebral palsy (congenital or acquired), and congenital developmental delay (e.g., physical, cognitive, emotional, speech and language).

Shi Zao Tang (十棗湯)

Yan Hua, Gan Sui, Da Ji, Da Zao

Shu Zuo Yin Zi (疏鑿飲子)

Ze Xie, Chi Xiao Dou, Shang Lu, Qiang Huo, Da Fu Pi, Jiao Mu, Mu Tong, Qin Jiao, Bing Lang, Fu Ling Pi, Sheng Jiang

Shui Lu Er Xian Dan (水陸二仙丹)

Qian Shi, Jin Ying Zi

Si Jun Zi Tang (四君子湯)

Ren Shen, Gan Cao, Fu Ling, Bai Zhu

Si Ling Tang (四苓湯)

Fu Ling, Bai Zhu, Zhu Ling, Ze Xie, Deng Xin Cao

Si Ni Tang (四逆湯)

Gan Cao, Gan Jiang, Fu Zi

Si Shen Tang (四神湯)

Fu Ling, Qian Shi, Bai Guo, Lian Zi	3 qian each
Shan Yao	5 qian
Yi Yi Ren	1 liang
Shan Zha	2 qian

Si Miao Wan (四妙丸)

Huang Bo, Cang Zhu, Niu Xi, Yi Yi Ren

Si Wu Tang (四物湯)

Dang Gui, Chuan Xiong, Bai Shao, Shu Di Huang

Tao Hong Si Wu Tang (桃紅四物湯)

Dang Gui, Chuan Xiong, Bai Shao, Shu Di Huang, Tao Ren, Hong Hua

Tao Ren Cheng Qi Tang (桃仁承氣湯)

Tao Ren, Da Huang, Gui Zhi, Gan Cao, Mang Xiao

Tearing on Exposure to Wind Formula (迎風落淚方 /Ying Feng Luo Lei Fang)

Ma huang	1.5 qian
Dan Shen, Cang Zhu, Fu Ling, Gan Cao	3 qian each
Chen Pi, Ban Xia, Mu Xiang	3 qian each
Sha Ren, Xi Xin, Wu Wei Zi	3 qian each
Bai Guo	4 qian
Rou Gui	5 qian

This original Yu Sheng formula contains the qi-boosting spleen-fortifying and qi-moving phlegm-transforming actions of **Xiang Sha**

Liu Jun Zi Tang and is similar to **Asthma Formula (Qi Chuan Fang)** except for the subtractions of Shan Yao and Xing Ren and the addition of Xi Xin. Xi Xin dispels wind and dissipates cold, frees the orifices and relieves pain, and warms the lung and transforms rheum; Ma Huang promotes sweating, resolves the exterior, and frees the nasal orifices; Wu Wei Zi constrains the lung and stabilizes panting; Bai Guo constrains the lung and dispels phlegm; and Rou Gui warms the kidney and supplements the spleen, resolves the exterior, and frees the channels. These medicinals complement the qi-boosting spleen-fortifying and qi-moving phlegm-transforming actions of **Xiang Sha Liu Jun Zi Tang**.

As its name indicates, this formula is specifically designed for the treatment of tearing on exposure to wind (**迎風落淚** yíng feng luò lèi), a classical TCM pathologic term that correlates with allergic rhinitis and other related pathoconditions of the sinuses. The underlying pathomechanism of tearing on exposure to wind is spleen yang vacuity with exterior pattern, which inhibits the spleen's capacity to absorb and diffuse nutrients throughout the entire body and results in a compromised immune system and inability to govern flesh. Dr. Lee explains that persistent and prolonged sneezing, nasal discharge, and post-nasal drip further irritates the lacrimal drainage system apparati, resulting in laxity of the lacrimal ducts upstream and/or clogged lacrimal puncta downstream that leads to excessive tearing (epiphora).

Ti Gang San (提肛散)

Chuan Xiong, Dang Gui, Bai Zhu, Ren Shen, Huang Qi, Chen Pi, Gan Cao, Sheng Ma, Chai Hu, Huang Qin, Huang Lian, Bai Zhi

Tiao Wei Cheng Qi Tang (調味承氣湯)

Da Huang, Gan Cao, Mang Xiao

Tong Jing Fang (通經方)

Cang Zhu	4 qian
Gan Cao	5 qian
Niu Xi, Xu Duan, Gu Sui Bu, Qian Cao	8 qian each

The Yu Sheng version is designed with similar therapeutic actions as its namesake **Tong Jing Wan**, but Dr. Lee has overhauled the composition choosing other medicinals with similar and complementary actions. Niu Xi dissipates stasis and quickens the blood, frees the channels and relieves pain, and supplements the liver and kidney; Xu Duan quickens the blood, joins sinew and bones, supplements the liver and kidney, and quiets the fetus; Gu Sui Bu quickens the blood, supplements the kidney, strengthens the sinew, and settles pain; and Qian Cao cools the blood and moves the blood. Cang Zhu has the action of drying dampness and fortifying the spleen to counteract the potential of digestion impairment and loose stools resulting from the blood-nourishing yin-enriching medicinals; and Gan Cao supplements the center and harmonizes the nature of medicinals. The addition of liver- and kidney-supplementing and sinew- and bone-strengthening medicinals complement the original formula's blood-breaking, channel-freeing, and pain-relieving actions.

Dr. Lee typically prescribes this formula for fractures, traumatic injuries, and osteoporosis, as well as adjuvant therapy for the side efforts of chemotherapy in bone and gynecologic cancer patients. It is also a commonly prescribed formula in Dr. Lee's cancer treatment protocol, specifically administered for malignant (or benign) tumors of the striated muscle and marrow (e.g., rhabdomyosarcoma, osteosarcoma) with its capacity to inhibit tumor-cell mediated angiogenesis and neovascularization, and the proliferation of cancer stem cells.

Tong Jing Wan (通經丸) – San Leng, E Zhu, Dang Gui, Chuan Xiong, Chi Shao, Chuan Shan Jia, Yan Hua, Liu Ji Nu

Wan Ling Dan (萬靈丹) – refer to **Bao An Wan Ling Dan (保安萬靈丹)**

Wen Dan Tang (溫膽湯)

Huang Qin, Zhi Shi	3 qian each
Chen Pi, Ban Xia, Fu Ling, Gan Cao	4 qian each
Zhu Ru	3 pieces
Da Zao	4 pieces

The Yu Sheng version is virtually the same as the original formula except for the addition of Huang Qin and the subtraction of Sheng Jiang. The heat-clearing dampness-drying action of Huang Qin complements this formula's overall qi-moving, phlegm-transforming, and harmonizing the gallbladder and stomach actions, making it suitable for the treatment of phlegm-heat with repletion heat or residual heat pattern pathoconditions.

Dr. Lee prescribes variants of this formula for a broad scope of ailments such as external contraction (e.g., common cold), insomnia, rhinitis, otitis, glaucoma, infertility (both male and female), and myasthenia gravis (damp-heat pattern type).

Wen Qing Yin (溫清飲)

Dang Gui, Chuan Xiong, Bai Shao, Shu Di Huang, Quang Qin, Huang Bo, Zhi Zi, Huang Lian

Wu Ling San (Calculi Formula) (五苓散 (結石方))

Rou Gui	2 qian
Yan Hu Suo, Mu Xiang, Huang Bo, Gan Cao	3 qian each
Cang Zhu, Zhu Ling, Fu Ling	5 qian each
Dang Gui	8 qian
Ze Xie	1 liang

This Yu Sheng version contains the essential components of the original formula except for replacing Gui Zhi with Rou Gui and Bai Zhu with Cang Zhu, and adding Dang Gui, Yan Hu Suo, Mu Xiang, Huang Bo, and Gan Cao. This formula includes large doses of Ze Xie for its water-inhibiting dampness-percolating and heat-draining actions, and large doses of Dang Gui for its blood-supplementing blood-quickening actions—a medicinal pair that promotes smooth muscle contractions of the bile ducts, kidneys, and urinary tract, thus resulting in the dislogdement and evacuation of calculi. Mu Xiang moves qi, relieves pain, and relaxes smooth muscle; and Yan Hu Suo quickens the blood, moves qi, and functions as a strong analgesic to promote evacuation of calculi and provide relief for pain. Huang Bo drains lower burner fire, dries dampness, resolves toxin, and disinhibits the gallbladder to treat inflammation.

As its name implies, Dr. Lee has specifically designed this formula for the treatment of calculi in the kidneys (nephrolithiasis) and other sites along the urogenital tract (e.g., urethra, bladder), bile ducts (gallstones/choledocholithiasis), and the pancreatic duct (pancreatolithiasis).

Wu Ling San (Nephritis Formula) (五苓散 (腎炎方))

Dang Gui	2 qian
Gan Jiang, Fu Zi, Huang Bo	3 qian each
Zhu Ling, Fu Ling, Cang Zhu, Ze Xie, Rou Gui	5 qian each
Huang Qi	1 liang

This Yu Sheng version contains the essential components of the original formula except for Rou Gui replacing Gui Zhi, Cang Zhu replacing Bai Zhu, and the addition of Dang Gui, Huang Qi, Gan Jiang, Fu Zi, and Huang Bo. Huang Qi supplements qi, disinhibits water and disperses swelling, increases myocardial contractility, promotes passage across membranes, and functions as a broad-spectrum antimicrobial, which complements Dang Gui's actions of supplementing and quickening the blood, as these medicinals combine to improve renal blood flow and filtration through the glomeruli. Rou Gui reinforces yang, greatly supplements life gate fire, conducts medicinals throughout the entire body, and promotes blood circulation, which complements Fu Zi's actions of reinforcing yang, supplementing the kidney and life-gate fire, freeing the twelve channels, and strengthening cardiac contractility, as these medicinals combine to increase stroke volume and reduce heart rate.

This formula warms kidney yang and promotes qi transformation and disinhibits water and percolates dampness for the treatment of inhibited urination, water swelling (edema), and water-damp collecting internally. Dr. Lee commonly prescribes this formula for the treatment of post-acute and chronic pathoconditions that present with proteinuria, edema, uremia, and hypoalbuminemia (e.g., nephrotic syndrome, glomerulonephritis, chronic kidney failure); pulmonary edema (e.g., intrinsic lung disease, congestive heart failure, kidney failure); and increased intracranial pressure (ICP).

Wu Wei Yi Gong San (五味異功散)

Ren Shen, Bai Zhu, Fu Ling, Gan Cao, Chen Pi, Sheng Jiang, Da Zao

Wu Zhu Yu Tang (吳茱萸湯)

Wu Zhu Yu, Ren Shen, Sheng Jiang, Da Zao

Xi Ji (洗劑/Vaginal Wash/Douche)

Long Dan Cao, She Chuang Zi, Xiong Huang, Liu Huang, Lu Gan Shi

This formula composition is similar to **Sai Ji (Vaginal Suppository)** except for the subtraction of Da Huang and the addition of Long Dan Cao and Lu Gan Shi. It is prescribed for various types of infections of the vulva and vaginal opening including including bacterial vaginosis (i.e., *Gardnerella vaginalis*), yeast (candidiasis), parasites (trichomoniasis), and sexually transmitted diseases (STDs) (e.g., genital herpes, gonorrhea, Chlamydia) that present with itching, irritation, and watery or viscous vaginal discharge.

This formula is typically prescribed as part of a therapeutic regimen that includes decocted formulas taken orally such as **Long Dan Xie Gan Tang**, **Jin Suo Gu Jing Wan**, or **Bu Zhong Yi Qi Tang**.

Xi Jiao Di Huang Tang (犀角地黃湯)

Xi Jiao (or Shui Niu Jiao), Sheng Di Huang, Shao Yao, Mu Dan Pi

Xian Fang Huo Ming Yin (仙方活命飲)/aka **Zhen Ren Huo Ming Yin (真人活命飲)**

Chen Pi, Tian Hua, Jin Yin Hua, Ru Xiang	3 qian each
Mo Yao, Fang Feng, Zao Jiao Ci, Dang Gui	3 qian each
Niu Bang Zi, Chi Shao, Bai Zhi, Gan Cao	3 qian each
Cang Zhu	4 qian
Sheng Shi Gao	1 liang

The Yu Sheng version is similar to the original formula except for the exclusion of Chuan Shan Jia, an endangered animal species that is now prohibited, and Zhe Bei Mu is either taken separately or added into the formula after decoction. Instead of Chuan Shan Jia, Dr. Lee includes Niu Bang Zi for its wind-coursing heat-dissipating, papule-outthrusting toxin-resolving, and swelling-dispersing actions; Sheng Shi Gao for its heat-clearing fire-draining actions; and Cang Zhu for its dampness-drying spleen-fortifying actions. These additions complement the blood-quickening channel passage-freeing and pus-expelling swelling-dispersing actions of Zao Jiao Ci, and provide an effective alternative for Chuan Shan Jia.

In TCM classical texts, this formula is classified as a "sore sage formula" for its heat-clearing toxin-resolving, swelling-dispersing hardness-breaking, and blood-quickening pain-relieving actions. It is traditionally prescribed for the treatment of acute and post-acute stage swelling and toxin of welling-abscesses (carbuncles, furuncles, boils) and sores in which there is localized redness, heat, swelling, and pain or generalized heat with mild aversion to cold. In addition to these types of external medicine pathoconditions, Dr. Lee prescribes this formula for pathoconditions such as innominate toxin swellings (both benign and malignant), cellulitis, appendicitis, postherpetic neuralgia (phantom pain), and pulmonary abscesses.

Xiang Sha Liu Jun Zi Tang (香砂六君子湯)

Dan Shen, Cang Zhu, Fu Ling	3 qian each
Gan Cao, Mu Xiang, Sha Ren	3 qian each
Chen Pi, Ban Xia	4 qian each

The Yu Sheng version is similar to the original formula except that Dan Shen replaces Ren Shen, Cang Zhu replaces Bai Zhu, and Sheng Jiang and Da Zao are subtracted. Dan Shen engenders blood and dispels stasis; and Cang Zhu fortifies the spleen and dries dampness, which is ideal for Taiwan's humid subtropical climate. Depending on the presenting signs, symptoms, and pattern, Dr. Lee may also add Ren Shen (powder) or Ren Shen/Chuan Qi Powder. Also, Sheng Jiang may be included as in the original formula for the treatment of morning sickness during the first trimester of pregnancy, and Gan Jiang may be included for the treatment of interior cold pattern pathoconditions.

This formula's qi-boosting spleen-fortifying and qi-moving phlegm-transforming actions are traditionally administered for pathoconditions involving spleen and stomach vacuity, dampness obstruction and qi stagnation, abdominal distention after food intake, acid reflux, and poor appetite. Some specific pathoconditions Dr. Lee typically prescribes this formula for are gastrointestinal reflux disease (GERD), gastritis, autoimmune diseases (e.g., SLE), ascites (e.g., hepatic disorders), renal disease (e.g., azotemia), and poor appetite and malnutrition during the late stages of cancer.

The qi-boosting spleen-fortifying and qi-moving phlegm-transforming actions of **Xiang Sha Liu Jun Zi Tang** form the foundation of the three formulas that treat the "allergic triad" manifestations of atopy—**Asthma Formula (Qi Chuan Fang)** treats the lung, **Atopic Dermatitis Formula (Yi Wei Xing Pi Fu Yan Fang)** treats the skin, and **Tearing on Exposure to Wind Formula (Ying Feng Luo Lei Fang)** treats the sinuses. These hyperallergic reactions may present as an inflammatory response in the upper respiratory tract (e.g., lungs, sinuses) or manifest on the skin.

In TCM theory, the spleen belongs to earth and engenders metal, governs the movement and transformation of the essence of grain and water, and also governs the flesh. The lung belongs to metal and governs qi, skin and hair, opens at the nose, and has an upward and outward diffusing movement, which carries moisture and nourishment to the skin.

Xiao Chai Hu Tang (小柴胡湯)

Huang Qin	3 qian
Dan Shen, Ban Xia, Gan Cao, Sheng Jiang	5 qian each
Chai Hu	6 qian
Da Zao	5 pieces

The Yu Sheng version is nearly identical to the original formula except for Dan Shen replacing Ren Shen. However, depending on the presenting signs, symptoms, and pattern, Ren Shen (powder) or Ren Shen/Chuan Qi Powder may also be included.

Traditionally, this is a commonly prescribed formula for the treatment of Shao Yang pattern pathoconditions (e.g., alternating heat and cold, fullness in the chest and rib-side, no desire for food and drink), general discomfort or pain in the hypochondriac region, heat entering the blood chamber, and pathoconditions of the liver, gallbladder, and spleen (e.g., hepatitis, cholecystitis, splenitis).

Dr. Lee's application of this formula can be classified into three broad categories: 1) Depressed heat (i.e., persistent low-grade fever) following external contraction (i.e., microbial infection), especially for pediatric patients and tuberculosis (TB) patients who have been administered antibiotic treatment; 2) Microbial infections, toxin (e.g., noxious chemicals), or autoimmune reactions leading to metabolic waste buildup that disrupts the capacity of the nervous system (specifically, the coordianted interactions of the CNS, ANS, and PNS) to regulate bodily functions and maintain homeostasis, thus resulting in dyscrasias (e.g., leukemia, hemophilia, multiple myeloma); and 3) For complex pattern pathoconditions that are difficult to diagnose and pathoconditions are in a transitional state which can be identified as half-interior half-exterior (midstage) pattern, this formula may be prescribed until a definitive diagnosis and/or pattern identification can be ascertained (e.g., whether a pathocondition is passing from the exterior into the interior or from the interior into the exterior).

Xiao Cheng Qi Tang (小承氣湯)

Da Huang, Hou Po, Zhi Shi

Xie Xin Tang (寫心湯)/aka **San Huang Xie Xin Tang (三黃瀉心湯)**

Da Huang, Huang Lian, Huang Qin

Xuan Fu Dai Zhe Shi Tang (旋覆代赭湯)

Xuan Fu Hua, Sheng Jiang, Ren Shen, Dai Zhe Shi, Gan Cao, Ban Xia, Da Zao

Xue Fu Zhu Yu Tang (血腹逐瘀湯)

Dang Gui, Sheng Di Huang, Tao Ren, Hong Hua, Zhi Ke, Chi Shao, Chai Hu, Gan Cao, Jie Geng, Chuan Xiong, Niu Xi

Xue Ku Fang (血枯方) – refer to **Blood Desiccation Formula**

Yan Nian Ban Xia Tang (延年半下湯)

Bing Lang, Jie Geng, Zhi Shi, Qian Hu, Ban Xia, Bie Jia, Ren Shen, Sheng Jiang, Wu Zhu Yu

Yang Dan Tang (陽但湯)

Rou Gui, Chi Shao, Sheng Cao, Sheng Jiang	5 qian each
Huang Qin	3 qian

Da Zao	5 pieces

This Yu Sheng version is virtually identical to the original formula, which is a derivative of **Gui Zhi Tang** (Gui Zhi, Bai Shao, Gan Cao, Sheng Jiang, Da Zao), except as is the case in many of Dr. Lee's other formulas Chi Shao is substituted for Bai Shao and Rou Gui for Gui Zhi.

Traditionally, this formula is prescribed for the treatment of wind strike cold damage, floating pulse, alternating heat (fever) and aversion to cold, sweating and aversion to wind, stiff neck, noisy nose (鼻鳴 bí míng) and dry retching. Its composition forms the foundation for Dr. Lee's therapeutic approach for the treatment of exterior wind-heat pattern pathoconditions of the sinuses, eyes, and skin. Dr. Lee typically does not prescribe **Gui Zhi Tang** decocting pieces for decoction on its own, but he may prescribe extract granules of this classic formula (or in combination with other formulas) for relatively mild external contraction wind-cold exterior vacuity pattern pathoconditions.

Yi Wei Xing Pi Fu Yan Fang (異位性皮膚炎方) – refer to **Atopic Dermatitis Formula**

Yin Qiao San (銀翹散)

Jin Yin Hua, Lian Qiao, Jing Jie, Dan Dou Chi, Jie Geng, Bo He, Niu Bang Zi, Gan Cao, Zhu Ye, Wei Gen

Ying Feng Luo Lei Fang (迎風落淚方) – refer to **Tearing on Exposure to Wind Formula**

You Gui Wan (右歸丸)

Shu Di Huang, Shan Yao, Gou Qi Zi, Tu Si Zi, Du Zhong, Lu Jiao Jiao, Shan Zhu Yu, Dang Gui, Fu Zi, Rou Gui

You Gui Yin (右歸飲)

Dang Gui, Fu Ling	2 qian each
Gou Qi Zi, Huang Bo, Gan Jiang	3 qian each
Sheng Di Huang, Shan Zhu Yu, Shan Yao	4 qian each

Cang Zhu, Du Zhong, Tu Si Zi	4 qian each
Fu Zi, Niu Xi, Rou Gui	5 qian each

The Yu Sheng version combines medicinals from **(Yu Sheng) Shen Qi Wan** and the original version of **You Gui Wan**, but adds medicinals to enhance its kidney yang-warming and -supplementing actions. Sheng Di Huang is included instead of Shu Di Huang, and Huang Bo, Gan Jiang, Cang Zhu, and Niu Xi are added. Along with providing blood-quickening stasis-dissipating, liver- and kidney-supplementing, and sinew- and bone-strengthening actions, Niu Xi and Du Zhong serve as channel conductors directing medicinals to the lower limbs. Huang Bo counteracts the heat of The Three Great Yang-Supplementers, and Cang Zhu dries dampness and fortifies the spleen to counteract the potential of digestion impairment and loose stools resulting from large doses of blood-nourishing yin-enriching and yang-supplementing medicinals.

Dr. Lee commonly prescribes this formula for a wide range of yang vacuity and depletion pattern pathoconditions such as lumbar and back pain (e.g., radiculopathy (sciatica) from herniated intervertebral disc, spondylolisthesis, spinal stenosis), limp knees and weak legs (e.g., various post-acute articular cartilage, ligament, and tendon injuries), congenital development disorders, and atopy (especially in male patients) (e.g., chronic stage asthma, tearing on exposure to wind, atopic dermatitis).

Yu Sheng Wan (育生丸)

Man Tuo Luo Hua	0.04 g/pill
Shan Yao	0.6 g/pill
Honey	

The principal medicinal in this pill is Man Tuo Luo Hua (aka Yang Jin Hua, Datura Flower, *Datura metel* L.), whose bioactive constituents are the anticholinergics scopolamine (hyoscine) and hyoscyamine (atropine). Shan Yao serves as a filler and diluent, and its balanced nature and qi-boosting spleen-supplementing and yin-nourishing actions provide a moderating effect on Man Tuo Luo Hua. Honey serves as a binder and preservative, and it supplements the center and moderates the nature of Man Tuo Luo Hua. Honey is boiled repeatedly until it solidifies into a gelatinous state and then the pulverized powder of these two medicinals are mixed into the honey, made into pills, and allowed to dry.

This is a commonly prescribed pill that Dr. Lee includes in the therapeutic regimen for a broad spectrum of pathoconditions. Dr. Lee explains that the underlying pharmacodynamics of this pill is its capacity to stimulate cerebral collateral circulation and rejuvenate the brain's self-regulating function. Cerebral circulation fluctuates in response to physical and mental activities and metabolic processes, and normally the brain is able to self-regulate (autoregulation) in order to maintain homeostasis. However, certain pathoconditions, as well as the process of aging, may lead to microvascular changes, decreased vascular density, and pericyte degeneration. These changes cause the brain to *misinterpret* the internal environment it holds dominion over, functioning imperceptively in a compromised state of dyshomeostasis.

Dr. Lee utilizes the actions of these properties to supplement the brain, remedy insomnia and depression, eliminate anxiety and stress, slow the degenerative process of aging and disease (e.g., dementia, Alzheimer's disease, Parkinson's disease), relieve all types of pain, check spasm, and stabilize panting (asthma). Its capacity to relax smooth muscle makes it effective for treating overactive bladder (females) and enlarged prostate (males) and for promoting the passage of urinary tract calculi and gallstones (using a large 1x dose of 4–6 pills for males and 4–8 pills for females accompanied by acupuncture). It is also prescribed as a part of Dr. Lee's cancer treatment protocol.

The efficacy of this pill is very much dose-related with large doses potentially causing side effects such as dry mouth, drowsiness, blurry vision, and confusion; thus, it is essential to limit the standard dosage to 1–3 pills per day.

Yue Bi Tang (越婢湯/Spleen-Effusing Decoction/Maidservant from *Yue* Decoction)

Ma Huang, Shi Gao, Sheng Jiang, Gan Cao, Da Zao

Yue Ju Wan (越鞠丸)

Cang Zhu, Xiang Fu, Chuan Xiong, Shen Qu, Zhi Zi

Zhen Wu Tang (真武湯)

Fu Ling, Shao Yao, Bai Zhu, Sheng Jiang, Fu Zi

Zhi Bo Di Huang Tang (知柏地黃湯)

Gan Cao, Huang Bo	3 qian
Zhi Mu, Shan Zhu Yu, Shan Yao, Fu Ling	4 qian each
Mu Dan Pi, Ze Xie, Niu Xi, Cang Zhu	4 qian each
Sheng Di Huang	8 qian

The Yu Sheng version is similar to the original formula except for Sheng Di Huang replacing Shu Di Huang and the addition of Niu Xi, Cang Zhu, and Gan Cao. Niu Xi quickens the blood, strengthens the sinews and bones, and is a channel conductor leading other medicinals downward; Cang Zhu supplements the spleen and dries dampness; and Gan Cao supplements the center and harmonizes the nature of medicinals. The combination of Huang Bo, Niu Xi, and Cang Zhu forms **San Miao Wan**, a commonly prescribed heat-clearing dampness-drying formula used for pathoconditions in the lower burner and lower limbs such as genitourinary damp-heat pouring downward and arthritic ailments.

Dr. Lee typically prescribes this yin-enriching fire-downbearing formula for effulgent yin vacuity fire and steaming bone pathoconditions such as osteomyelitis, pulling of the sinews and inhibited bending and stretching (e.g., musculoskeletal sprains, strains, and tears; osteoarthritis), bone fractures, heel pain syndrome, tuberculosis, yin vacuity cough (aka dryness cough), epilepsy, diabetes, genitourinary tract disorders, seminal emission, and menopausal symptoms.

This is an essential formula for acute and sub-acute muskuloskeletal injuries (e.g., arthritic, traumatic, autoimmune) manifesting in swelling and inflammation, because of its capacity to promote self-repair and prevent the potential development of further degeneration (e.g., fibrosis, enthesopathy) that may arise as a result of complications from aspiration, bleeding, or administration of anti-inflammatory agents.

Zhi Gan Cao Tang (炙甘草湯)

Gan Cao, Ren Shen, Gui Zhi, Sheng Jiang, E Jiao, Sheng Di Huang, Mai Men Dong, Ma Ren, Da Zao

Zhi Zi Bo Pi Tang (梔子柏皮湯)

Shan Zhi Zi, Huang Bo, Gan Cao

Zhi Zi Chi Tang (梔子豉湯)

Zhi Zi, Xiang Chi

Zuo Gui Yin (左歸飲)

Dang Gui	2 qian
Gou Qi Zi, Fu Ling, Gan Cao	3 qian each
Sheng Di Huang, Shan Zhu Yu, Shan Yao	4 qian each
Tu Si Zi, Du Zhong, Cang Zhu	4 qian each
Niu Xi	5 qian

The Yu Sheng version is similar to the original formula except for replacing Shu Di Huang with Sheng Di Huang and adding Niu Xi, Du Zhong, and Tu Si Zi. Niu Xi quickens the blood and frees the channels, supplements the liver and kidney, strengthens the sinews and bones, conducts fire (blood) downward, and conducts medicinals downward to the lumbus and lower limbs; Du Zhong supplements the liver and kidney, strengthens sinew and bones, and conducts medicinals downward to the lumbus and lower limbs; and Tu Si Zi supplements the kidney and secures essence. These additions enhance this formula's essence-replenishing and blood-supplementing actions and complement it with kidney yang-supplementing medicinals that target the lumbus and lower limbs.

In the early years of Dr. Lee's clinical practice, he would prescribe this formula for post-acute and chronic stage lumbar pain (e.g., degenerative disc disease) and limp knees and weak legs (e.g., articular cartilage, ligament, and tendon injuries of the lower limbs) in which heat pattern (inflammation) was still pronounced and for patients with yin vacuity constitutions. Nowadays, Dr. Lee seldom prescribes this formula, often choosing to use **Zhi Bo Di Huang Tang** variants instead.

BIBLIOGRAPHY

Bensky, Dan, Steve Clavey, Erich Stoger. *Chinese Herbal Medicine: Materia Medica* (3rd Edition). Eastland Press, 2015.

Chang, Hsian-che; Tsai, Gui-hua. *Processing of Traditional Chinese Medicine Materia Medica* [Zhong Yao Pao Zhi Xue] Second Edition (Chinese). Taichung, Taiwan (R.O.C.): China Medical University, 2003.

Chen, Shi-gong. *Orthodox Manual of External Medicine* [Wai Ke Zheng Zong] (Chinese). China: Qing Dynasty (1617).

Cheng, Wu-ji. *The Clear Rationale of Cold Damage* [Shang Han Ming Li Lun] (Chinese). China: Jin Dynasty (1156).

Chinese Materia Medica [Zhong Hua Ben Cao] (Chinese). Shanghai, China: Shanghai Science Technology Publication, 1998.

Chinese Materia Medica Grand Dictionary [Xin Bian Zhong Yao Da Ci Dian] (Chinese). Taipei, Taiwan (R.O.C.): Xin Wen Feng Publishing Co., Ltd., 1982.

Clinical Applications of Traditional Chinese Medicinals [Zhong Yao Lin Chuang Ying Yong] (Chinese). Taipei, Taiwan (R.O.C.): Cheers Books Co., 1988.

Deng, Tie-tao. *Traditional Chinese Medicine Diagnostics* [Zhong Yi Zhen Duan Xue] (Chinese). Taipei, Taiwan (R.O.C.): Jyin Publishing Co., 2003.

Fundamentals of Chinese Medicine [Zhong Yi Ji Chu Xue] (Chinese). Taipei, Taiwan (R.O.C.): Cheers Books Co., 1994.

Harrison's Principles of Internal Medicine 19th Edition. McGraw-Hill, 2015.

Hong, Zhen-hui. *Dictionary of Chinese Medicine* [Zhong Guo Yi Xue Ci Dian] (Chinese). Taipei, Taiwan (R.O.C.): Li De Publishing Co., Ltd., 1983.

Huang, Wei-san. *Science of Acupuncture and Moxibustion* [Zhen Jiu Ke Xue] (Chinese). Taipei, Taiwan (R.O.C.): Zheng Zhong Publishing Co., Ltd., 1985.

Ke Qin. *Collected Writings on the Renewal of the 'Treatise on Cold Damage'* [Shang Han Lun Su Ji] (Chinese). China: Ming Dynasty (1674).

Keisetsu, □tsuka, *Thirty Years of Kampo Diagnosis and Treatment* [Han Fang Zhen Liao San Shi Nian] (Chinese). Tainan, Taiwan (R.O.C.): Zheng Yan Medical Publications, 1959.

Kou, Zong-yi. *Expanded Herbal Foundation* [Ben Cao Yan Yi] (Chinese). China: Song Dynasty (1116)

Lee, Chen-yu. *Neuropathy: Traditional Chinese Herbal Treatment in a Modern Medical Environment.* tr. Daniel L. Altschuler. Taipei, Taiwan (R.O.C.): Cheers Books Co., 2005.

Lee, Chen-yu. *Traditional Chinese Medicine Treatment of Common Liver Diseases* [Chang Jian Gan Bing Zhong Yi Liao Fa] (Chinese). Taipei, Taiwan (R.O.C.): Cheers Books Co., 2001.

Li, Dong-yuan. *Treatise on the Spleen and Stomach* [Pi Wei Lun] (Chinese). China: Jin Dynasty (1249).

Li, Nian-e. *Essential Knowledge of Internal Medicine* [Nei Jing Zhi Yao] (Chinese). China: Ming Dynasty (1642).

Li, Shi-zhen. *Herbal Foundation Compendium* [Ben Cao Gang Mu] (Chinese). China: Ming Dynasty (1590).

Li, Shi-zhen. *Supplement to the Herbal Foundation* [Ben Cao Gang Mu Shi Yi] (Chinese). China: Ming Dynasty (1590).

Ma, Jian Zhong. *Chinese Medicine Internal Medicine* [Zhong Yi Nei Ke Xue] (Chinese). Taipei, Taiwan (R.O.C.): Zheng Zhong Publishing Co., Ltd., 1986.

Neal, Anthony J., Peter J. Hoskin. *Clinical Oncology Basic Principles and Practice* (Third Edition). London, UK: Arnold, 2003.

Oswald, Cyril, Frank Delaigue. *Les Hommes de l'Art* (French). You-Feng (Librairie), 2013.

Taber's Cyclopedic Medical Dictionary (23rd Edition). Philadelphia, PA (U.S.A.): F.A. Davis Company, 2017.

Tang, Zong-zai. *Treatise on Blood Syndromes* [Xue Zheng Lun] (Chinese). China: Qing Dynasty (1884).

Chinese Materia Medica Grand Dictionary [Zhong Yao Da Ci Dian] (Chinese). Taipei, Taiwan (R.O.C.): Xin Wen Feng Publishing Co., Ltd., 1982.

The Divine Husbandman's Herbal Foundation Canon [Shen Nong Ben Cao Jing] (Chinese). China: est. Qin or Han Dynasty.

The Yellow Emperor's Inner Canon [Huang Di Nei Jing] (Chinese). China: Eastern Han Dynasty.

Wang, Ang. *Medical Formulas Gathered and Explained* [Yi Fang Ji Jie] (Chinese). China: Qing Dynasty (1682).

Wang, Ang. *The Essential Herbal Foundation* [Ben Cao Bei Yao] (Chinese). China: Qing Dynasty (1694).

Wang, Qing-ren. *Correction of Errors in Medical Classics* [Yi Lin Gai Cuo] (Chinese). China: Qing Dynasty (1830).

Wiseman, Nigel and Ye, Feng. *A Practical Dictionary of Chinese Medicine* (Second Edition). Brookline, Massachusetts: Paradigm Publications, 1998.

Wu, Qian. *Essential Teachings on Acupuncture and Moxibustion* [Ci Jiu Xin Fa Yao Jue] (Chinese). China: Qing Dynasty (1742).

Wu, Qian. *Essential Teachings on Miscellaneous Diseases* [Za Bing Xin Fa] (Chinese). China: Qing Dynasty (1742).

Wu, Qian. *The Golden Mirror of Medicin*e [Yi Zong Jin Jian] (Chinese). China: Qing Dynasty (1742).

Yakazu, D□mei. *Kampo Prescriptions Explained* [Han Fang Chu Fang Jie Shuo] (Chinese). Tainan, Taiwan (R.O.C.): Zheng Yan Medical Publications, 1966.

Yang, Ji-zhou. *The Great Compendium of Acupuncture and Moxibustion* [Zhen Jiu Da Cheng] (Chinese). China: Ming Dynasty (1601).

Young, Wei-chieh. Annotated Explanations of The Yellow Emperor's Inner Classic: Basic Questions [Huang Di Nei Jing Su Wen Yi Jie] (Chinese). Taipei, Taiwan (R.O.C.): Chih-Yuan Publishing Co., Ltd., (1994).

Young, Wei-chieh. Annotated Explanations of The Yellow Emperor's Inner Classic: The Spiritual Pivot [Huang Di Nei Jing Ling Shu

Yi Jie] (Chinese). Taipei, Taiwan (R.O.C.): Chih-Yuan Publishing Co., Ltd., (2006).

Young, Wei-chieh. *Practical Applications: Chinese Medicinal Formulas* [Shi Yong Zhong Yi Fang Ji Xue] (Chinese). Taipei, Taiwan (R.O.C.): Le Qun Cultural Publications, 1992.

Yun Tie-qiao, *Research on Treatise On Cold Damage* [Shang Han Lun Yan Jiu] (Chinese). China: 1923.

Zhang, Bo-yu. *Traditional Chinese Medicine Internal Medicine* [Zhong Yi Nei Ke Xue] (Chinese). Taipei, Taiwan (R.O.C.): Jyin Publishing Co., 1989.

Zhang, De-yu. *True Meaning of the Herbal Foundation* [Ben Cao Zheng Yi] (Chinese). China: Qing Dynasty (1828).

Zhang Ji [Zhong-jing]. *On Cold Damage and Miscellaneous Diseases* [Shang Han Za Bing Lun] (Chinese). China: Eastern Han Dynasty.

Zhang Xi-chun. *Records of Chinese Medicine with Reference to Western Medicine* [Yi Xue Zhong Zhong Can Xi Lu] (1918-1934) (Chinese). China: Chinese Medicine Classics Publications, 2016.

American Cancer Society
https://www.cancer.org/

American Society of Clinical Oncology
https://www.cancer.net/

Mayo Clinic
https://www.mayoclinic.org/

MSD (Merck) Merck Manuals Professional Edition
https://www.msdmanuals.com/professional

McMaster Pathophysiological Review
http://www.pathophys.org/

Mesothelioma | Cancer Research UK
https://www.cancerresearchuk.org/

中醫世家 [Zhong Yi Shi Jia] (a Chinese language TCM databank)
http://www.zysj.com.cn/

醫砭 [Yi Bian] (a Chinese language TCM databank)

http://yibian.hopto.org/

ABOUT THE AUTHOR

Scott Herbster has spent the better part of the past 25 years in Taiwan and China immersed in Chinese culture and pursuing related studies in literature, philosophy, religion, music, martial arts, and traditional Chinese medicine (TCM).

From 1993 to 1996, he learned Mandarin at Normal Taiwan University Mandarin Training Center; from 2001 to 2007, he precepted under the tutelage of Dr. Lee Chen-Yu at the Yu Sheng Chinese Medicine Clinic; and from 2007 to 2012, he studied in the Postbaccalaureate Chinese Medicine program at China Medical University in Taichung, Taiwan, which included a Western medicine clerkship at Tri-Service General Hospital and TCM internships at Taipei Municipal Heping Hospital, Taipei City Hospital (Kunming TCM Branch), and Taipei City Hospital (Linsen TCM Branch).

Upon completion of his Chinese medicine degree in 2012 to the present, he has had the honor and privilege of returning to assist Dr. Lee in the clinical setting as well as compiling and translating academic papers, case study presentations, and now this three-volume series of correspondences.

ABOUT THE EDITORS

Marc Wasserman studied under Dr. Lee Chen-Yu from 2004 through 2014. During those years, he worked directly with patients in the clinic while also assisting Dr. Lee with research, translation, and publication projects. He and Dr. Lee often travelled together, making presentations at various international medical conferences.

Marc is a graduate of the doctoral program at Liaoning University of Traditional Chinese Medicine, a prestigious medical school in northeastern China. He is the first American of non-Asian heritage to complete the program. He holds a visiting professorship with Liaoning University of Traditional Chinese Medicine, and is an adjunct professor at Virginia University of Oriental Medicine.

Currently, Dr. Wasserman runs a small clinic in Hunt Valley, Maryland. For more information on his practice, please visit www.flowhealthclinic.com

Seth Shamon received his Master's in Acupuncture and Oriental Medicine from Maryland University of Integrative Health (formerly Tai Sophia Institute) in 2015. After that time, Seth practiced acupuncture and herbal medicine in Washington DC for two-and-a-half years, treating over 7,000 patients for a wide range of conditions.

In 2018, Seth moved to Taiwan to further his studies in Chinese medicine and Chinese language. After witnessing and being impressed with Dr. Lee's clinical approach, he became involved with this book, bringing to the project his analytical drive for perfection and his past academic experience as a student of German philosophy (and of physics and mathematics).

Made in the USA
Middletown, DE
12 July 2020

12585804R00201